TRENDS IN DIETARY CARBOHYDRATES RESEARCH

TRENDS IN DIETARY CARBOHYDRATES RESEARCH

M. V. LANDLOW
EDITOR

Nova Science Publishers, Inc.
New York

For permission to use material from this book please contact us:
Telephone 631-231-7269; Fax 631-231-8175
Web Site: http://www.novapublishers.com

LIBRARY OF CONGRESS CATALOGING-IN-PUBLICATION DATA
Trends in dietary carbohydrates research / M.V. Landow, editor.
p. ; cm.
Includes bibliographical references and index.
ISBN 1-59454-798-X
1. Carbohydrates in human nutrition. 2. Carbohydrates--Metabolism. 3. Animal nutrition. I. Landow, M. V.
[DNLM: 1. Dietary Carbohydrates. 2. Animal Nutrition. 3. Diet. 4. Dietary Carbohydrates--adverse effects. QU 75 T794 2006]
QP701.T64 2006
612'.01578--dc22 2005033921

Published by Nova Science Publishers, Inc. ✢New York

CONTENTS

Preface vii

Chapter 1 Macronutrient Intakes in the United States and the Diet Quality of Adults Eating Low to High Amounts of Carbohydrate: NHANES 1999-2002 **1**
Shanthy A. Bowman and Alvin Nowverl

Chapter 2 Sources of Carbohydrates in the Diet and Relationship to Obesity and Dental Caries **23**
Jennifer M. MacKeown

Chapter 3 Associations between Carbohydrate Intake and Risk for Coronary Heart Disease, Insulin Resistance and the Metabolic Syndrome **55**
Maria Luz Fernandez and Marcela Vergara-Jimenez

Chapter 4 The Effect of Carbohydrate Supplementation during the First of Two Prolonged Cycling Bouts on Immunoendocrine Responses **71**
Tzai-Li Li and Michael Gleeson

Chapter 5 Pharmacokinetics and its Relevance to Diet **91**
V. K. Katiyar and Somna Mishra

Chapter 6 Carbohydrate Effects on the Efficiency of Utilization of Ruminal Ammonia Nitrogen for Milk Protein Synthesis in Dairy Cows **109**
Alexander N. Hristov

Chapter 7 Effect of Carbohydrate Supplementation on Performance in Rats Exposed to Hypobaric Hypoxia **141**
Alka Chatterjee, Shashi Bala Singh, and W. Selvamurthy

Chapter 8 Effects of Prebiotics in Dog and Cat Nutrition: A Review **179**
M. Hesta, J. Debraekeleer, G. P. J. Janssens and R. De Wilde

Index **221**

PREFACE

Carbohydrates present in food comprising digestible sugars and starches and indigestible cellulose and other dietary fibers. The former are the major source of energy. The sugars are in beet and cane sugar, fruits, honey, sweet corn, corn syrup, milk and milk products, etc.; the starches are in cereal grains, legumes, tubers, etc. In patients with hepatic forms of porphyria, a person should consume at least 350 mg of carbohydrate per day, or the carbohydrates should make up 60-65% of the daily consumption. This new book examines and presents new research of the complexity, effects and nutritional aspects of dietary carbohydrates.

The federal dietary guidance aims to promote the health of Americans and to reduce the risk for major chronic diseases through better diet and physical activity. The federal government conducts nationally representative dietary surveys as part of its nutrition monitoring activities. Chapter 1 examines the diet of 17,107 Americans, 2 years of age and above, who provided complete, reliable one-day dietary data in the National Health and Nutrition Examination Survey (NHANES) 1999-2002 conducted by the Centers for Disease Control and Prevention's (CDC) National Center for Health Statistics (NCHS). The study had two focus areas. The first area examined the macronutrient profile of U.S. population and six age-gender groups: children 2-5 years; children 6-11 years; males, 12-19 years; females, 12-19 years; adult males, ages 20 years and over; and adult females, ages 20 years and over. The percent energy from carbohydrate ranged from 49% to 56% among the six groups. However, children 11-19 years of age obtained a higher percent of energy from added sugars than adults (21% vs.16%). The grain products were the top source of dietary fiber followed by vegetables. The mean percent of total calories from saturated fat among the groups (11%-12%) was above the level recommended by the federal dietary guidance (less than 10%). In children, milk and milk products group, and in adults, meat, poultry, fish and eggs group were the top sources of saturated fat. The second study area compared the diet quality of adults (n=8,983) in the four quartiles based on their percentage of total energy from carbohydrate. After adjusting for age and gender in regression models, the adults in the highest carbohydrate quartile had the lowest energy, saturated fat, and cholesterol intakes. They chose low fat foods from milk and meat groups. They ate more whole grains and citrus fruits, melons, and berries, foods that were good sources of dietary fiber. However, the dietary fiber intakes of all four quartiles were far below the recommended level of 14 grams per 1,000 kilocalories. The study showed that children and adults could increase the nutritional quality of their diet and also simultaneously decrease their energy intake by controlling intakes of foods and beverages high in added sugars and/or saturated fat and by increasing intake of whole grains, legumes, fruits, and vegetables, foods that are rich in dietary fiber and micronutrients and also relatively low in energy content.

Two of the most prevalent chronic diseases in both developed and developing countries are dental caries and obesity. Over the years there has been a marked increase in the number of children, adolescents and young adults becoming obese and developing many of the health problems associated with obesity, now considered an international epidemic. Dental caries is an infectious disease that involves all age groups. However, adolescence is a period in which the risk for dental caries remains especially high. Adolescents have unique needs and concerns in regard to both dental caries and obesity. Among these concerns is the adolescent diet which contains high amounts of carbohydrate snack foods, such as carbonated beverages and confectionery containing significant amounts of sugar, Carbohydrates are thus major components of our food. They are important as body energy stores and, besides fat, are major determinants of daily energy intake. Both sugar and soft drink (carbonated and non-carbonated) consumption have increased dramatically over the years, particularly among adolescents, with teens consuming more added sugar as a percentage of energy than any other group. This is partly due to the consumption of a westernized diet in developed countries, and an increase in urbanization, characterised by a nutrition transition, in developing countries. Research studies have linked both dental caries and obesity either positively or negatively to carbohydrate intake in the form of starch (complex and/ or refined) and added sugars. However, the findings are only consistent with the view that frequency and amount of sugar intake are a necessary link in the etiology of dental caries, but this role is not as strong as it was in the pre-fluoride era. A combination of both starch and sugar appear to have the highest cariogenic effect. In contrast, research studies on the association between sugar intake and obesity have not been able to show a strong positive relationship, but provide support that consumption of carbohydrate based foods with a high fibre content is associated with reduced body mass index (BMI) and weight loss. The subject of "carbohydrates in research" is extremely vast. Epidemiological studies are continually taking new directions and focus as a result of earlier findings. It is therefore impossible to cover all aspects of this topic in one chapter and thus the aim of chapter 2 is to provide only a brief overview of past and present epidemiological research on carbohydrates with regard to the analysis of consumption patterns in terms of food sources of carbohydrates rather than nutrients. This has an increasingly important place in nutrition research, creating many future research challenges. Further more, the altering trends in many of the western type diseases, including dental caries and obesity, two of the most prevalent diseases associated with carbohydrate intake, make identification of food sources of carbohydrates, and different customary eating patterns which may contribute to the development of these diseases, of topical importance

Because the incidence of obesity has increased dramatically over the past 20 years, finding the most appropriate diets for losing weight has become a major issue. It is also well established that overweight individuals have a higher risk of developing insulin resistance, coronary heart disease (CHD) and diabetes type II. The amount of carbohydrate in the diet may play a significant role in the maintenance of body weight and in reducing the risk factors for chronic disease. Dietary carbohydrates are indeed at the core of the debate regarding healthy diets that promote weight loss and decrease biomarkers for heart disease and the metabolic syndrome. Very low, moderate or high carbohydrate diets have been studied in their effects on body weight, dyslipidemias, insulin sensitivity, plasma glucose, leptin levels, inflammatory cytokines and adhesive molecules. Very low carbohydrate diets have been reported to effectively reduce body weight and improve plasma lipids and insulin sensitivity in studies of short duration between 4 to 24 weeks. Moderate and high carbohydrate diets have also been shown to have beneficial effects on anthropometrics and other cardiovascular risk factors depending on the duration of the study and the investigated population. Overall the controversies of the findings depend on the type of study (parallel versus randomized crossover) the duration of the intervention, the assessed subjects (normal versus diabetic or hyperlipidemic) and the retention of subjects, which appeared to be poor in the majority of the cases. All these factors still continue to make it difficult to interpret the available data and to reach conclusive statements regarding the relationship between dietary carbohydrate and chronic disease. It is the purpose of chapter 3 to evaluate a variety of clinical interventions conducted in the past 5 years in which dietary carbohydrate was one of the main variables under investigation. The effects of different dietary interventions varying in the amount of dietary carbohydrate on symptoms associated with the metabolic syndrome, insulin resistance and increased risk for CHD are discussed.

The purpose of chapter 4 was to examine the effect of carbohydrate feeding during the first of two 90-min cycling bouts (EX1 started at 09:00 and EX2 started at 13:30) at 60% $\dot{V}O_{2\,max}$ on leukocyte redistribution, *in vitro* lipopolysaccharide (LPS)-stimulated degranulation and phorbol-12-myristate-13-acetate (PMA)-induced oxidative burst by blood neutrophils and plasma interleukin-6 and stress hormone responses. Subjects ($n = 9$) consumed a 10% w/v carbohydrate (glucose) or placebo beverage during EX1: 500 mL just before exercise and 250 mL every 20 min during exercise, which were completed in a counterbalanced order and separated by at least 4 days. Venous blood samples were taken 5 min before exercise and immediately post-exercise for both trials. The main findings of the present study were that ingestion of carbohydrate compared with placebo during EX1 1) maintained higher plasma glucose concentration throughout the experimental protocol; 2) blunted the responses of plasma adrenaline, adrenocorticotrophic hormone and cortisol during EX2; 3) attenuated circulating leukocytosis and monocytosis throughout the experimental protocol, neutrophilia during the recovery interval, and lymphocytosis during EX2; 4) lessened the decline in LPS-stimulated degranulation and PMA-induced oxidative burst on per neutrophil basis from 3 h post-EX1 onwards; but 5) did not affect changes in plasma interleukin-6. These findings suggest that carbohydrate ingestion during EX1 increases carbohydrate availability during both bouts of exercise; has a limited effect on immunoendocrine response during EX1 but attenuates plasma stress hormone responses during EX2; and blunts the delayed neutrophilia and concurrent decline in neutrophil functions on a per cell basis after EX1. Hence, athletes may benefit from consuming carbohydrate at the earliest opportunity when performing repeated bouts of endurance exercise in a single day.

To understand the effect of a drug and the further response of the body, it is very important to realize what there effects can be and how they can be measured as described in chapter 5. Therefore a thorough study is usually conducted. Generally it is done by 'in vivo' experiments on animals. These drugs exert different effects and side effects on the body and are measured regularly at different time intervals. After a drug is introduced into a biological system it is subject to a number of processes whose rates control the concentration of drug in that elusive region known as the "site of action", thus affecting its onset, its duration of action and intensity of biological response. The food taken by human being is called diet. In general terms, an adequate diet is one which permits normal growth, maintenance and reproduction.

Ammonia is a major source of N for microbial protein synthesis in the rumen and consequently, milk protein synthesis in lactating ruminants. In chapter 6, the effect of carbohydrate (CHO) type on ruminal fermentation, microbial protein synthesis, and the efficiency of utilization of ruminal ammonia nitrogen (N) for milk protein synthesis were studied in two in vivo experiments with lactating dairy cows. Ammonia N was labeled with ^{15}N through continuous intraruminal infusion (Exp. 1) or pulse dosing (Exp. 2) of a 20 at. % exc. $(^{15}NH_4)_2SO_4$. Recovery of ^{15}N in milk protein was determined gravimetrically. The experiments involved four ruminally and duodenally cannulated, mid- to late-lactation Holstein dairy cows. Experimental designs were cross-over (Exp. 1), or Latin square (Exp. 2). In Exp. 1 treatments were ruminally fermentable starch and sugars (RFSS; barley and molasses) vs. ruminally fermentable neutral detergent fiber (RFNDF; corn, beet pulp, and brewers grains). In Exp. 2, treatments were corn dextrose (GLU), corn starch (STA), fiber (control; NDF, white oat fiber), and a CHO mix (25% of each, apple pectin, GLU, STA, and NDF; PEC). Ruminal ammonia concentration was lowered by RFNDF in Exp. 1. There was no effect of diet on ruminal pH, volatile fatty acid (VFA) concentrations, or microbial protein flow to the duodenum. The proportion of milk protein N originating from ruminal microbial N was greater for RFNDF than for RFSS. Cumulative recovery of ^{15}N in milk protein was 13% greater for RFNDF than for RFSS. In Exp. 2, ruminal pH was decreased by GLU, STA, and MIX compared with NDF. Concentration of ammonia in ruminal fluid and ammonia N pool size were decreased by GLU and STA. Acetate, *iso*-butyrate, *iso*-valerate, and total VFA concentration in the rumen were also decreased, and butyrate was increased by GLU compared with the other CHO. Microbial N flow to the duodenum was lower for NDF than for the other CHO. Flow of microbial N formed from ammonia was greater for STA compared with GLU and NDF. The proportion of bacterial N synthesized from ammonia in the rumen was greater with STA than with NDF and MIX and was the lowest for GLU. Irreversible ammonia loss and flux were also lowered by GLU compared with STA and NDF. As percent of the dose given, cumulative secretion of ^{15}N ammonia in milk protein was greater for STA than for GLU or NDF. Data from these two experiments indicate that diets differing in concentration of ruminally available starch and sugars and fiber produced similar level and pattern of fermentation acids and did not affect microbial protein synthesis in the rumen. Increased concentration of ruminally available starch and sugars enhanced ^{15}N-ammonia capture by ruminal bacteria, but overall transfer of ^{15}N-ammonia into milk protein was greater when cows were fed the ruminally fermentable fiber diet. The provision of readily fermentable energy as dextrose or starch in Exp. 2 decreased ammonia levels in the rumen through inhibited production of ammonia and enhanced incorporation of preformed feed amino acids, or through enhanced uptake of ammonia for microbial protein synthesis. Rapidly fermentable in the rumen energy decreases ammonia production, flux, and may decrease ammonia nitrogen cycling, but the overall efficiency of ammonia utilization for milk protein synthesis can be only increased by enhancing ruminal microbial ammonia uptake.

In chapter 7, the effect of a carbohydrate supplement, offered as a diet option, on feeding behavior, body weight gain and endurance exercise was studied in young and old rats exposed to hypobaric hypoxia. Male albino rats (n=47) were randomly divided into hypoxic supplemented and control groups; and a normoxic control group. They were trained to run in the Runimex for 5 days, and subsequently, the hypoxic groups were exposed to simulated high altitude equivalent to 6096 m for 11 days continuously. Food and water intakes, body weight and exercise performance were recorded before and during the exposure period. Blood glucose, and muscle and liver glycogen levels were assayed at the end of the exposure period. Blood samples were taken at the end of the exposure period for total cholesterol, HDL-Cholesterol, LDL-Cholesterol and triglyceride levels. Hypobaric hypoxia resulted in a significant decrease in food and water intakes, body weight, and blood glucose and a deterioration in exercise performance compared to the basal and normoxic group values. With the exception of one supplemented group that showed a significant decrease, there was no significant change in the total cholesterol during the hypoxic exposure. HDL-Cholesterol concentrations were significantly decreased by the end of the exposure period in all the hypoxic groups. The VLDL-Cholesterol + LDL-Cholesterol concentrations were significantly decreased in the older batch while it was significantly increased in the younger batch of animals. The plasma triglycerides showed a tendency to decrease in all the groups. The carbohydrate supplement did not ameliorate the hypoxia-induced loss in body weight, but however, significantly ameliorated the decrement in performance in the supplemented rats compared to the hypoxic control group.

Prebiotics are substrates for bacteria already present in the large intestine. An overview is given in chapter 8 on the effects of prebiotics on the gastrointestinal (GI) tract (faecal characteristics, flora, digestibility, gastrointestinal dimensions and potential side effects), metabolism (lipid, carbohydrate and nitrogen metabolism), immune system and palatability in dogs and cats. Potential clinical benefits and topics for future research are discussed.

In: Trends in Dietary Carbohydrates Research
Editor: M. V. Landlow, pp. 1-22
ISBN 1-59454-798-X

Chapter 1

MACRONUTRIENT INTAKES IN THE UNITED STATES AND THE DIET QUALITY OF ADULTS EATING LOW TO HIGH AMOUNTS OF CARBOHYDRATE: NHANES 1999-2002

Shanthy A. Bowman* and Alvin Nowverl
USDA, Agricultural Research Service, Beltsville Human Nutrition Research Center
Community Nutrition Research Group, Beltsville, MD

ABSTRACT

The federal dietary guidance aims to promote the health of Americans and to reduce the risk for major chronic diseases through better diet and physical activity. The federal government conducts nationally representative dietary surveys as part of its nutrition monitoring activities. This study examines the diet of 17,107 Americans, 2 years of age and above, who provided complete, reliable one-day dietary data in the National Health and Nutrition Examination Survey (NHANES) 1999-2002 conducted by the Centers for Disease Control and Prevention's (CDC) National Center for Health Statistics (NCHS).

The study had two focus areas. The first area examined the macronutrient profile of U.S. population and six age-gender groups: children 2-5 years; children 6-11 years; males, 12-19 years; females, 12-19 years; adult males, ages 20 years and over; and adult females, ages 20 years and over. The percent energy from carbohydrate ranged from 49% to 56% among the six groups. However, children 11-19 years of age obtained a higher percent of energy from added sugars than adults (21% vs.16%). The grain products were the top source of dietary fiber followed by vegetables. The mean percent of total calories from saturated fat among the groups (11%-12%) was above the level recommended by the federal dietary guidance (less than 10%). In children, milk and milk products group, and in adults, meat, poultry, fish and eggs group were the top sources of saturated fat.

* Author for corresspondence. Shanthy A. Bowman, Nutritionist, USDA, Agricultural Research Service, Beltsville Human Nutrition Research Center, Community Nutrition Research Group, 10300 Baltimore Avenue, Beltsville, MD 20705-2350; e-mail: bowmans@ba.ars.usda.gov; Phone: 301-504-0619

The second study area compared the diet quality of adults (n=8,983) in the four quartiles based on their percentage of total energy from carbohydrate. After adjusting for age and gender in regression models, the adults in the highest carbohydrate quartile had the lowest energy, saturated fat, and cholesterol intakes. They chose low fat foods from milk and meat groups. They ate more whole grains and citrus fruits, melons, and berries, foods that were good sources of dietary fiber. However, the dietary fiber intakes of all four quartiles were far below the recommended level of 14 grams per 1,000 kilocalories.

The study showed that children and adults could increase the nutritional quality of their diet and also simultaneously decrease their energy intake by controlling intakes of foods and beverages high in added sugars and/or saturated fat and by increasing intake of whole grains, legumes, fruits, and vegetables, foods that are rich in dietary fiber and micronutrients and also relatively low in energy content.

INTRODUCTION

The federal dietary guidance aims to promote the health of Americans and to reduce the risk for major chronic diseases through better diet and physical activity. The Dietary Guidelines for Americans, 2005 [1,2] recommend eating a variety of foods within and among the basic food groups, grains, fruits, vegetables, dairy, and meat, fish, and poultry without exceeding energy requirements. The guidelines encourage individuals to increase daily intake of fruits, vegetables, whole grains, and nonfat or low-fat milk and milk products and recommend limiting intake of foods high in saturated fats, cholesterol, added sugars and sodium. The key to making healthful food choices is to achieve nutritional adequacy without consuming excess energy, because consuming excess energy for a prolonged period of time will place a person on positive energy balance and will subsequently lead to weight gain. A person whose body weight continues to increase could eventually become overweight or obese. Obesity, a preventable health condition, affects the quality of life.

The federal government conducts nationally representative dietary surveys as part of its nutrition monitoring activities. This study examines the diet of 17,107 Americans, ages 2 years and over, who provided complete and reliable day-1 dietary interview data in the National Health and Nutrition Examination Survey (NHANES) 1999-2002 conducted by the Centers for Disease Control and Prevention's (CDC) National Center for Health Statistics (NCHS) [3,4]. Dietary data was collected through interviewer-assisted, 24-h recall method. The NHANES 1999-2002 dietary data was the most recent data at the time this chapter was written.

One of the major objectives of NHANES is to study the relationship between diet, nutrition, and health [5,6]. Some of the other major objectives of NHANES are: to estimate the number and percent of persons in the U.S. population and designated population subgroups with selected diseases and risk factors, to monitor trends in the prevalence, awareness, treatment, and control of selected diseases, to monitor trends in risk behaviors and environmental exposures, to explore emerging public health issues and new technologies, and to establish and maintain a national probability sample of baseline information on health and nutritional status.

The NHANES survey design is a stratified, multistage probability sample of the civilian noninstitutionalized U.S. population [5,6]. The stages of sample selection are as follows: selection of Primary Sampling Units (PSUs) which are counties or small groups of contiguous counties; segments within PSUs consisting of a block or group of blocks containing a cluster of households; households within segments; and one or more participants per household.

This chapter has two focus areas. The first area examines the macronutrient profile of U.S. population and six age-gender subgroups: children 2-5 years; children 6-11 years; adolescent males, 12-19 years; adolescent females, 12-19 years; adult males, ages 20 years and over; and adult females, ages 20 years and over. The second study area compares the diet quality of adults (n=8,983) in the quartile groups based on their percentage of total energy from carbohydrate.

The NHANES over-sampled low-income persons, adolescents 12-19 years of age, individuals 60 years of age and over, African Americans, and Mexican Americans [5,6]. Therefore, survey design effects were used in the data analyses so that the results would be nationally representative of the population subgroups studied. SUDAAN software was used for data analyses (SAS-Callable SUDAAN for Solaris, release 8.0.1, Research Triangle Institute, Research Triangle Park, North Carolina, USA.).

Macronutrient Intake

The mean macronutrient intakes of the U.S. population ages 2 years and over and for specific age and gender groups are in table 1. Overall, about half the day's total energy came from carbohydrate, about one-third from total fat, and about one-sixth from protein. The percent total energy from carbohydrate ranged from 49 percent to 56 percent among the six groups. However, children 11-19 years of age obtained a much higher percent of energy from added sugars than adults (21% vs.16%). Individuals 18 years of age and older should keep total fat intakes between 20 percent and 35 percent, children 4 to 18 years of age between 25 percent and 35 percent, and children 2 to 3 years of age between 30 percent and 35 percent of total energy [1,2,7]. The mean percentage of total energy from total fat was within the dietary recommendation, but the mean percentage of total energy from saturated exceeded the recommended 10 percent for all six groups analyzed. The recommended Adequate Intake (AI) for fiber is 14 grams per 1,000 kilocalories [1,7]. The mean dietary fiber intakes were below half the recommended level for all age groups.

In order to assess the changes, if any, in energy and macronutrient intakes from the mid-1990s, an analysis of U.S. Department of Agriculture's (USDA's) Continuing Survey of Food Intakes by Individuals conducted in1994-1996 and the Supplemental Children's Survey conducted in 1998 (CSFII 1994-1996, 1998) [8-10] was carried out. Energy and macronutrient intakes reported in the NHANES and the CSFII were compared.

The energy increase was not appreciable in children 2-11 years (about 40-60 kilocalories more in NHANES). However, a notable increase in the energy intake was observed between the adults in the two surveys. In the CSFII, males 20 years and over reported 2,456 kilocalories intake and females 20 years and over reported 1,647 kilocalories intakes. It should be noted that the observed increase of 136 kilocalories for men and 184 kilocalories for women could be due to a combination of true increase in the energy intake between the two survey periods and due the differences in the survey methodology. The U.S. daily average added sugars consumption increased from 82 grams in the CSFII to 92 grams in the NHANES. Increase in added sugar intakes were seen across all age groups. However, while there were differences in energy intakes, the percentages of total energy from carbohydrate, total fat, and protein were similar in both surveys, for the six age-gender groups, implying that the mean energy increase resulted from proportional increase in carbohydrate, total fat, and protein.

Food Groups and Macronutrients

The food coding system used in the NHANES 1999-2002 was the same as that of the CSFII. Therefore, the CSFII food groups were used to categorize foods reported eaten in the NHANES [9]. In the CSFII, total milk and milk products included fluid milk, milk drinks, yogurt, milk desserts, cheese, sour cream, half-and-half, and whipped cream. It excluded butter and milk and milk products that were ingredients in food mixtures coded as a single food item and tabulated under a different food group. For example, cheese in pizza was tabulated under total grain products. The total grain products group included yeast bread rolls, cereals, rice, pasta, ready-to-eat cereals, quick breads, pancakes, cakes, cookies, pastries, pies, crackers, popcorn, pretzel, corn chips and grain mixtures such as pizza, egg rolls, tacos, spaghetti with sauce and frozen meals in which the main course was a grain mixture. Total fruits group included fruits and juices, dried fruits, and other fruits; and excluded fruits that were ingredients in food mixtures coded as a single item and tabulated under another food group. For example, apples in apple pie were tabulated under total grain products.

Tables 2-7 include energy and macronutrients from selected major food groups for the six age-gender groups studied. The reader may note that all food groups are not included in the tables, and therefore, the sum of mean energy and nutrients from food groups will not equal the mean energy and nutrients for each age-gender group in table 1.

Several similarities were noted in the food and nutrient patterns among the six age-gender groups. Also, there were a few striking differences. In very young children's (2-5 years) diet, by weight, milk and milk products ranked first followed by total beverages, grain products, and total fruits. For all other age groups, total beverages ranked first by weight. The total beverages group included alcoholic beverages and nonalcoholic beverages such as coffee, tea, soft drinks, and fruit drinks. This group did not include fluid milk, milk drinks, fruit juice, vegetable juices, and water.

In addition to being the top contributor to the total food amount consumed per day, the total beverages group was also the third highest energy provider in the diet of adolescents (tables 4-5) and adults (tables 6-7), providing 15 percent of total energy in adolescent males' and men's diet, 13 percent in adolescent females' diet, and about 12 percent in women's diet. In 2-5 years olds' diet, the total beverages provided about 7 percent of total energy and in 6-11 years olds' diet about 9 percent. A high proportion of energy from total beverages was from carbohydrate, specifically from added sugars and a part of the energy came from alcohol present in alcoholic beverages.

Table 1. Mean[1] energy and macronutrient intakes per individual, by age-gender, NHANES 1999-2002

Energy and macronutrients	Age-gender groups						
	All individuals	2-5 years	6-11 years	Males, 12-19 years	Females, 12-19 years	Males, 20 years and over	Females, 20 years and over
Sample size (N)	17,107	1,521	2,098	2,244	2,261	4,229	4,754
Energy (Kcals)	2,163±11	1,633±19	1,999±33	2,675±36	1,985±26	2,592±23	1,831±16
Total fat (g)	80.0±0.5	58.0±0.9	73.4±1.4	95.7±1.7	71.7±1.2	96.4±1.0	68.4±0.7
Saturated fatty acids (g)	26.8±0.2	21.6±0.4	26.0±0.4	33.8±0.6	24.8±0.4	31.7±0.4	22.3±0.3
Polyunsaturated fatty acids (g)	16.1±0.1	10.1±0.2	13.7±0.4	17.6±0.4	14.3±0.3	19.3±0.3	14.6±0.2
Protein (g)	78.5±0.5	55.2±0.7	66.5±0.9	92.4±1.8	65.4±0.9	96.9±0.8	67.5±0.8
Carbohydrate (g)	276±2	228±3	274±5	360±5	274±4	314±4	235±2
Dietary fiber (g)	15.0±0.2	10.6±0.2	12.3±0.2	15.2±0.5	12.0±0.2	17.7±0.3	14.1±0.3
Added sugars (g)	91.6±1.8	66.5±2.3	95.0±3.1	141±3.6	104±2.6	103±2.4	75±2.0
% energy from carbohydrate	52±0.2	56±0.3	55±0.3	54±0.4	56±0.3	49±0.3	52±0.3
% energy from added sugars	16.5±0.3	16.2±0.5	18.8±0.4	21.3±0.6	20.9±0.4	15.5±0.3	15.7±0.4
% energy from total fat	33±0.2	32±0.3	33±0.2	32±0.3	32±0.4	33±0.3	33±0.2
% energy from saturated fat	11±0.1	12±0.2	12±0.1	11±0.1	11±0.1	11±0.1	11±0.1
% energy from polyunsaturated fat	6.7±0.04	5.6±0.09	6.1±0.09	5.9±0.08	6.4±0.09	6.7±0.1	7.1±0.1
% energy from protein	15±0.1	14±0.1	13±0.1	14±0.2	13±0.1	15±0.1	15±0.1

[1] Mean±SEM

Table 2. Mean[1] macronutrient intakes from selected food groups by children 2-5 years of age, NHANES 1999-2002

Food groups	Food amount and Macronutrients							
	Food amount (g)	Energy (Kcals)	Carbo-hydrate (g)	Dietary fiber (g)	Added sugars (g)	Total fat (g)	Saturated fat (g)	Protein (g)
Total grain products	242±6	587±9	93±1.4	4.8±0.11	16.6±0.6	17.8±0.41	4.9±0.1	14.8±0.3
Total vegetables	88±3	114±6	16±0.7	1.9±0.08	1.3±0.2	5.0±0.3	1.4±0.1	2.2±0.1
Total fruits and fruit juices	236±11	124±5	31±1.2	1.8±0.1	1.2±0.1	< 0.5	< 0.1	1.1±0.04
Total milk and milk products	450±20	326±14	32±1.5	0.4±0.03	8.9±0.6	14.7±0.6	9.0±0.4	17.0±0.7
Total meat, poultry, fish, and eggs	114±5	240±10	8±0.5	0.6±0.05	0	14.5±0.7	4.8±0.2	17.9±0.6
Seeds, nuts, and legumes	17±1	38±3	3±0.3	0.9±0.1	0	2.3±0.2	0.7±0.03	2.8±0.1
Total sugars and sweets	33±3	69±5	16±1.0	0.2±0.02	12.4±0.9	<1.0	< 1.0	< 1.0
Total beverages	299±13	114±6	29±1.5	< 0.1	25.6±1.3	< 0.1	< 0.1	< 0.1

[1]Mean±SEM

Table 3. Mean[1] macronutrient intakes from selected food groups by children 6-11 years of age, NHANES 1999-2002

Food groups	Food amount and Macronutrients							
	Food amount (g)	Energy (Kcals)	Carbo-hydrate (g)	Dietary fiber (g)	Added sugars (g)	Total fat (g)	Saturated fat (g)	Protein (g)
Total grain products	325±8	802±16	121±2.6	6.3±0.14	21.2±0.8	26.3±0.5	7.7±0.2	21.5±0.5
Total vegetables	98±4	130±5	18±0.6	2.1±0.09	1.3±0.2	5.9±0.27	1.6±0.07	2.4±0.09
Total fruits and fruit juices	170±9	87±4	22±1.1	1.4±0.07	1.1±0.1	< 0.5	< 0.5	< 1
Total milk and milk products	385±11	302±9	31±0.9	0.6±0.05	10.5±0.6	13.3±0.4	8.2±0.3	15.1±0.5
Total meat, poultry, fish, and eggs	150±6	320±13	11±0.7	0.7±0.07	0	19.5±1.0	6.4±0.3	24.2±0.8
Seeds, nuts, and legumes	16±2	39±4	3±0.4	0.8±0.10	0	2.5±0.3	0.5±0.06	1.6±0.2
Total sugars and sweets	44±3	106±7	23±1.6	0.3±0.02	18.6±1.4	1.7±0.12	< 1	< 1
Total beverages	478±19	178±7	45±1.8	0	41.0±1.6	0	0	0

[1]Mean±SEM

Table 4. Mean[1] macronutrient intakes from selected food groups by adolescent males 12-19 years of age, NHANES 1999-2002

Food groups	Food amount and Macronutrients							
	Food amount (g)	Energy (Kcals)	Carbo-hydrate (g)	Dietary fiber (g)	Added sugars (g)	Total fat (g)	Saturated fat (g)	Protein (g)
Total grain products	378±14	975±23	145±3.7	7.9±0.20	24.2±1.3	32.6±0.9	9.6±0.3	26.8±0.8
Total vegetables	135±8	187±10	25.4±1.3	2.9±0.15	1.5±0.2	8.7±0.5	2.4±0.1	3.4±0.2
Total fruits and fruit juices	168±12	82±6	19.9±1.4	1.1±0.08	< 1	<0.5	0	<1
Total milk and milk products	399±20	328±14	30.3±1.6	0.6±0.05	9.3±0.7	15.7±0.7	9.7±0.4	17.0±0.7
Total meat, poultry, fish, and eggs	242±9	501±15	17.6±0.9	1.2±0.08	1.3±0.08	28.6±0.8	9.5±0.3	41±1.3
Seeds, nuts, and legumes	23±4	46±5	4.1±0.7	1.2±0.19	0	2.3±0.3	0.5±0.06	2.1±0.3
Total sugars and sweets	35±3	108±6	22.8±1.5	0.3±0.03	18.5±1.3	2.0±0.2	0.9±0.09	0.6±0.06
Total beverages	1,082±56	400±22	93.6±3.9	0	84.3±3.3	0	0	0

[1]Mean±SEM

Table 5. Mean[1] macronutrient intakes from selected food groups by adolescent females 12-19 years of age, NHANES 1999-2002

Food groups	Food amount and Macronutrients							
	Food amount (g)	Energy (Kcals)	Carbo-hydrate (g)	Dietary fiber (g)	Added sugars (g)	Total fat (g)	Saturated fat (g)	Protein (g)
Total grain products	292±9	744±19	110±3	5.8±0.2	18.9±0.7	25.0±0.9	7.4±0.3	20.3±0.7
Total vegetables	125±5	150±7	21±1.0	2.5±0.11	0.9±0.07	6.8±0.4	1.8±0.1	2.9±0.1
Total fruits and fruit juices	165±8	85±5	21±1	1.3±0.09	1.3±0.4	< 0.5	0	< 1
Total milk and milk products	268±11	237±9	22±1.0	0.4±0.03	7.4±0.4	11.6±0.4	7.2±0.3	12.1±0.5
Total meat, poultry, fish, and eggs	160±6	324±12	12±0.6	0.8±0.05	0.9±0.08	18.3±0.7	5.8±0.2	26.7±0.9
Seeds, nuts, and legumes	16±2	32±3	3±0.3	0.7±0.07	0	2.0±0.2	0.4±0.04	1.4±0.1
Total sugars and sweets	36±2	104±5	21±1.2	0.3±0.02	16.2±0.9	2.4±0.2	1.1±0.08	0.8±0.06
Total beverages	736±26	261±10	64±2	0	58.1±2.3	0	0	0

[1]Mean±SEM

Table 6. Mean[1] macronutrient intakes from selected food groups by males 20 years of age and over, NHANES 1999-2002

Food groups	Food amount and Macronutrients							
	Food amount (g)	Energy (Kcals)	Carbo-hydrate (g)	Dietary fiber (g)	Added sugars (g)	Total fat (g)	Saturated fat (g)	Protein (g)
Total grain products	337±8	815±18	124±3	7.5±0.2	18.5±0.7	26.2±0.7	7.4±0.2	22.8±0.6
Total vegetables	206±5	197±5	28±0.6	4.0±0.10	1.1±0.1	8.4±0.3	2.2±0.1	4.4±0.1
Total fruits and fruit juices	175±8	95±4	22±0.9	1.8±0.07	0.9±0.1	0.6±0.03	0.1±0.01	1.0±0.04
Total milk and milk products	275±8	255±6	23±0.7	0.4±0.08	7.8±0.3	12.7±0.4	7.8±0.2	13.4±0.4
Total meat, poultry, fish, and eggs	289±5	567±9	18±06	1.4±0.06	1.2±0.07	32.2±0.6	10.5±0.2	49.1±0.6
Seeds, nuts, and legumes	41±2	87±4	7±04	2.1±0.1	0.5±0.06	5.2±0.3	1.0±0.1	2.5±0.1
Total sugars and sweets	26±1	84±3	17±0.7	0.3±0.02	14.4±0.6	1.7±0.1	0.8±0.04	0.6±0.04
Total beverages	1,584±36	415±11	73±2	0	56.9±2.2	0	0	0

[1]Mean±SEM

Table 7. Mean[1] macronutrient intakes from selected food groups by females 20 years of age and over, NHANES 1999-2002

Food groups	Food amount and Macronutrients							
	Food amount (g)	Energy (Kcals)	Carbo-hydrate (g)	Dietary fiber (g)	Added sugars (g)	Total fat (g)	Saturated fat (g)	Protein (g)
Total grain products	267±5	627±8	97±1	6.0±0.1	15.8±0.5	19.7±0.3	5.5±09	17.1±0.3
Total vegetables	185±5	150±3	22±0.5	3.5±0.1	0.8±0.05	6.1±0.2	1.6±0.05	3.9±0.1
Total fruits and fruit juices	165±7	89±4	22±0.9	1.8±0.07	0.9±0.06	0.6±0.03	0.10±0.01	1.2±0.04
Total milk and milk products	226±7	200±5	19±05	0.3±0.02	6.5±0.2	9.4±0.3	5.8±0.2	10.7±0.3
Total meat, poultry, fish, and eggs	186±3	350±7	18±0.6	1.4±0.06	0.7±0.04	32.2±0.6	10.5±0.2	49.1±0.6
Seeds, nuts, and legumes	29±2	55±3	5±0.3	1.4±0.09	0.4±0.04	3.2±0.2	0.6±0.03	2.5±0.1
Total sugars and sweets	23±1	72±3	15±0.6	0.2±0.02	12.1±0.5	1.5±0.1	0.7±0.06	0.5±0.03
Total beverages	1,037±25	217±5	43±2	0	36.2±1.6	0	0	0

[1]Mean±SEM

Often, foods high in added sugars are high in energy and low in essential micronutrients [1,11]. Therefore, added sugars increase the energy content of foods and beverages without increasing micronutrient content. As a result, added sugars exert a dilution effect on the micronutrient quality of the total diet [12]. Bowman found that persons in the CSFII 1994-1996 (n=14,709), who had more than 18 percent of total energy intake from added sugars (high added sugars group), consumed 189 kilocalories more energy than persons who had less than 10 percent of energy from added sugars (low added sugars group) (2,049 kcals vs. 1,860 kcals). In spite of the higher energy intake, person in the high added sugars group had significantly lower intakes of vitamin A, thiamin, riboflavin, vitamin C, Vitamin E, niacin, folate, vitamin B6, vitamin B12, calcium, phosphorus, magnesium, iron, zinc, and copper than persons in the low added sugars group. Moreover, a smaller percentage of them met the 1989, Recommended Dietary Allowances (RDAs) for the 14 micronutrients listed above. The high added sugars group's fruits, vegetables, and dietary fiber intakes were lower than that of persons in the low added sugars group. But they drank about 16 ounces (2 cups) more nondiet soft drinks than the low added sugars group [12]. A study by Krantz *et al.* showed that preschoolers in the CSFII 1994-1996, 1998 who obtained more than 16 percent of total energy from added sugars, had low calcium intakes [13].

A study by Bowman, comparing energy intakes from beverages by adolescent females 12-19 years of age, showed that adolescents who drank milk, but did not drink soft drinks had lower energy intakes but higher calcium, phosphorus, and magnesium intakes than those who drank both milk and soft drinks. Moreover, adolescents who drank soft drinks but did not drink milk had the highest energy intake from beverages and very low calcium, magnesium, and phosphorus intakes [14]. Therefore, beverages' role as energy providers in the American diet is especially important when energy contribution comes with low or meager micronutrients contribution.

Overweight and obesity are on the increase among U.S. children and adults. Bray and colleagues [15], using USDA's national food consumption surveys from 1960 to 1998, looked at the food consumption patterns of children 2 years and older. They found that the consumption of high fructose corn syrups (HFCS), which is an added sugar, increased by more than 1000 percent between 1970 and 1990. HFCS is the sole caloric sweetener in soft drinks in the U.S. HFCS also represents more than 40 percent of caloric sweeteners added to foods and beverages. Bray and colleagues state that because fructose, unlike glucose, does not stimulate insulin secretion or enhance leptin production, there is a possibility of excess energy intake through over-consumption of foods high in HFCS leading to weight gain.

According to the CDC, 66 percent adults and 15 percent children are overweight [16,17]. Body weight gain results when an individual consumes energy above one's energy requirement. Because, beverages such as nondiet soft drinks and nondiet fruit drinks are high in added sugars and low in micronutrients and are also consumed in high amounts by children and adults, controlling intakes of such beverages is a way to control energy intake without compromising diet quality.

Next to the total beverages group, total grain products group was the second highest source of added sugars for all age groups. The total grain products were also the top source of day's energy. It is an expected outcome, because the grain products are the major source of carbohydrate in the U.S. diet, and Americans get about half their daily energy from carbohydrate. Among the grain products, bakery products such as cakes, cookies, pastries, and pies contain a significant amount of added sugars and total fat, and therefore are high in energy. However, the grain products are also good or substantial food sources of several micronutrients such as magnesium, iron, calcium, phosphorus, copper, folate, thiamin, vitamin A, riboflavin, niacin, vitamin B6, and vitamin B12 [1,2]. By choosing grain products that are rich in micronutrients but relatively low in added sugars and total fat would provide energy control without adversely affecting nutrient quality of the total diet.

The total sugars and sweets group ranked third in added sugars contribution. This group included jams, jellies, preserves, marmalades, candies, chocolates, popsicles, ices, chewing gum, gelatin desserts, sugars, syrups, and honey [9]. The total sugars and sweet group did not include sugars that were ingredients in food mixture coded as a single food item and included under another food group. For example, sugar present in baked goods such as cakes, cookies, pies, and pastries are included under grain products, and sugar in carbonated soft drinks is included under beverages group [9]. The mean intakes of total sugars and sweets group ranged from 23 grams to 44 grams for different age groups. In spite of small mean intakes, the total sugars and sweets food group provided between 69 kilocalories and 108 kilocalories per day (table 2-7). A reduction in daily energy intake by 100 kilocalories will equal a reduction of 36,500 kilocalories per year, or about 10 pounds weight loss. Individuals who would like to reduce their energy intake should choose sparingly from the sugars and sweets group. Because this food group is not a good source of essential micronutrients, reducing intakes of sugars and sweets will not adversely affect the diet quality.

Milk and milk products provided added sugars. However, only 11-14 percent of total energy from milk and milk products came from added sugars. Among the milk products group, dairy desserts and flavored milk were the sources of added sugars. The milk products are rich sources of calcium, phosphorus, and magnesium that are needed for bone health [1,2]. They are also rich in vitamins such as riboflavin, folate, vitamin A, and vitamin D. Milk consumption has declined in the past three decades across all age groups, especially in children and adolescents, with a simultaneous increase in soft drink consumption [11,14]. Sugar-sweetened beverages, especially soft drinks are popular with children. Choosing sugar-sweetened beverages over milk would reduce calcium intake [14,18]. Marshall and colleagues [18] looked at the diet of 645 children 1-5 years of age in the Iowa Fluoride Study. They found that milk intake was inversely associated with soft drink and juice drinks intakes. Johnson and colleagues [19], using USDA's CSFII 1994-1996 and 1998 data, looked at flavored milk and soft drink intakes of U.S. children. They found that children who drank flavored milk had higher total milk and calcium intakes and lower soft drink and fruit drink intakes than children who did not consume flavored milk. Drinking flavored milk did not increase the percentage of energy from added sugars, because children who drank flavored milk and children who did not drink flavored milk had similar percent energy from added sugars. That reason being, the food and beverage sources of added sugars between the two groups of children differed, but the proportion of energy from added sugars to the total energy did no differ. Johnson *et al.* concluded that flavored milk could be a nutritious alternative to high-energy, low-nutrient beverages.

Today, childhood obesity is on the rise. Therefore, parents of young children should be cognizant of the amount of added sugars present in beverages and foods. Because added sugars add extra energy to foods and beverage without a significant addition of micronutrients, it is important to choose foods and beverages that are low in added sugars or contain no added sugars. It essential that children develop healthful food habits, because food habits formed in childhood are likely to continue through adulthood. Parents influence their children's food habits development [20,21]. Parents who make healthful food choices for themselves are more likely to have a positive influence on their children's food choices than parents who do not make healthful food choices [22].

In general, foods that are good sources of dietary fiber are also nutritious. Fruits, vegetables, legumes, lentils, and whole grains products are high in dietary fiber and relatively low in energy content. Eating foods high in fiber will also help reduce energy intake thus facilitating body weight maintenance or weight loss. However, adding fat or sugars during cooking or processing to the above foods will increase their energy content. Slavin [23] in a recent review of studies on dietary fiber and body weight found strong evidence in epidemiological studies that dietary fiber intake prevented obesity. There was an inverse association between dietary fiber intake and body mass index [weight (kg) /height (m^2)] and body fat. In intervention studies, the results were mixed, but in general, addition of dietary fiber reduced food intake.

High fiber intake reduces the risk of coronary heart disease (CHD) [1]. In a pooled analysis of 10 prospective cohort studies from the U.S. and Europe, Pereira and colleagues, over 6-10 year of follow-up, found that intakes of dietary fiber from cereals and fruits were inversely associated with risk of CHD [24]. Oh *et al.* examined the associations of dietary carbohydrate, glycemic index, and glycemic load with stroke risk among 78,779 women who were free of cardiovascular disease and diabetes in 1980. The 18-year follow-up study findings showed that high refined-carbohydrate intakes were associated with hemorrhagic stroke risk, especially among overweight women, and cereal fiber intake was associated with lower risk of total and hemorrhagic stroke [25].

Total grain products were the top dietary source of fiber, followed by total vegetables, and fruits and fruit juices. Whole grains products contain bran, germ, and endosperm in the proportion as present in nature. Because bran is high in fiber, whole grains are good sources of dietary fiber. The Dietary Guidelines for Americans, 2005 [1,2] recommend that half the grain intake should be from whole grains. Whole-wheat flour, bulgur, brown rice, oatmeal, whole cornmeal, millets, and grain products containing whole grain flour are good sources of dietary fiber.

In children's (2-19 years) diet, milk and milk products group was the highest provider of saturated fat, and in adults' diet it was total meat, fish, poultry, and eggs group. Also, a substantial amount of saturated fat came from total grain products. Increased intake of saturated fat increases the risk of cardiovascular disease (CVS) [1]. The Dietary Guidelines for Americans, 2005 recommend consuming less than 10 percent of total energy from saturated fat for adults having LDL cholesterol below 130ml/dL and less than 7 percent of total energy for adults having LDL cholesterol 130 ml/dL or more [1,2]. Individuals could reduce saturated fat intake by trimming visible fat from meat, removing skin off chicken, replacing whole milk with skim milk, choosing low fat yogurt and low fat cheese over full fat versions, and by reducing intakes foods containing butter, hydrogenated fats and shortening. By following the above listed saturated-fat-reduction strategies, individuals could make nutritious food choices from meat, milk, and grain groups while keeping saturated fat intake within the recommended level.

ADULTS' DIET QUALITY BY CARBOHYDRATE-ENERGY QUARTILES

Energy intake in excess of energy expenditure, over a prolonged period of time, will result in weight gain [26]. Many American's use diet plans ranging from very low to high carbohydrate levels to lose weight. Independent of the macronutrient composition, weight loss is due to energy restrictions [27]. It is important to note, while energy restriction is desirable in weight management, achieving nutritional adequacy is also crucial. The second area of this chapter evaluates the nutritional quality of diets of adults who obtained low to high percentage of energy from carbohydrate. The Acceptable Macronutrient Distribution Range (AMDR) for carbohydrate is between 45 and 65 percent of total energy [7].

There were 8,983 adults, ages 20 years and over with reliable food intake records, in the NHANES 1999-2002. The adults were grouped into quartiles based on the percentage of total energy obtained from carbohydrate. The percentages of total energy from carbohydrate from the first (low) to fourth (high) quartile ranged between: 0% to less than 42.7%, 42.7% to less than 50.6%; 50.6% to less than 58.0%, and 58.0% and above. The weighted percentages of adults from the first to fourth quartiles were: 25.06%, 24.98%, 24.81%, and 25.15% respectively. Their mean intakes of energy and macronutrients (tables 8 and 9), nutrient densities defined as nutrient per 1,000 kilocalories of total energy intake (table 10), 1992, USDA Food Guide Pyramid food group servings (table 12), and food sources of macronutrients (table 13) were estimated. Alpha =0.05 a priori level of significance was used to consider two means different (tables 8-10, 12).

Table 8 includes unadjusted mean intakes of U.S. adults and adults in the four carbohydrate quartiles. Mean cholesterol and sodium values are included, because there are limits placed on their daily intakes. It is recommended that adults consume less than 2,300 mg of sodium per day [1,2]. Caffeine was included in table 8 because, by weight, beverages ranked first in total food amount consumed by adults, and most of the caffeine consumed came form beverages.

The adults in the fourth quartile had the lowest mean energy intake (1,968 kcal). They consumed 227 kilocalories less than the U.S. average (2,195 kcal). Notable differences in the energy intakes, ranging from 223 kilocalories to 374 kilocalories, existed between the fourth quartile adults and others. The total fat, saturated fat, polyunsaturated fat, monounsaturated fat, and protein intakes decreased, and carbohydrate, dietary fiber, and added sugars increased from the first to fourth quartiles.

Striking differences in the macronutrients consumption patterns between the first and fourth quartile were noted. Especially, the differences in saturated fat and added sugars intakes were noteworthy. The fourth quartile ate only about half the amount of total fat, saturated fat, and mono- and polyunsaturated fats consumed by the first quartile adults. Also, the fourth quartile had mean percent energy from total fat and saturated fat within the recommended levels, and the respective percentages for the first quartile were above the recommended levels. An opposite trend was noted with added sugars. The fourth quartile consumed more than twice as much added sugars as the first quartile. The mean percent added sugars energy consumed by the fourth quartile was at the high end of IOM's recommendation (less than 25% of total energy). Therefore, many adults in this quartile would have exceeded the recommended upper limit for added sugars.

The Recommended Dietary Allowance (RDA) for carbohydrate is 130 grams per day for all individuals [1,7]. The mean carbohydrate intakes of all four quartile groups were well above this level. Although it is relatively easy to meet the RDA for carbohydrate, to meet the fiber recommendation of 14 grams per 1,000 kilocalories, an intake of carbohydrate at about 55 percent of total energy would be necessary.

The mean cholesterol intakes were above the recommended upper limit (300 mg) for the first two quartiles. It was due to high consumption of cholesterol containing foods such as eggs, meat, and poultry. All four quartiles had mean sodium intakes above the recommended level (less than 2,300 mg per day). Most foods prepared away from home, such as fast food, pizza, and restaurant foods and many processed foods including soups, salty snacks, cereal-based snacks such as corn chips, breads, frozen dinners, salad dressings and condiments such as pickles and soy sauce are high in sodium. Moreover, using salt at the table would further increase sodium intake.

Caffeine intake decreased with an increase in carbohydrate energy because the fourth quartile adults drank less coffee than the first quartile adults (mean coffee intakes: 399g, 351g, 315g, and 234g from quartiles 1-4 respectively). The nondiet soft drink consumption ranged from 179g for the first quartile to 510g for the fourth quartile and the mean caffeine from 14mg to 44mg respectively.

Table 9 includes mean energy, macronutrients, cholesterol, and sodium intakes from regression models controlling for age and gender variations. Except for energy intake, no appreciable differences were seen between the adjusted and unadjusted means of all the other variables analyzed. The first and the fourth quartiles' unadjusted (table 8) and adjusted mean (table 9) energy intakes differed. The reason for the differences could be due to the fact that there were more males than females in the first quartile and more females than males in the fourth quartile. Adjusting for gender differences reduced the differences in energy intakes between the two quartiles. In spite of the differences between the adjusted and unadjusted means, the fourth quartile still had the lowest energy intake and the differences in the energy intakes between adults in fourth quartiles and adults in the other three quartiles ranged from 205 to 277 kilocalories.

Nutrient density (amount of nutrient per 1,000 kilocalories) for macronutrients and selected micronutrients are in table 10. As expected, total fat, saturated fat, polyunsaturated fat, monounsaturated fat, protein, and cholesterol densities decreased, and carbohydrate, dietary fiber, and added sugars densities increased from the first to fourth quartile. Moreover, the nutrient densities of each quartile were significantly different from that of the adjacent quartiles. This finding implied that there were notable differences in the food selection patterns among adults in each quartile. Some of their food choices affected their diet quality adversely. For example, the adults in lower quartiles chose foods high in saturated fat, while adults in the third and fourth quartiles chose foods high in added sugars. Also, in spite of high carbohydrate intake, the mean dietary fiber intake of adults in the fourth quartile was only about two thirds of IOM's recommendation of 14 grams per 1,000 kilocalories.

Among micronutrients, sodium, phosphorus, selenium, zinc, and vitamin B12 densities decreased, and calcium, magnesium, potassium, iron, and vitamin C densities increased from the first to fourth quartile. In spite of significant differences in energy densities, further analyses of data (not in tables) showed that the mean phosphorus, selenium, vitamin B12, vitamin B6, vitamin C and riboflavin were close to or above the RDAs for all four quartiles [28-30]. The mean iron intake ranged from 14.4 mg to 16.2 mg and was fairly adequate.

Grain products such as ready-to-eat cereals and yeast breads are among the top iron sources in the American diet. Magnesium intakes ranged from 270 mg to 292 mg, which may be fairly adequate for women but not for men. The RDAs for magnesium are between 310–320 mg for women and 400-420 mg for men [28,29]. The grain products, especially whole grains are major source of magnesium. Importantly, all quartile groups consumed between 752 mg and 923 mg calcium, a range well below the recommended 1,000-1,200 mg per day Adequate Intake of for adults [28,29].

The low calcium intake was explained by low milk and dairy servings intakes by all four quartiles (table 11). Fruit intakes were also low, except for the fourth quartile adults who had more than two servings of fruits. Nutritious fruits such as citrus fruits, melons, and berries made up half the total fruit intake for the four quartiles. Although statistically different, whole grains intakes and dairy intakes among the four quartiles were very low. Overall, adults' diets were low in whole grains, fruits, and milk (dairy). The Dietary Guidelines for Americans, 2005 recommend that Americans consume daily 3 ounces (equivalent of 3 servings) of whole grains, 3 cups of nonfat or low-fat milk or equivalent amounts of nonfat or low-fat yogurt or low-fat cheese (equivalent of 3 dairy servings), and 21/2 to 61/2 cups (equivalent of 5 to 13 servings) of fruits and vegetables combined. The actual number of fruits and vegetables servings within the recommended range depends upon a person's energy requirement. There was a substantial difference in the meat, poultry, fish, and eggs intakes among the quartiles. The adults in the first quartile ate more than twice the amount from this group than adults in the fourth quartile, which explained the high saturated fat intake of first quartile adults.

Table 12 provides an analysis of major food group sources of energy, saturated fat and added sugars. The latter two nutrients should be consumed in moderation, therefore were included in the table. An awareness of food sources of the two nutrients will help consumers who would like to improve their diet quality and/or reduce their day's energy intake without compromising nutritional quality. There were differences in the food sources of total fat and saturated fat among the four quartiles. The meat, poultry, fish, and eggs group was the highest total fat source in the diet of first quartile, and the grain products were the top souce in the diets of fourth quartile adults. The second and third quartiles obtained more or less the same amount of total fat from these two food groups. Also, the meat, poultry, fish, and eggs group was the highest saturated fat source followed by the milk and milk products in the diet of first quartile. The adults in the other three quartiles obtained approximately equal amounts of saturated fat from three food groups: the meat, poultry, fish, and eggs group, the grain products, and the milk and milk products.

Moreover, the adults in the fourth quartile chose foods lower in total fat and saturated fat than the adults in the first quartiles. They consumed less total fat and saturated fat per 100 grams of meat, milk, and grain groups than the adults in the fourth quartile. Although the adults in the first quartile obtained more energy from total beverages than the adults in the fourth quartile, per 100 grams of beverages, the fourth quartile consumed more energy than the first quartile. That is, the fourth quartile drank more energy dense beverages than the first quartile. The fourth quartile's added sugars intake from total beverages was three times more than that of the first quartile adults.

Table 8. Mean[1] intakes of energy and nutrients by adults, 20 years and over, grouped by percent carbohydrate energy quartiles, NHANES 1999-2002 (unadjusted means)

	All adults	Percentage of total energy from carbohydrate			
		Quartile 1 (<= 42.7%)	**Quartile 2 (> 42.7% to <=50.6%)**	**Quartile 3 (> 50.6% to <=58.0%)**	**Quartile 4 (> 58.0%)**
Energy (kcals)	2,195±15	2,341±39[a]	2,283±23[a]	2,191±24[b]	1,968±25[c]
Total fat (g)	82±0.6	104±1.6[a]	92±1.3[b]	78±1.0[c]	53±0.9[d]
Saturated fat (g)	27±0.3	34±0.7[a]	30±0.5[b]	26±0.4[c]	17±0.3[d]
Polyunsaturated fatty acids (g)	17±0.2	21±0.4[a]	19±0.3[b]	16±0.3[c]	12±0.2[d]
Monounsaturated fatty acids (g)	31±0.3	39±0.6	34±0.6[b]	29±0.4[c]	20±0.4[d]
Carbohydrate (g)	273±2	208±4[a]	266±3[b]	297±3[c]	319±4[d]
Dietary fiber (g)	15.8±0.2	13.5±0.3[a]	15.8±0.2[b]	16.6±0.3[c]	17.4±0.5[c]
Added sugars (g)	88±2	51±2[a]	80±2[b]	100±2[c]	120±5[d]
Protein (g)	82±0.6	100±1.4[a]	88±1.0[b]	77±1.0[c]	61±1.0[d]
% total energy from total fat	33.1±0.2	40.7±0.3[a]	36.0±0.25[b]	31.9±0.2[c]	23.9±0.2[d]
% total energy from saturated fat	10.8±0.1	13.2±0.1[a]	11.8±0.1[b]	10.5±0.1[c]	7.6±0.1[d]
% total energy from polyunsaturated fat	6.9±0.1	8.3±0.1[a]	7.4±0.1[b]	6.7±0.1[c]	5.2±0.1[d]
% total energy from monounsaturated fat	12.3±0.1	15.2±0.1[a]	13.4±0.1[b]	11.8±0.1[c]	8.7±0.1[d]
% total energy from carbohydrate	50.4±0.2	35.4±0.2[a]	46.7±0.1[b]	54.2±0.1[c]	65.3±0.2[d]
% total energy from added sugars	15.6±0.3	8.3±0.2[a]	13.4±0.3[b]	17.3±0.4[c]	23.4±0.7[d]
% total energy from protein	15.2±0.1	17.9±0.2[a]	16.0±0.1[b]	14.4±0.1[c]	12.6±0.2[d]
Cholesterol (mg)	286±3	407±9[a]	322±5[b]	254±6[c]	159±3[d]
Sodium (mg)	3,433±32	3,786±73[a]	3,692±53[a]	3,418±53[b]	2,843±51[c]
Caffeine (mg)	199±6	225±8[a]	210±10[a]	194±9[b]	166±10[c]

[1]Mean±SEM. Means with different superscripts are significantly different at $p < 0.05$.

Table 9. Mean[1] energy and nutrient intakes by adults, 20 years and over, grouped by percent carbohydrate energy quartiles and adjusted for age and gender, NHANES 1999-2002

	Percentage of total energy from carbohydrate			
	Quartile 1 (<= 42.7%)	**Quartile 2 (> 42.7% to <=50.6%)**	**Quartile 3 (> 50.6% to <=58.0%)**	**Quartile 4 (> 58.0%)**
Energy (kcals)	$2,283 \pm 34^{a\,b}$	$2,282 \pm 22^{a}$	$2,211 \pm 26^{b}$	$2,006 \pm 24^{c}$
Total fat (g)	103 ± 1.5^{a}	91.6 ± 1.3^{b}	79 ± 1.0^{c}	54.5 ± 0.9^{d}
Saturated fat (g)	33.4 ± 0.6^{a}	30.2 ± 0.5^{b}	26.1 ± 0.4^{c}	17.5 ± 0.3^{d}
Polyunsaturated fatty acids (g)	20.8 ± 0.4^{a}	18.7 ± 0.3^{b}	16.1 ± 0.25^{c}	11.7 ± 0.22^{d}
Monounsaturated fatty acids (g)	38.6 ± 0.6^{a}	34.3 ± 0.6^{b}	29.3 ± 0.4^{c}	20.1 ± 0.4^{d}
Carbohydrate (g)	201 ± 3.2^{a}	266 ± 2.6^{b}	300 ± 3.5^{c}	234 ± 3.9^{d}
Dietary fiber (g)	13.2 ± 0.3^{a}	15.8 ± 0.2^{a}	16.7 ± 0.3^{b}	17.7 ± 0.5^{b}
Added sugars (g)	49 ± 1.6^{a}	80 ± 2.2^{b}	102 ± 2.7^{c}	121 ± 4.2^{d}
Protein (g)	97.9 ± 1.4^{a}	88.4 ± 0.9^{b}	77.8 ± 1.0^{c}	62.2 ± 1.1^{d}
Cholesterol (mg)	401 ± 8.3^{a}	322 ± 5.2^{b}	256 ± 5.7^{c}	164 ± 3.3^{d}
Sodium (mg)	$3,702 \pm 69^{a}$	$3,690 \pm 48^{a}$	$3,444 \pm 56^{b}$	$2,901 \pm 53^{c}$

[1]Mean±SEM. Means with different superscripts are significantly different at $p < 0.05$.

Table 10. Mean[1] micronutrient intakes per 1,000 kilocalories of energy intake by adults, 20 years and over, grouped by percent carbohydrate energy quartiles, NHANES 1999-2002 (unadjusted means)

	All adults	Percentage of total energy from carbohydrate			
		Quartile 1 (<= 42.7%)	Quartile 2 (> 42.7% to <=50.6%)	Quartile 3 (> 50.6% to <=58.0%)	Quartile 4 (> 58.0%)
Total fat (g)	36.8±0.2	45.2±0.3[a]	40.0±0.3[b]	35.5±0.2[c]	26.5±0.2[d]
Saturated fat (g)	11.9±0.1	14.6±0.1[a]	13.1±0.1[b]	11.7±0.1[c]	8.5±0.1[d]
Polyunsaturated fatty acids (g)	7.7±0.1	9.3±0.1[a]	8.3±0.1[b]	7.3±0.1[c]	5.8±0.1[d]
Monounsaturated fatty acids (g)	12.3±0.1	15.2±0.1[a]	13.4±0.1[b]	11.8±0.1[c]	8.7±0.1[d]
Carbohydrate (g)	126±0.5	88±0.5[a]	117±0.1[b]	136±0.1[c]	163±0.5[d]
Dietary fiber (g)	7.6±0.10	5.9±0.10[a]	7.3±0.1[b]	7.9±0.1[c]	9.3±0.2[d]
Added sugars (g)	39±0.8	21±0.6[a]	33±0.7[b]	43±0.9[c]	58±1.8[d]
Protein (g)	38.1±0.2	44.7±0.4[a]	39.9±0.3[b]	36.1±0.3[c]	31.5±0.4[d]
Cholesterol (mg)	133±1	186±3[a]	146±2[b]	119±2[c]	80±2[d]
Sodium (mg)	1,600±9	1,677±14[a]	1,650±16[a]	1,595±15[b]	1,480±23[c]
Calcium (mg)	395±4	369±5[a]	409±5[b]	409±7[b c]	392±7[c]
Phosphorus (mg)	615±3	642±4[a]	633±4[b]	607±6[c]	577±6[d]
Magnesium (mg)	135±1	128±1[a]	132±1[b]	134±1[c]	144±3[d]
Potassium (mg)	1,326±10	1,282±12[a]	1,325±12[b]	1,321±14[b]	1,376±25[c]
Selenium (mg)	51±0.3	58±0.6[a]	53±0.6[b]	49±0.4[c]	44±0.5[d]
Iron (mg)	7.3±0.1	6.4±0.1[a]	7.0±0.1[b]	7.6±0.1[c]	8.3±0.2[d]
Zinc (mg)	5.5±0.05	6.1±0.09	5.6±0.08[b]	5.4±0.07[b]	5.1±0.13[c]
Vitamin C (mg)	47±1.3	32±0.8[a]	41±1.3[b]	49±1.5[c]	66±2.7[d]
Vitamin B12 (mcg)	2.4±0.05	2.9±0.10[a]	2.5±0.11[b]	2.2±0.05[c]	2.1±0.07[c]
Riboflavin (mg)	0.98±0.01	0.96±0.01[a]	1.01±0.01[b]	0.99±0.01[c]	0.97±0.02[a c]
Vitamin B6 (mg)	0.89±0.01	0.87±0.01[a]	0.85±0.01[a]	0.87±0.02[a]	0.94±0.02[b]

[1]Mean±SEM. Means with different superscripts are significantly different at $p < 0.05$.

Table 11. Mean[1] intakes of Pyramid food groups by adults grouped by percent carbohydrate energy quartiles, NHANES 1999-2002 (unadjusted means)

	All adults	Percentage of total energy from carbohydrate			
		Quartile 1 (<= 42.7%)	Quartile 2 (> 42.7% to <=50.6%)	Quartile 3 (> 50.6% to <=58.0%)	Quartile 4 (> 58.0%)
Total grains servings (number)	6.66±0.08	5.54±0.12[a]	6.92±0.10[b]	7.36±0.11[c]	6.83±0.12[b]
Whole grain servings (number)	0.83±0.02	0.57±0.03[a]	0.79±0.03[b]	0.94±0.05[c]	1.03±0.03[c]
Total fruit servings (number)	1.57±0.06	0.87±0.05[a]	1.33±0.06[b]	1.71±0.08[c]	2.35±0.11[d]
Citrus, melons, and berries servings (number)	0.76±0.04	0.46±0.03[a]	0.67±0.04[b]	0.82±0.05[c]	1.10±0.07[d]
Total vegetable servings (number)	3.3±0.05	3.5±0.08[a]	3.5±0.09[a]	3.2±0.06[b]	2.9±0.10[c]
Milk servings (number)	0.92±0.02	0.76±0.03[a]	1.05±0.04[b]	1.01±0.03[b]	0.87±0.03[c]
Total dairy servings (number)	1.55±0.03	1.55±0.05[a]	1.79±0.06[b]	1.61±0.05[a]	1.27±0.04[c]
Lean meat from meat, poultry, and fish (oz)	4.9±0.06	7.4±0.14[a]	5.3±0.09[b]	4.1±0.07[c]	2.8±0.07[d]

[1]Mean±SEM. Means with different superscripts are significantly different at $p < 0.05$.

Table 12. Mean energy and macronutrient intakes from selected food groups by adults, 20 years and over, grouped by percent carbohydrate energy quartiles, NHANES 1999-2002

		Percentage of total energy from carbohydrate			
		Quartile 1 (<= 42.7%)	Quartile 2 (> 42.7% to <=50.6%)	Quartile 3 (> 50.6% to <=58.0%)	Quartile 4 (> 58.0%)
Total grain products	Food amount[1] (g)	229±8	313±8	333±7	329±7
	Energy (kcals)	566	760	805	739
	Total fat (g)	20	26	25	20
	Saturated fat (g)	5.8	7.4	7.1	5.2
	Added sugars (g)	10.6	17.3	20.7	19.9
Total vegetables	Food amount[1] (g)	211±6	199±8	186±6	185±9

Table 12. Mean energy and macronutrient intakes from selected food groups by adults, 20 years and over, grouped by percent carbohydrate energy quartiles, NHANES 1999-2002 (Continued)

		Percentage of total energy from carbohydrate			
		Quartile 1 (<= 42.7%)	Quartile 2 (> 42.7% to <=50.6%)	Quartile 3 (> 50.6% to <=58.0%)	Quartile 4 (> 58.0%)
	Energy (kcals)	194	184	171	141
	Total fat (g)	9	8	7	5
	Saturated fat (g)	2.4	2.1	1.9	1.3
	Added sugars (g)	1.0	1.0	0.8	0.8
Total fruits and fruit juices	Food amount[1] (g)	92±6	146±7	189±10	251±12
	Energy (kcals)	49	78	103	138
	Total fat (g)	0.5	0.5	0.6	0.6
	Added sugars (g)	0.4	0.7	1.2	1.3
Total milk and milk products	Food amount[1] (g)	212±7	282±10	268±8	236±8
	Energy (kcals)	231	256	233	185
	Total fat (g)	13.4	12.8	10.8	7.0
	Saturated fat (g)	8.2	7.8	6.7	4.3
	Added sugars (g)	5.2	7.7	7.8	7.7
Total meat, poultry, fish, and eggs	Food amount[1] (g)	326±7	264±6	212±6	138±4
	Energy (kcals)	687	503	389	237
	Total fat (g)	41	28	21	12
	Saturated fat (g)	13	9	7	4
Total sweets and sugars	Food amount[1] (g)	15±1	22±1	28±2	34±2
	Energy (kcals)	50	71	90	98
	Added sugars (g)	8	12	15	18
Total beverages	Food amount[1] (g)	1,527±42	1,263±35	1,201±37	1,205±44
	Energy (kcals)	366	277	272	331
	Added sugars (g)	23	39	52	71

[1]Mean±SEM

The first quartile consumed a very high amount (505g) of total alcoholic beverages. The second to fourth quartile adults consumed 198g, 78g, and 38g of total alcoholic beverages respectively. From the first to fourth quartile, adults obtained 252 kcal, 99 kcal, 40 kcal, and 18 kcal energy respectively from total alcoholic beverages. Alcohol provides energy (7kcal/g). Therefore, reducing alcoholic beverages intake will reduce energy intake.

CONCLUSION

The study showed that there are several strategies children and adults could use to further increase their nutritional status with a simultaneous decrease in energy intake. Children, especially adolescents, and the adults in the fourth-carbohydrate quartile could decrease energy intake by reducing added sugars intake. They should be cognizant of the type and amount of beverages they choose to drink, because the beverage group (excludes 100% fruit juices, milk and milk drinks) is the third highest energy provider in the American diet and the top added sugars provider in most children's, adolescents', and at least 25 percent of adults' diet. Americans could choose low calorie beverages and water instead of sugar-sweetened beverages that are high in energy and low in micronutrients. Persons by drinking lowfat milk, skim milk, or soy-based milk at meals instead of sugar-sweetened beverages could increase the nutritional quality of the meals while decreasing energy intake.

The study also showed that the American diet while being high in added sugars, a form of carbohydrate generally associated with foods and beverages high in energy and low in micronutrients, was low in dietary fiber, also a class of carbohydrate associated with nutritious foods with relatively low energy content. Increasing whole grains, legumes, fruits, and non-starchy vegetables would increase fiber intake. However, when increasing fiber intake, it is important not to simultaneously increase energy and saturated fat intakes by adding butter, sour cream, and other fats high in saturated fat to grain products and vegetables. Persons may eat a high carbohydrate diet by choosing foods rich in fiber and low in added sugars (whole grains, legumes, fruits, and vegetables), low in saturated fat (grains, fruits, vegetables, legumes, lean meat and nonfat milk and milk products), and low in energy for the prevention of heart disease, certain types of cancers, and obesity.

In April 2005, the USDA unveiled MyPyramid, an interactive food guidance system based on the Dietary Guidelines for Americans, 2005 recommendations [31]. It is available at: http://www.MyPyramid.gov. MyPyramid Plan tool available at this site would enable consumers to obtain personalized information on their grains, fruits, vegetables, milk, and meat and beans groups requirements per day and how to choose foods from each of the five groups. The recommendations are based on energy requirements for age, gender, and physical activity status. The MyPyramid Tracker tool helps consumers assess their food intake and physical activity status. Americans are encouraged to use information from the new food guidance system and plan personal strategies to improve their diet quality, increase nutritional status, and to increase energy expenditure through increased physical activity. They may also use the MyPyramid tools for successful weight management.

REFERENCES

[1] The Dietary Guidelines Advisory Committee. 2005. Report of the Dietary Guidelines Advisory Committee on the Dietary Guidelines for Americans, 2005 - to the Secretary of Health and Human Services and the Secretary of Agriculture. Prepared for the committee by the Agricultural Research Service, U.S. Department of Agriculture. August 2004. Washington, DC.

[2] U.S. Department of Health and Human Services and U.S. Department of Agriculture. *Dietary Guidelines for Americans 2005*. Washington, DC. 2005. Available at: http://www.healthierus.gov/dietaryguidelines.

[3] National Center for Health Statistics. The *NHANES 1999-2000 Data Files, Data, Docs, Codebooks, SAS Code*. Hyattsville, MD. Available at: http://www.cdc.gov/nchs/about/major/nahnes/nhanes99_00.htm

[4] National Center for Health Statistics. The *NHANES 20019-2002 Data Files, Data, Docs, Codebooks, SAS Code*. Hyattsville, MD. Available at: http://www.cdc.gov/nchs/about/major/nahnes/nhanes01_02.htm

[5] National Center for Health Statistics. The *NHANES 1999-2000 Public Data Release File Documentation*. Hyattsville, MD. Available at: http://www.cdc.gov/nchs/data/nhanes/gendoc.pds

[6] National Center for Health Statistics. The *NHANES 2001-2002 Public Data Release File Documentation*. Hyattsville, MD. Available at: http://www.cdc.gov/nchs/dat/nhanes/nhanes_01_02/general_data_release_doc.pdf

[7] Institute of Medicine. *Dietary Reference Intakes for Energy, Carbohydrate, Fiber, Fat, Fatty Acids, Cholesterol, Protein, and Amino Acids*. National Academies Press, Washington, DC. 2002.

[8] U.S. Department of Agriculture, Agricultural Research Service, Food Survey Research Group. The Continuing Survey of Food Intakes by Individuals and the Diet and Health Knowledge Survey, 1994-96. CD-Rom data, Beltsville, Maryland, USA. U.S. Department of Agriculture; 2000.

[9] U.S. Department of Agriculture, Agricultural Research Service. *Food and Nutrient Intakes by Individuals in the United States, by Sex and Age, 1994-96. 1998.* Nationwide Food Surveys Report No. 96-2. Beltsville, Maryland, USA.U.S. Department of Agriculture; 2000.

[10] Tippett, KS, Cypel, YS (Eds.): *Design and operation: The Continuing Survey of Food Intakes by Individuals and the Diet and Health Knowledge Survey, 1994-96*. 1998. Nationwide Food Survey Report, No. 96-1. Beltsville, Maryland, USA.U.S. Department of Agriculture; 1998.

[11] Popkin, BM; Nielsen, SJ. The sweetening of the world's diet. *Obes Res*, 2003,11(11),1325-1332.

[12] Bowman, SA. Diets of individuals based on energy intakes from added sugars. *Fam Econ Nut Rev*, 1999,12(2),31-37.

[13] Krantz, S; Smicklas-Wright, H,;Siega-Riz, AM; Mitchel, D. Adverse effect of high added sugar consumption on dietary intake in American preschoolers. *J Pediatr*, 2005,146,105-111.

[14] Bowman, SA. Beverage choices of young females: changes and impact on nutrient intakes. *J Am Diet Assoc*, 2002,102(9),1234-1239.

[15] Bray, GA; Nielsen, SJ; Popkin, BM. Consumption of high-fructose corn syrup in beverages may play a role in the epidemic of obesity. *Am J Clin Nutr*, 2004,79(4):537-543.

[16] Flegal, KM; Carroll, MD; Ogden, CL; Johnson, CL. Prevalence and trends in obesity among US adults, 1999-2000. *JAMA*, 2002,288(14),1722-1727.

[17] Hedley, AA; Ogden, CL; Johnson, CL; Carroll, MD; Curtin, LR; Flegal, KM. Prevalence of overweight and obesity among US children, adolescents, and adults, 1999-2002. *JAMA*, 2004,291(23),2847-2850.

[18] Marshall, TA; Eichenberger-Gilmore, JM; Broffitt, B; Sumbo PJ, Levy SM. Diet quality in young children is influenced by beverage consumption. *J Am Coll Nutr*, 2005,24(1):65-75.

[19] Johnson, RK; Frary, C; Wang, MQ. The nutritional consequences of flavored-milk consumption by school-aged children and adolescents in the United States. *J Am Diet Assoc*, 2002,102(6),853-856.

[20] Hursti, UK. Factors influencing children's food choice. *Ann Med* 1999,31 Suppl 1:26-32.

[21] Benton, D. Role of parents in the determination of the food preferences of children and the development of obesity. *Int J Obes*, 2004,28:858-69.

[22] Fisher, JO; Mitchell, DC; Smiciklas-Wright, H; Mannino, ML; Birch, LL; Meeting calcium recommendations during middle childhood reflects mother-daughter beverages choices and predicts bone mineral status. *Am J Clin Nutr*, 2004,79(4):698-706

[23] Slavin JL. Dietary fiber and body weight. *Nutrition*, 2005,21(3):411-418.

[24] Pereira, MA; O'Reilly, E; Augustsson, K; Fraser, GE; Goldbourt, U; Heitmann, BL, et.al. Dietary fiber and risk of coronary heart disease: a pooled analysis of cohort studies. *Arch Inter Med*, 2004,164(4):370-376.

[25] Oh, K; Hu, FB; Cho, E; Rexrode, KM; Stampfer, MJ; Manson, JE; Liu, S; Willett, WC. Carbohydrate intake, glycemic index, glycemic load, and dietary fiber in relation to risk of stroke in women. *Am J Epidemiol*, 2005,161(2):161-169

[26] Report of Joint WHO/FAO Expert Consultation on Diet, Nutrition, and the Prevention of Chronic Diseases. *WHO Technical Report Series* 916. Geneva: World Health Organization; 2003.

[27] Freedman, MR; King, J; Kennedy, E. Popular diets: a scientific review. *Obes Res*, 2001,9,Supplement 1:1S-40S.

[28] Institute of Medicine. *Dietary Reference Intakes: Applications in Dietary Assessment*. Washington, DC. 2002.

[29] Institute of Medicine. *Dietary Reference Intakes for Calcium, Phosphorus, Magnesium, Vitamin D, and Fluoride*. National Academies Press, Washington, DC. 1997.

[30] Institute of Medicine. *Dietary Reference Intakes for Thiamin, Riboflavin, Niacin, Vitamin B6, Folate, Vitamin B12, Pantothenic Acid, Biotin, and Choline*. National Academies Press, Washington, DC. 1998.

[31] U.S. Department of Agriculture. MyPyramid. Available at: *http://www.MyPyramid.gov*. Washington, DC.

In: Trends in Dietary Carbohydrates Research
Editor: M. V. Landlow, pp. 23-53
ISBN 1-59454-798-X

Chapter 2

SOURCES OF CARBOHYDRATES IN THE DIET AND RELATIONSHIP TO OBESITY AND DENTAL CARIES

Jennifer M. MacKeown*

South African Medical Research Council (MRC)/Health and Development Research Group; Johannesburg; South Africa

ABSTRACT

Two of the most prevalent chronic diseases in both developed and developing countries are dental caries and obesity. Over the years there has been a marked increase in the number of children, adolescents and young adults becoming obese and developing many of the health problems associated with obesity, now considered an international epidemic. Dental caries is an infectious disease that involves all age groups. However, adolescence is a period in which the risk for dental caries remains especially high. Adolescents have unique needs and concerns in regard to both dental caries and obesity. Among these concerns is the adolescent diet which contains high amounts of carbohydrate snack foods, such as carbonated beverages and confectionery containing significant amounts of sugar, Carbohydrates are thus major components of our food. They are important as body energy stores and, besides fat, are major determinants of daily energy intake. Both sugar and soft drink (carbonated and non-carbonated) consumption have increased dramatically over the years, particularly among adolescents, with teens consuming more added sugar as a percentage of energy than any other group. This is partly due to the consumption of a westernized diet in developed countries, and an increase in urbanization, characterised by a nutrition transition, in developing countries. Research studies have linked both dental caries and obesity either positively or negatively to carbohydrate intake in the form of starch (complex and/ or refined) and added sugars. However, the findings are only consistent with the view that frequency and amount of sugar intake are a necessary link in the etiology of dental caries, but this role is not as strong as it was in the pre-fluoride era. A combination of both starch and sugar appear to have the highest cariogenic effect. In contrast, research studies on the association between sugar intake and obesity have not been able to show a strong positive

* Correspondence: Dr. J. M. MacKeown PhD, Senior Scientist, MRC/Health and Development Research Group, Environment and Health Research Office, P. O. Box 87373, Houghton, 2041, Johannesburg, South Africa; Tel: +27 (0)11 6437367; Fax: +27 (0)11 6426832; e-mail address: jenny.mackeown@mrc.ac.za

relationship, but provide support that consumption of carbohydrate based foods with a high fibre content is associated with reduced body mass index (BMI) and weight loss.

The subject of "carbohydrates in research" is extremely vast. Epidemiological studies are continually taking new directions and focus as a result of earlier findings. It is therefore impossible to cover all aspects of this topic in one chapter and thus the aim is to provide only a brief overview of past and present epidemiological research on carbohydrates with regard to the analysis of consumption patterns in terms of food sources of carbohydrates rather than nutrients. This has an increasingly important place in nutrition research, creating many future research challenges. Further more, the altering trends in many of the western type diseases, including dental caries and obesity, two of the most prevalent diseases associated with carbohydrate intake, make identification of food sources of carbohydrates, and different customary eating patterns which may contribute to the development of these diseases, of topical importance.

Classification and Functions of Carbohydrates

Carbohydrates are the major components of our food and the complex varieties, in particular, have been the nutrient most promoted by nutritionists during the last 20-25 years [1]. Not so long ago, the classification of carbohydrates was regarded as relatively straightforward. It was understood that carbohydrates were either available or unavailable and a series of simple dietary rules could be applied. It was thought that available carbohydrates were digested to glucose, fructose and galactose along the gastrointestinal tract and completely absorbed within the small intestine. The main function of carbohydrates was therefore to provide the body with energy. The rate of digestion was believed to depend on the chain length of the carbohydrate and the fibre content of the diet. This belief produced an over-simplified classification of "simple sugars" and "complex carbohydrates".

It was assumed that available carbohydrates were inert and passed through the gastrointestinal tract unaltered. In the colon, their role was to increase faecal mass and decrease transit time, thus diluting and speeding excretion of potentially harmful substances. They were not regarded as an energy source.

Carbohydrates haven't changed, but what we know about them has. Research over the past decade has shown that carbohydrate classification is far more complex than this. Additional properties have been identified and functions are more clearly understood. [2]

In deciding how to classify dietary carbohydrates the primary problem is to reconcile their various chemical divisions with their numerous physiological functions. However, the Food and Agricultural Organisation of the United Nations (FAO) and the World Health Organisation (WHO) recommended that carbohydrates be classified according to their degree of polymerization (molecular weight) [3,4,5], as shown in Table 1. [4].

The main functions of the sugars are to supply energy and spare protein for use as an energy source, preventing ketosis, regulation of blood glucose and imparting flavour and sweetness to foods. Dietary fibre adds mass to the stool which eases elimination. Soluble fibre also controls blood glucose and lowers serum cholesterol. [6]

Dietary Guidelines for Carbohydrates

Dietary guidelines are designed to maintain an adequate intake of nutrients, including carbohydrates, to protect against diet related disease. Current population dietary guidelines advocate an increased intake of carbohydrate to more than 55% of the dietary energy intake, which should mainly be derived from starch. Added sugars intake should only contribute about 10% of the total energy intake [7]. One rationale in advising a moderate intake of added sugars is the role sugars play in promoting dental caries. A second is the low nutrient density of many sugary foods which makes high consumption of sugary foods incompatible with eating a nutritious diet at an energy level that maintains a healthful weight [8] However, very few meet these recommendations. The diets of the American population were scored according to the dietary guidelines and in particular "eat a variety of foods". Results indicated that only 1-3% eat the recommended number of servings from all the food groups on a given day. Fruit are the most commonly omitted food group. Intakes of specific types of vegetables (ie. dark green, deep yellow) and grains (whole grains) are well below that recommended and, intakes of total fat and added sugars exceed current recommendations [9].

Table 1 Classification of carbohydrates according to their degree of polymerization [4] (reproduced from the Current Carbohydrate Developments education pamphlet with permission from the South African Sugar Association (SASA))

Class	Sub-group	Components	Food sources
Sugars	Monosaccharides	Glucose	Fruit, vegetables, sugar, honey, milk products, ceteals
		Fructose	Fruit, vegetables, honey
		Galactose	Milk products
	Disaccharides	Sucrose (glucose + fructose)	Fruit, vegetables, sugar, honey
		Lactose (glucose + galactose)	Milk products
		Maltose (glucose + glucose)	Malt products, some cereals
	Polyols (sugar + alcohol)	Sorbitol	Alternative nutrient sweetener
Oligosaccharides	Malto-oligosaccharides	Maltodextrins	Some cereals
	Other oligosaccharides	Raffinose, Starchyose	Legumes
Polysaccharides	Starch	Amylose, Amylopectin, modified starch	Cereals, grains, vegetables, legumes
	Non-starch polysaccharides	Insoluble NSP (cellulose, hemicellulose)	Wholewheat cereals and grains, bran, vegetables

Food Sources of Carbohydrates in the Diet

Carbohydrates are the single most important source of food energy in the world comprising some 40-80% of the total food energy intake depending on cultural considerations and economic circumstances [4, 10]. They are also important sources of a variety of nutrients including protein, vitamins, minerals and phytochemicals (such as flavenoids) [11, 12]. As a result it seemed appropriate to determine the variety and types of carbohydrate sources consumed in both developing and developed countries. In fact, as early as 1985 Fanelli and Stevenhagen [13] considered the analysis of consumption patterns in terms of food rather than nutrients to play an increasingly important role in nutrition research.

Developed Countries

Contribution of Carbohydrates to Total Intake

Most of the studies on carbohydrate sources in developed countries have concentrated on sugars (mono- and disaccharides), in contrast to starches, as the main contributor to carbohydrate intake and have also shown a general increased intake of these sugars over the years, with adolescents consuming more added sugar as a percentage of energy than any other group [8].

In the United States the mean percent of energy from total sugars minus lactose was 18% according to the data from the 1987-1988 US Department of Agriculture Nationwide Food Consumption Survey, being slightly lower in the European Union at 15.2% [14]. The intake of caloric sweetener increased by 74kcal/day between 1962 and 2000. Data showed an 83kcal/day increase of caloric sweetener consumed and a 22% increase in the proportion of energy from caloric sweetener [15]. Among US male and female adolescents average intakes of added sugar contributed 20% of total energy intake, with children aged 6-11 years following a close second with added sugars contributing nearly 19%. The major sources of added sugars for 6-17 year old American children contributed 90% of childrens' and adolescents' total added sugar intake [8]. Children aged 2 years and older consumed the equivalent of 82g carbohydrate per day from added sweeteners accounting for 16% of the total energy intake, with adolescents having the highest intake [8].

The National Nutrition Survey in 1995 of Australian children and adolescents aged 2-18 years [16] found refined sugar to represent approximately 14% of their total energy intake and showed the top 100 foods to represent means of 85% and 82% of total sugar intake for boys and girls, respectively, being slightly lower than that found for American children [8]. Mean daily intakes of refined sugar ranged from 26.9 to 78.3g/day for the Australian 2-18 year old girls, representing 6.6-14.8% of total energy intake. Corresponding figures for boys were 27.0 to 81g/day and 8.0-14.0%, respectively.

An earlier study among 11-14 year old northern English children found sugar intake higher than in Australia at 118g/day, representing 21% of the total energy intake and 43% of the total carbohydrate intake [17]. However, in all these studies intakes of sugar over time (trends) must be viewed within the context of varying definitions, changes in food composition, changes in dietary intake methods and acknowledged increases in the underreporting of intake, [18] not forgetting that the majority of sugar consumed by humans is hidden in processed foods. [19].

It is evident from research findings that sugars are probably the most important contributors of total carbohydrates in the diets of all populations and across all age and gender groups, but the actual food sources of these sugars need to be identified, together with other sources of carbohydrates.

Individual Carbohydrate Sources in the Diets

Beverages are major contributors to the total amount of sugar consumed in developed countries and have featured very prominently as important sources of added sugars and/or carbohydrates [20] Much of the change in children and adolescents added sugar intakes can be attributed to changes in both fruit and beverage consumption patterns.[21] and evidence is accumulating that the consumption of regular soft drinks has increased in recent years, [22,23] indeed more rapidly than any other food group during the 1990's, [24] particularly among children [21] and adolescents [22]. Lytle *et al.* found that as children progressed from childhood to early adolescence both the prevalence and frequency of milk and fruit juice intake decreased, whereas soft drink intake more than tripled, [25] with the percentage contribution of soft drinks to added sweeteners peaking at age 18-34 years [8]. Based on USDA Food Consumption Survey data, Morton and Guthrie [26] found increased intake of regular soft drink to be one of the major changes in children's diets between 1989-1991 and 1994-1995. Using the same data set Chanmugam *et al* [27] found that consumption of soft drinks by adults also increased during the same period. Trends between 1977/78 and 1994/98 in the prevalence, amounts and sources of soft drink consumption were examined among American youth age 6 to 17 years from three national surveys: the Nationwide Food Consumption survey 1977/78 and the combined Continuing Survey of Food Intakes by Individuals 1994/96 and the Supplemental Children's Survey 1998. The prevalence of soft drink consumption increased 48% from a prevalence of 37% in 1977/78 to 56% in 1994/98. Mean intakes of soft drinks more than doubled over this time period [28]. Guthrie *et al.* [8] also investigated the major sources of added sugars in the diets of American children ages 6-17. These included non-diet soft drinks, fruitade drinks, sugars and sweets, sweetened grains, sweetened dairy products and presweetened cereals. Together these contributed 90% of childrens' and adolescents' total added sugars intake with non-diet soft drinks contributing the greatest percentage of added sugars to the diets of children; 22% for children ages 6-11 and 37% and 41% for adolescent females and males, respectively [8]. For people aged 2 years and over four items; namely regular soft drinks, sugar/sweets; sweetened grains and fruitades/drinks contributed almost 75% of the intake of added sweeteners, of which regular soft drinks accounted for one third. However, differences across age and gender groups in the sources of added sweeteners were found, but the findings generally emphasise the importance of regular soft drinks as sources of added sweeteners in the diets of Americans [8].

Foods from the grains group were also important contributors to the intake of added sweeteners for the American population. Concern has been expressed about the intake of presweetened cereals, especially by children. However, grains were actually larger contributors of added sweeteners, many of which are high in fat. Grain intake has been increasing in recent years but unfortunately little of this intake is whole grain [8].

An early study in 1981 found the average daily total sugar consumption for the total sample of 5-12 year old American children was 134.3g with the food group milk contributing on average the greatest number of grams of sugar. Other food groups making significant contributions were cakes, cookies, pies, and other desserts, sweetened beverages, fruits and fruit juices. Spline distribution indicated the food groups most likely to be consumed at levels resulting in excessive amounts of sugars intake were sweetened beverages, cakes, cookies, pies and other desserts and fruit juices [29].

Sweetened beverages such as soft drink and in particular cola –type and cordials were also substantial sources of refined sugar intake among 2-18 year-old Australian children. Of the 10 highest sources of refined sugars for each age group, sweetened beverages, especially the cola type beverages were the most prominent. [16].

From the German national Food Consumption Survey on persons aged 4 years and older, table sugar, confectionery, ice-cream, biscuits cakes and pastries and preserves, dairy products and non alcoholic beverages were the main sources of sucrose with varying importance in different age groups [30].

In the United Kingdom among 11-14-year-old northern English children sugars were derived from a variety of food sources with confectionery being the largest source. Snacks accounted for 65% of the sugars intake, but only 46% of the total energy intake [17]. More recently the food and nutrient intake of members of a birth cohort study in the UK was evaluated when young children in 1950 and investigated differences from present day childrens' diet. Compared to 1992/93, the 1950 diet contained substantially more bread and vegetables and less sugar and soft drinks giving a higher starch and fibre content.[31]. Another recent study in the UK reporting the first national survey in the UK to assess the diets of British children at 14 months indicated that bread and cereal were consumed frequently. Fifty percent of the children ate raw fruit, 51% ate cooked vegetables, 76% drank cows milk daily, but the consumption of sweetened drinks such as cordials and carbonated beverages was also very common among this young age group [32].

The trends in food related behaviour among 9-11 year old French children during three consecutive surveys (1993, 1995 and 1997) showed the most preferred foods to be rich in sugar and/or fat (fried potatoes, ice-cream, nut spread, chocolate, cake) [33].

Large scale national surveys among Norwegian adolescents were conducted in 1985, '89, '93 and '97 as part of the WHO International Study, Health Behaviour in School-aged Children. The results showed a strong increase in the daily intake of soft drinks and sweets from 11-15 years in each survey year [34].

The US Department of Agriculture Continuing Surveys of Food Consumption by Individuals (CSFII) has provided valuable information on the sources of carbohydrates consumed by the American population. The top 10 sources of carbohydrates consumed by young children in the 1989-1991 survey were bread, soft drinks/sodas, milk, ready-to- eat cereals, cakes/cookies, quick breads/doughnuts, syrups, jams, fruit drinks, pasta and potatoes [35]. However, nearly one quarter of all vegetables consumed by American children and adolescents 2-18 years of age who were respondents in the 1989-1991 survey were French fries. Their intakes of all fruit and dark green and/or deep yellow vegetables were very low compared with the recommendations. Only one in five children consumed five or more fruit and vegetable servings per day [36]. The average whole grain consumption ranged from 0.8 servings per day for preschool children to 1.0 serving per day for these adolescents. Ready-to-eat (RTE) cereals, corn and other chips, and bread were found to be the major food sources of whole grains accounting for 30.9%, 21.7% and 18.1% of whole grain intake, respectively [37].

Data including the 1994-1996 and 1998 surveys showed that the mean daily intakes of 100% fruit juices increased with increase in age. At age 5 mean intake of fruit drinks exceeded that of 100% fruit juice. Carbonated soft drink intake exceeded that of 100% fruit juice at age 5 and of milk at age 13. By age 13 adolescents drank more carbonated soft drinks than 100% fruit juice, milk and fruit drinks and ades [38]. It also showed that children and adolescents who consumed more added sugars are predicted to consume more grains [39].

However, data has indicated that the consumption of sugar sweetened beverages, sugars and sweets and sweetened grains has a negative impact on the diet quality [40]. Only 45% of the children who participated in the 1994-96 and 1998 surveys aged 4 and 6 years and 32% of 7-10 year olds consumed adequate fibre to meet the "age+ 5 rule ". Those who met this rule did so by consuming significantly more high and low fibre bread and cereals, fruit, vegetables, legumes, nuts and seeds. The children with low intakes of dietary fibre suggests they are at risk for future chronic disease. [41]. Data from the Dortmund Nutritional and Anthropometric Longitudinally designed (DONALD) Study evaluated the effect of intake of added sugars on intakes of nutrients and food groups. With the exception of "sugary foods" and beverages ($P<0.0001$) and dairy (NS), intake of all other food groups also decreased with increasing intake of added sugars ($P<0.0001$) among German children aged 2-18 years. [42].

Thus an increased intake of added sweeteners may displace more nutrient dense foods [26,43,44]. Morton and Guthrie [26] found the diets of children in 1994 –1995 were higher in energy than reported in 1989-1991, but nutrient intakes were generally similar.

Research studies [43,45,46] have also found that soft drinks tend to displace milk in the diets which has negative implications on diet quality. Data collected on children 2-18 years as part of the 1994 Continuing Survey of Food Intakes by Individuals (CSFII) was analysed to determine whether carbonated soft drinks consumption was associated with consumption of milk, fruit juice and the nutrients concentrated in these beverages. Children in the highest soft drink consumption category consumed less milk and fruit juice compared with those in the lowest consumption category [43].

Low nutrient density foods consumed by children from the third National Health and Nutrition Examination Survey (1988-1994) contributed more than 30% of their daily energy intake with sweeteners and desserts jointly accounting for nearly 25%. Intakes of total energy from carbohydrates and fat related positively, but percentage of energy from protein and dietary fibre related inversely to the reported number of low nutrient density (LND) foods ($P<0.05$). High LND food reporting was related to high energy intake but lower amounts of the 5 major food groups and most micronutrients [47].

Among ten year old American children with increasing sugar intake there was a significant linear decrease in mean intakes of protein, fat, saturated fat, starch, cholesterol, sodium, vitamin B6 and E, thiamin, niacin, iron and zinc and a significant linear increase in mean intakes of carbohydrates, fructose, lactose, sucrose, vitamin D and calcium. Eating patterns reflected the differing nutrient intakes with high sugar consumers having significantly higher intakes of total candy, beverages and milk and fewer intakes of meat and cheese than lower consumers [48].

However, if on the other hand added sweeteners were consumed in addition to more nutritious food the diet may be excessive in energy, thereby promoting obesity. However meta-analysis of studies of energy compensation in response to energy manipulation using liquid and solid foods indicates that compensation for increases in energy from carbohydrates ingested in fluids is significantly less than for solids which results in the potential for increased total energy intake [49].

Developing Countries

Information on individual food sources of nutrients, and carbohydrate sources in particular, is very scanty or completely lacking in developing countries Dietary histories of 4 and 5-year old rural black, urban black, Indian and white children in the Gauteng Province in South Africa were analysed to determine which foods consumed were the major macronutrients and energy contributors and what percentage of group total each food provided. Bread, milk, sugar and margarine were the main energy sources common to all groups. The main contributors of carbohydrates were maize-meal porridge, bread, sugar, potato and milk for the rural and urban black communities. For the Indian and white communities bread, sugar, milk, cooldrink (carbonated beverages) and cordials (non-carbonated beverages) were the main contributors of carbohydrates. Sugar, cooldrink, cordials and sweets were the main contributors of added sugars for all the groups with sugar contributing the highest percentage (24% of the total amount consumed for the urban Indian and white communities, 40-62% for the urban and rural black communities, respectively) The rural blacks, however consumed the lowest intake of dietary fibre. [50]. An earlier study in Cape Town, South Africa, also found rural blacks to consume the lowest intake of dietary fibre [51]. However, previous studies in South Africa have shown the reverse with the rural blacks consuming the highest fibre intake and the urban group the lowest [52].

The total amount of individual food items consumed by these 4 and 5-year old South African children differed markedly between the communities. When the food items were ranked in descending order according to the percentage of the total amount consumed, tea (generally consumed with sugar) was ranked the top item for both rural and urban blacks (23.5% and 18.2%, respectively) and milk was the top item for the urban Indians and whites (11.4% and 19.7%, respectively). Stiff-maize meal porridge was consumed in the largest amount by the rural and urban black communities (18.4% and 8.9%, respectively), rice by the Indians (3.5%) and bread by the whites (2.4%). Cooldrinks (carbonated beverages), cordials (non-carbonated beverages) and added sugar were the only added sugars that ranked within the top 25 food items, with the highest intake of cooldrink (carbonated beverages) by the Indians (11.2%) [53].

In South Africa studies have also been conducted in Ndunakazi, a rural area in KwaZulu, Natal Province. Subjects have included infants up to 24 months of age, [54,55,56], preschoolers [55], and school children. [55,57]. Almost 98% of preschool and school children consumed sugar every day and almost 30% consumed biscuits, sweets, crisps and savoury snacks at least 4 times per week. Fifty-five percent consumed maize-meal porridge every day, followed by 38% and 21% consuming rice with beans and bread on a daily basis, respectively. Samp with beans and rice were consumed by more than 40% at least 4 days per week. On the other hand milk was seldom or never consumed by the majority of children [55].

The diet consumed by the primary school children comprised a limited number of food items. Fruit and vegetable consumption was low. Phutu (a stiff maize-meal porridge), bread, biscuits, potatoes, mealie (corn), savoury snacks, sweets/chocolates, rice, cooldrinks (carbonated beverages) and rice with beans were consumed by 50-100% of the children at least 4 times per week. Breakfast cereals consumption was seldom or never consumed by the children [57].

Among the infants 4-24 months maize-meal porridge, nutromeal (specially developed maize-meal based porridge), rice, rice with beans, and potatoes were the most popular items consumed on most days of the week. The childrens' food intake reflected a high intake of carbohydrate rich foods and irregular intakes of fruit and vegetables [54]. The food items consumed by these young rural children. 43 reported in a 24 hour dietary recall, were ranked in descending order according to the number of consumers. Soft maize-meal porridge, sugar, beans (legumes), rice, phutu (a stiff maize-meal porridge) were reported for more than 50% of the children. Formula milk, phutu (a stiff maize-meal porridge), beans (legumes) soft maize-meal porridge and rice contributed more than 5% of the childrens' total energy intake. It was noted that an infant cereal was given as the first solid food to 50% of the children and 81% had received an infant cereal at some stage, usually at an early age, but the duration for the use of infant cereals was short, on average 3 months [56].

In addition to this rural area, Ndunakazi, in KwaZulu-Natal, children from the black community 4-24 months of age were included in the study from two urban areas in the Gauteng Province of South Africa – Soweto and the northern suburbs of Johannesburg and Sandton to determine the variety and frequency of consumption of food items, including cariogenic items consumed by these children. Significant differences were found in the food items consumed between the rural and urban groups, with most of the items showing the rural group to be significantly different from both urban groups. Soft maize-meal porridge was consumed by the highest percentage of children in the rural and urban Soweto groups (73%). For the children who consumed the various food items among the carbohydrates the rural children consumed stiff maize-meal porridge, soft maize-meal porridge and Nestum infant cereal most frequently (5.6-7.3 times per week), while the urban Soweto children consumed soft maize meal porridge, Maltabella porridge and oats porridge more than 6 times per week. For the urban Johannesburg children bread and soft maize meal porridge were the most frequently consumed food items. Within the sugars group; sugar was consumed most frequently by the rural children (5.8 times per week) in addition to cooldrinks (carbonated beverages), cordials (non-carbonated beverages), sweets and jelly. [58].

In 1988 a study was conducted on 11-year old rural and urban children in two regions of Southern Africa, KwaZulu-Natal Province of South Africa and Namibia, to determine the variety of food items consumed. The KwaZulu urban children consumed the largest variety with 65 items contributing 80% of the total group intake and Namibian urban consumed the fewest (43). Maize-meal porridge was ranked the top item for all groups except for the KwaZulu urban group where tea was ranked the top item. Starches (maize-meal, bread, dried beans, rice and samp) predominated in the food choices for all the groups. Among the sugars, cordials (non-carbonated beverages), cooldrinks (carbonated beverages) and sugar per se were the popular choices. However, the choice and amounts of foods consumed differed between the regions being specific to the particular region [59]. Steyn *et al.* [60] found similar items, maize-meal porridge, tea, bread and chicken consumed in the largest amount by 11-14 year old rural Pedi children in Lebowa, an area in Northern Gauteng Province of South Africa.

In a west Indian island (Antigua) 41% of all energy was obtained from foods consumed as snacks between lunch and dinner and 8% of all energy was obtained from morning snacks.

Principal snack foods included soft drinks, fresh fruit and unsweetened fruit juices, sweets and chocolates, sugar and sugar based products. Over 33% of the daily energy intake, 50% of carbohydrate intake and almost 66% of added sugar are obtained from snacks [61]. An earlier study in the same region investigated the pattern of sugar consumption in samples of 12-year-old and 15-19-year-old adolescents The frequency of total sugary food and drink episodes for children was 3.16 and 3.71 for adolescents, respectively. This was mainly accounted for by the consumption of sugary items at meals. Students mainly consumed sweetened drinks at meals especially at breakfast and ate sugary foods between meal times, particularly between lunch and dinner. Sweetened tea and juice were the most popular drinks and confectionery was the most popular snack [62].

In summary, although there are common sources of carbohydrates in both developed and developing countries, studies have shown that differences in the importance of individual food sources of carbohydrates exist between and within countries and between age groups, genders etc., with many of the sources conveying traditional food customs and beliefs. However in all the studies investigated sugar and soft drinks, both carbonated and non-carbonated, have been shown to predominate as important sources of carbohydrate in the diet. The studies have also shown the importance of these food sources to change over time and with increasing age. It is clear though that the studies are specific to the particular area and community and cannot be extrapolated to other countries or communities.

Knowledge of the basic food types generally consumed by the population is essential for the development of any nutrition education programme and government policy. This is especially the case in South Africa and possibly in most other developing countries with heterogenous populations with great cultural diversity, where information on individual items is scanty or completely lacking. In a rapidly changing society with altered food habits, nutritional problems and the demands of todays professional practices there is a need for nutritional surveys on the actual food items consumed by populations at regular intervals that will provide valid information on food types and dietary changes [63,64].

Children and adolescents with poor diet quality, as suggested through the consumption of high intakes of sugars, may be at risk for a multitude of health problems such as obesity, heart disease, dental caries and osteoporosis as well as other chronic diseases that occur later in life [65].

Carbohydrates in Relation to Diseases

Two of the most prevalent chronic diseases linked to carbohydrate intake in both developed as well as developing countries are dental caries [66] and obesity [67,68, 69]. As mentioned previously, consumption of added sugars has increased steadily as documented by both supply data and nationwide food consumption survey data and diets high in sugars have been associated with various health problems including dental caries, dyslipidaemias, obesity, bone loss and fractures and poor diet quality [70]. It has also been suggested that larger portion sizes of foods low in fat and commercial energy dense foods and beverages could be important factors in maintaining high energy intake, causing over consumption and enhancing the prevalence of obesity in the population [71]. Obesity, in turn, and physical inactivity are precursors to the development of a number of chronic conditions, including hypertension,

Type II diabetes, cancer and hypercholesterolaemia, being components of the metabolic syndrome [72,73]. Diabetes, which is related to obesity (and a diet high in sugar and fat) has been linked to increases in oral disease [74].

Adolescence is a time of accelerated growth with increasing caloric needs. A strong attraction for the taste of sugar and its availability have detrimental consequences for the adolescent's dentition as well as their general health. Obesity and its associated maladies are additional issues for consideration during adolescence [75].

Obesity

Prevalence

Energy balance and macronutrient balance are the cornerstones upon which any theories of obesity must be built. Obesity can only occur when energy intake remains higher than energy expenditure for an extended period of time. However the macronutrient composition of the diet can also affect energy balance. [76].

The prevalence of obesity has risen dramatically throughout the world in the past few decades and now poses a major public health problem, the literature being quite overwhelming supporting this statement [67,68,69,77,78,79,80,81,82,83].

Overweight increased approximately twofold in the 20 year period from 1974 to 1994, with the largest increases observed among 19-24-year-olds. The annual increases in weight and obesity that occurred from 1983 to 1994 were 50% higher than those from 1973 to 1982 [84]. The overall age-adjusted prevalence of adult obesity (BMI>30) was 30.5% in 1999-2000 compared with 22,9% reported in the National Health and Nutrition Examination Survey (NHANES) III in the 1988-1994 cohort. The prevalence of adult overweight (BMI>25) rose in the same period from 55.9% to 64.5% [85]. During this same period, the NHANES reported significant changes in the percent of adolescents (ages 12-19) who were overweight (at or above the 95th percentile of BMI for age): 15.5% in 1999-2000 compared to 10.5% in 1988-1994 [86]. Currently, approximately 1 in 4 children and 1 in 2 adults are overweight, prevalence rates that have increased by 50% since 1960 [87]. A recent article by Mokdad *et al.* [88] highlights an even more extensive problem emerging in the next decade. The WHO estimates that 1 billion people around the world are now obese or overweight and that westernization of diets has been part of the problem. Fruits, vegetables and whole grains are being replaced by readily accessible foods high in saturated fat, sugar and refined carbohydrates [79]. From a cross-sectional survey of junior high school students in Tapei it was concluded that from 1980 to 1994 body weight increased dramatically over body height and the prevalence of obesity increased significantly, especially among boys while the percentage of overweight children did not vary. Overall this study indicates that obesity and the adverse effects of being overweight is no longer just a problem of western countries [89]. Thus the marked increase in the number of children, adolescents, young adults and adults becoming obese and developing many of the health problems associated with obesity is now an international epidemic [72,77,79,82,90].

The development of obesity has been associated with four critical periods, namely intrauterine life, infancy, the period of adiposity rebound (ages 5-7years) and adolescence [91] but, the association between poor diet quality and the increased incidence of childhood obesity, is by far the most emergent concern [86]. Recently a new national composite index on the health and wellbeing of American children (the Foundation for Child Development and Index of Child Well-Being) identified obesity as the "single most widespread health problem facing children today" [92]. The prevalence of childhood obesity is on the rise in the USA and has reached epidemic proportions [93]. An estimated 1 in 4 children in the United States is overweight, while 11% are obese [84]. As a percentage this means that approximately 20% of children and adolescents are overweight as defined by a BMI greater than the 85th percentile [93]. In fact, over the past three decades the prevalence of overweight has tripled among US children ages 6-11 years and adolescents, 4% to 15% and 5% to 16%, respectively [86]. Among 14-15 year old adolescents from the French West Indies 20% presented a BMI over the chosen thresholds for overweight and obesity. Foods rich in animal fats and carbohydrates were prevailing [94].

There is a consistent body of literature demonstrating the importance of weight gain during childhood and adolescence being predictive of adult obesity, [95] with physical activity and the environment during adolescence serving as strong predictors of adult obesity [79,96,97]. Children who are overweight tend to remain so up to 20 years of age and in general they have a 1.5 to twofold higher risk for becoming overweight adults [84]. Despite the magnitude of this problem, little attention has been given to tackling this problem during adolescence [85].

There is thus abundant evidence to support the international nature of the problem, with data from several developed countries reporting increases in overweight among their children and adolescents [98,99,100].

However, the problem has now "immigrated " to developing countries and is no longer localized in developed countries [77,80,83, 98].

Using identical cut-offs for BMI, the prevalence of childhood overweight in Russia, Brazil South Africa and China ranged from 10.5% to 25.6% (based on the 85th percentile) [101]. South Africa is a developing country with a predominantly black population in which the prevalence of obesity is high among adult African women [102,103]. but low among African girls [104,105].

Childhood stunting has been suggested as a factor contributing to high rates of adult obesity in developing countries [101,106] and was common among the children surveyed in Russia, Brazil,China and South Africa, affecting 9.2-30.6% of all children. A recent national study of South African children found that stunting remained the most common nutritional disorder affecting 21.6% of children ages 1-9 years, whereas 6% were classified as overweight as defined by a z score of >2 for weight for age [105]. Stunted girls seemed to be at risk of greater fat deposition especially in the abdominal area [83] and this could be a contributing factor to developing one or more of the components of the metabolic syndrome in later life. Cameron and Getz [107] described a gain in fat among South African adolescent girls occurring after peak height velocity. However, there is a lack of data on body composition and, in particular, the prevalence of stunting, overweight and obesity among sub-Sahara African children, especially for girls ages 10-15 years [105]. In the past stunted children in developing countries grew up under conditions of food shortage and had little opportunity to become obese. The nutrition transition is associated with shifts in dietary composition and activity patterns that may lead to the development of overweight [77].

In North Africa the etiology of obesity is not well understood and few studies shed any light on its development. However, a study was undertaken to compile what is known about the prevalence of obesity and its determinants in Morocco and Tunisia. Overall levels of obesity identified by BMI > or = 30kg.m(2) were 12.2% in Morocco and 14.4% in Tunisia and overweight increased with age and seemed to take hold in adolescence, particularly among girls. Fat intake (31% of total energy intake) is high in Tunisia and carbohydrate (65%-67%) is high in Morocco [108].

It is clear therefore that overweight children whether from developed or developing countries are at risk of serious health, economic and quality of life consequences [109]. Overweight youth are 2.4 times as likely to have a high serum total cholesterol level and 43.5 times likely to three cardiovascular risk factors [84]. Thus it is important to identify those most likely to have high BMIs and take steps to both maintain weight and prevent the onset of obesity. This strategy is most effective when applied to young people as it easier to form healthy living habits at a young age. Even small improvements can have large benefits to society [109].

Although the total energy intake of the children has remained the same, and the macronutrient density of the diet has changed, the percentage of energy from fat has decreased while that from carbohydrate and protein has increased. Children have been consuming lower amounts of fats/oils, vegetables/soup, bread/grains, mixed meats, desserts, candy and eggs and increasing amounts of fruits/fruit juices, beverages, poultry, snacks, condiments and cheese. Changes in specific eating patterns may explain the increase in adiposity among children [84]. Among 9-10-year-old American children percentage of energy in the diet was inversely related to adiposity. These findings suggest that the macronutrient intake of children, particularly dietary fat and carbohydrate intake, may play a role in adiposity, independent of the influence of total energy intake [110].

Relationship between Carbohydrate Intake and Obesity

One reason for the increase in obesity and lifestyle diseases all over the world is the change in dietary components. This nutrition transition is characterized by improvement in dietary variation but also by increase in the content of fat and sugar. Urbanisation leads to over-consumption by increasing market access to fatty and sugary foods, including fast foods. Globalisation increases the consumption of sweet soda pops, biscuits and snacks. It has also been proposed that the population in developing countries is more vulnerable towards these dietary changes in regard to obesity and chronic diseases [111].

Historically carbohydrates have been thought to play only a minor role in promoting weight gain and in predicting the risk of development of chronic disease. Most of the focus has been on reducing total dietary fat. During the last 20 years fat intake decreased, while the number of individuals who were overweight or developed a chronic condition have dramatically increased. Simultaneously, the energy from carbohydrates has also increased [112]. One in five American children is overweight, despite a decrease in total fat consumption. [87,113]. In an attempt to combat this problem the Federal Government and various official medical agencies have advocated decreasing intake of total fat and sugar, while increasing consumption of complex carbohydrates [87]. This has sparked an interest in the carbohydrate composition of the diet, including the glycemic index (GI). Carbohydrates can be classified by their post-prandial glycemic effect, called the glycemic index. Carbohydrates with a high glycemic index produce substantial increases in blood glucose and insulin levels after ingestion. Within a few hours after their consumption, blood glucose levels begin to decline rapidly due to an exaggerated increase in insulin secretion. A profound state of hunger is created. The continued intake of high-glycemic load meals is associated with an increased risk of chronic diseases such as obesity, cardiovascular disease and diabetes [112], the epidemic of which is increasing among children, adolescents and adults [114] and increasing markedly for obese children after puberty [115]. Overweight is the most powerful modifiable risk factor for Type II diabetes.

There is accumulating evidence to support the hypothesis that whole grain consumption is associated with reduced risk of incident Type II diabetes [114] with an ad libitum reduced glycemic index diet appearing to be a promising alternative to a conventional diet in treating obese adolescents [115]. The prolonged satiety associated with low GI foods may prove an effective method for reducing energy intake and achieving long term weight control [113,116].

On the other hand other dietary patterns, among several other factors, are associated with the likelihood of a high BMI. Total weight of food and beverage intake has been positively associated with the likelihood of a high BMI among young children. Also the higher the proportion of energy from protein and fat, the higher the likelihood that a child will have a high BMI [117]. Concern has also been expressed about the apparent increasing consumption of added sugars and their possible role in displacing or diluting nutrients in the diet and contributing to the epidemic of obesity in developed countries. One of the 2000 Dietary Guidelines for Americans states " Choose beverages and foods to moderate your intake of sugars" [118].

Free sugars promote a positive energy balance. Some short term experiments in humans confirm that total energy intake increases when energy density of the diet is increased, whether by free sugars or fat [119,120]. Drinks rich in free sugars increase overall energy intake by limiting appetite control. There is thus less of a compensatory reduction of food intake after consumption of high sugar drinks than when additional foods of equivalent energy content are provided [121].

Children with a high consumption of soft drinks rich in free sugars are thus more likely to be overweight and gain excess weight [122].Diets limited in free sugars have been shown to reduce total energy intake and induce weight loss, even when people are encouraged to replace sugars with starches and non starch polysaccharides [123,124].

Recent research has confirmed an association between the consumption of sugar sweetened beverages with the increased risk of childhood obesity [122]. Excessive sweetened drink consumption by children aged 6-13 years displaced milk from the children's diet. Because children failed to reduce consumption of solid foods to compensate for the caloric contribution of sweetened drinks, higher daily energy intakes were observed. Consequently the greater the sweetened drink consumption the greater the weight gain (1.12+/- 0.7kg) [125]. However, among children aged 6-19 from the US Department of Agriculture Continuing Survey of Food Intake by Individuals (CSFII) 1994-1996, 1998 it was found that BMI was positively associated with consumption of diet carbonated beverages and negatively associated with consumption of citrus juice. BMI was not associated with the consumption of milk, regular carbonated beverages, regular or diet fruit drinks/ades or non citrus juices [126],

In Canada it was found that obese children and adolescents consumed more servings of meat and alternatives, grain products, sugar sweetened drinks and potato chips which contributed to a higher energy, fat and sugar intake compared to non-obese children and adolescents. The consumption of meat servings and sugar sweetened drinks was positively correlated with percent body fat. [127].

Sugars provide a strong pleasant sweet taste and at the same time deliver energy when ingested. Their effects on food intake and selection may therefore be a result of both their hedonic and their physiologic features. The theory that appetite signals arising from sugars are different from those arising from other carbohydrates because of sugars' sweetness has led to the hypothesis that sugars are a cause of excessive energy intake and obesity. However there are only a few studies that support this. [128,129]. New epidemiological studies provide evidence that sugar consumption as well as carbohydrate consumption is associated with leanness, not obesity and there is no basis for a causative association between sugar intake and obesity. Thus there is no evidence to support the hypothesis that sugar is unique among carbohydrates as a dietary component affecting food intake [128,129]. A recent study among 6-7year old children from four Spanish cities found bakery products, sweetened soft drinks and yoghurt to supply 15.5, 1.0 and 5.6% of the total energy intake, respectively. Higher consumption of these three foods was associated with greater energy intake but not with higher BMI. It was concluded that the impact of the consumption of bakery products, sweetened soft drinks and yoghurt on the quality of diet of Spanish children was only modest, although it may contribute to aggravating certain unhealthy characteristics of their diet particularly excess energy and sugars [130]. A longitudinal study in Australia on 2-15 year old children was conducted to investigate the relationship between food energy and macronutrient intake and body fatness assessed up to 7 times. It was found that the current level of body fatness of the child and parental adiposity are more important predictors than dietary intake variables of risk of children becoming or remaining overweight as they grow [131].

Several studies suggest that the consumption of ready-to-eat cereals (RTE) can improve the macronutrient intake status in various populations [67.68.69] and that regular consumption of RTE cereals is associated with healthy weight and a healthy lifestyle [69,132, 133] together with reduced BMI and/or weight loss [67,68,69,132,133]. Albertson [68] also found that frequent cereal eaters (consumed RTE cereals over 8 times in 14 days) had lower BMI's than non frequent cereal eaters consistently across age and gender. Increased consumption of RTE cereal was positively associated with an increase in dietary fibre. Higher intakes of fibre may induce more satiation and may help people control body weight. The differences between the breakfast habits of obese/overweight (those with BMI above the 75th percentile) and normal weight school children (those with a BMI below the 75th percentile) were analysed. It was found that obese subjects and in particular females, omitted breakfast more frequently and took significantly smaller quantities of cereals than did normal weight subjects. In addition obese subjects took lower quantities of carbohydrates This may be a reflection on the diet as a whole that is less adequate [132].

Summary

There is epidemiological evidence supporting the role of sucrose and other free sugars in the global epidemic of obesity. On the other hand new epidemiological studies provide evidence that sugar consumption as well as carbohydrate consumption is associated with leanness, not obesity and there is no basis for a causative association between sugar intake and obesity. However, reducing the intake of sugars may make a useful contribution along with other measures in reducing the risk of obesity and its clinical consequences. Suggesting an appropriate upper limit requires judgement based on dietary and disease patterns, but has been guided by the association between free sugars and dental caries [134].

Dental Caries

Prevalence

A decline in the prevalence of dental caries over three decades has occurred without a significant change in the consumption of fermentable carbohydrates, and in many countries 80% of the caries is present in only 20% of the population, [135]. Caries prevalence data from studies in all European countries between 1990 and 1995 showed a general trend towards a decline for children and adolescents. However, in several countries with already low caries prevalence in primary teeth, there was no further decrease. Regarding the permanent dentition, further reductions were observed in the 12-year age group, these being even more evident at the ages of 15-19 years. In some central and eastern European countries caries prevalence in children and adolescents was high, but few data were available on young adults [136]. However, the report by the British Nutrition Foundation Task Force reports that the improvements in the levels of caries in the UK are halting and remain unacceptably high in some 'risk groups'. It states that a two pronged attacked ie. reduced frequency of consumption of sugary foods and use of fluoride is necessary to address the problem [137] but, despite improved trends in the level of dental caries in developed countries, dental caries remains prevalent and is increasing in some developing countries undergoing nutrition transition [138]. According to the recently published demographic and health survey undertaken by the South African Department of Health in 1998, dental problems are of great concern among South Africans [139]. It is widespread among the communities, but it also displays wide variation in prevalence and severity across communities, the prevalence of dental caries approaching 90% in most adult South African communities [140].

Development of Caries

Dental caries is a highly prevalent chronic disease [66]. It is a bacterially based disease and when in progress, acid produced by bacterial action on dietary fermentable carbohydrate diffuses into the teeth and dissolves carbonated hydroxyapaptite mineral – a process called demineralization. Pathological factors including acidogenic bacteria (mutans streptococci and lactobacilli), salivary dysfunction as well as dietary carbohydrates are related to caries progression Protective factors which include salivary calcium, phosphate and proteins, salivary flow, fluoride in saliva and antibacterial components or agents can balance, prevent or reverse dental caries [141]. The classic literature on the topic, with studies readily recognizable by name – The Vipeholm Study [142], Turku Sugar Study [143], World War II Food Rationing [144,145,146] and Hopewood House [147], to mention a few, still forms the basis of our understanding of the etiology of dental caries [148].

Although dental caries involves all age groups, adolescence is a period in which the risk for dental caries remains especially high. Many factors some unique to the teenage years, contribute to the initiation and progression of dental caries in this age group. One factor with the potential for being significant is the adolescent diet, especially the high consumption of sugars. One product that tends to contribute to the amount of sugar ingested is carbonated beverages. Many soft drinks also contain significant amounts of caffeine. Regular caffeine ingestion may lead to increased or habitual usage. It is suggested that the combination of the consumption of highly sweetened soft drinks and habitual usage of caffeine may significantly increase a susceptible adolescent's potential for developing dental caries [149].

Sugars and other Factors Related to Caries Development

With regard to diet, a dynamic relation still exists between sugars and oral health [150] and numerous lines of evidence have conclusively established the role of sugars in the etiology of dental caries and the importance of sugars as the principal dietary substrate that drives the caries process has not been scientifically challenged. While sugars appear to differ little in acidogenic potential, sucrose has been given special importance as the sole substrate for synthesis of extracelluālr glucans [148]. Evidence from human intervention studies, epidemiological studies, animal studies and experimental studies have shown an association between the amount and frequency of free sugar intake and dental caries [139]. However, many other factors affect the caries process, including the form of food or fluid, the duration of exposure, nutrient composition, sequence of eating, salivary flow, presence of buffers and oral hygiene as shown in Figure 1. Since the introduction of fluoride, the incidence of caries worldwide has decreased, despite increases in sugar consumption. Other factors in addition to sugar, such as fermentable carbohydrates [139], the presence of buffers in dairy products, the use of sugarless chewing and the consumption of sugars as part of the meal rather than between meals may reduce the risk of caries [150] but, because of the complexity of the caries process, the potential cariogenicity of specific food items is difficult to assess [151].

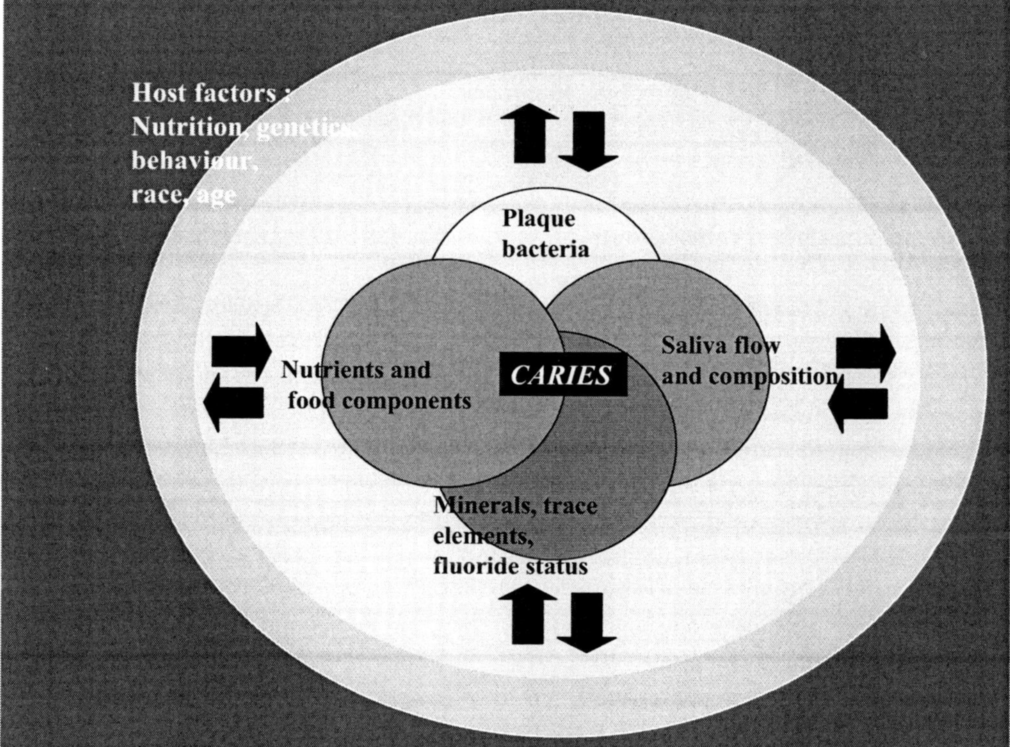

Figure 1. Factors in the development of dental caries

Sugar/caries relationship

Existing Evidence of Sugars in Relation to Dental Caries

The understanding that sugars are an important etiologic factor in dental caries has been with us since the dawn of civilized man, but the controversy surrounding this subject is a more recent phenomenon. The subject has been the focus of several recent review articles and considerable debate with some authors reaching different conclusions from basically the same studies. This existing evidence has come form classic studies, mentioned previously, national surveys, systematic reviews and other evidence (animal studies, in situ studies, plaque pH studies and laboratory studies) [148] each of which will be discussed in more detail.

National Surveys

Evidence is provided from national surveys comparing caries experience and sugar supply data that have established a sugar caries relationship at the population level. However, it is also evident from the later surveys that the nature of this relationship has changed in most industrialized countries. The use of fluoride in all forms has resulted in a dramatic decrease in caries prevalence. The weakening of this relationship in industrialized countries may also be explained by the high level of sugar consumption by the majority of the population and the well known problem of obtaining accurate data on sugar intake [152,153,154], which leaves little room to establish a clear relationship. This relationship is further complicated by the wide variation in sugar consumption patterns among individuals. Comparison of the relationship between sugar consumption and caries among different countries is also limited by the reliability of sugar consumption data and caries data [148].

Systematic Reviews

Many epidemiologic studies, shown in Table 2 [148], have evaluated the relationship between sugar consumption and caries risk. The topic has recently been the subject of a systematic review by Burt and Pai [155] conducted as part of of the NIH/NIDCR Consensus Development Conference on Diagnosis and Management of Dental Caries throughout life. This review specifically addressed the question : "in the modern age of extensive fluoride exposure, do individuals with a high level of sugar intake experience greater caries severity relative to those with a lower level of intake?" Thirty six papers with a quality score of 55 or higher were rated for the strength of the relationship between sugar and caries and were used as the basis for their conclusions. Only 2 papers found a strong relationship, 16 found a moderate relationship and 18 found the relationship to be weak-to-none. Based on the reviews it was concluded that while the relationship between sugar consumption and caries is not as strong as it was in the prefluoride era, restriction of sugar consumption still has an important role in caries prevention. It is thus obvious that the role of sugar in the etiology of caries should be revised and the diet as a whole considered. South African studies have investigated the diet as whole in relation to dental caries incidence, including energy, macro-and micronutrients specifically among urban black preschool children. However, in all the studies the association of nutrient intake, including sugar, with caries incidence was found to be weak and isolated and therefore not clinically relevant among this group of children [156,157,158].

Table 2. Review articles on the relationship between sugar (diet) and dental caries [148] (reproduced from reference 148 with permission from the author: Prof. DT. Zero)

Authors	Main conclusions
Marthaler (1967 [162]	foodstuffs containing simple sugars are far more cariogenic than common starchy foods
Newbrun (1969) [159]	called for the specific elimination of sucrose or sucrose containing foods rather than restricting total carbohydrate consumption
Bibby (1975) [163]	snack foods share importance with sucrose in caries causation
Sreebny (1982a) [164]	total consumption and frequency of intake contribute to dental caries; lacking evidence about the precise definition of the relationship
Newbrun (1982a) [165]	compelling evidence that the proportion of sucrose in a food is one important determinant of its cariogenicity
Sheiham (1983) [166]	sugar is the principal cause in industrialized countries: recommended that sugar consumption be reduced to 15kg/person/year or below
Shaw (1983) [167]	studies in animals consistent with the clinical evidence on the relationship between sugar and caries
Rugg-Gunn (1986) [168]	cariogenicity of starchy foods is low; the addition of sucrose to cooked starch is comparable to similar quantities of sucrose; fresh fruits appear to have low cariogenicity
Bowen and Birkhed (1986) [169]	frequency of eating sugars is of greater importance than total sugar consumption
Walker and Cleaton-Jones (1989)[170]	degree of incrimination of sugar as a cause of caries is grossly exaggerated; questioned prediction of reduction in caries from decreases in sugar and snack intake
Marthaler (1990) [154]	in spite of dramatic reduction in caries due primarily to widespread use of fluoride, sugars continue to be the main threat to dental health
Rugg-Gunn (1990) [171]	dietary modification involving restriction on the frequency and amount of extrinsic sugars can be more effective than other control measures
Konig and Navia (1995) [172]	acknowledged the relationship between frequency and sugar intake and caries; recommended removing the focus away from elimination of sugar and towards improved oral hygiene and use of fluoride toothpaste
Ruxton et al (1999) [173]	evidence strongly supports formulation of advice on frequency of consumption, not amount
Konig (2000) [160]	dental health problems do not require any dietary recommendations other than those required for maintenance of general health
van Loveren (2000) [161]	if good oral hygiene is maintained and fluoride supplied frequently; teeth will remain intact even if carbohydrate containing food is frequently eaten
Sheiham (2001) [66]	sugars, particularly sucrose, are the most important dietary cause of caries, the intake of extrinsic sugars greater than 4 times a day increases caries risk; sugar consumption should not exceed 60g/day foe teenagers and adults and proportionally less for younger children

Although the original claim that "Sucrose is the Arch Criminal of Dental Caries" [159] has been softened over the years it continues to be the most common form of added sugar in the diet. This has led some authors to conclude that recommendations to restrict sugar consumption may no longer be necessary [160,161]. Clearly fluoride has raised the threshold at which the caries process will progress to frank cavitation in that a higher cariogenic diet can be tolerated before caries occurs in many individuals. However, fluoride has its limits and caries remains a serious problem for economically disadvantaged individuals and a rising problem in many developing countries where sugar consumption is increasing.

A weakening of the sugar/caries relationship may also be explained by the many technical, biological, behavioural and genetic factors. These studies are not without limitations: Most studies have used different dietary assessment methods which have only rarely been validated. The role of sugar in the etiology of caries is complex as sugar is seldom eaten in a pure form. The cariogenicity of foods can be modified by many factors including the amount and type of carbohydrate (sucrose versus other starch combinations), protective components (proteins, fats, calcium, phosphate, fluoride) and physical and chemical properties (liquid vs solid, retentiveness, solubility, pH, buffering capacity). While some studies have measured frequency of ingestion, most studies do not account for other behaviours associated with food consumption such as eating sequence in relation to other foods, eating before bedtime, late night snacks and behaviours after food ingestion such as oral hygiene. In addition environmental, genetic, social. economic, political and educational factors may confound the relationship between sugar consumption and caries if not controlled for [148].

Other Evidence

Other indirect evidence in support of the role of sugars in caries comes from animal studies, in situ studies, plaque pH studies and laboratory studies. The main use of these model systems has been to evaluate the cariogenic potential of individual food items with the aim of ranking them which is something that cannot be done in human clinical trials due to the impact of a highly variable background diet. The cariogenic potential of a food is influenced by its properties, most importantly its sugar content, the presence of protective factors and the consumption patterns such as the frequency of consumption [174,175], which further divided the possible factors that can influence the cariogenicity of foods into food factors (amount and type of carbohydrate, food pH and buffering power, food consistency and retention in the mouth, eating pattern etc.) and cultural and economic factors [148].

While the ability to rank foods based on their relative cariogenic potential seems desirable, there are several problems with this approach. Both the human plaque acidity models and animal caries models do not account for how foods are actually consumed, in regard to the frequency of ingestion, patterns of ingestion, or relationship of the dietary intake to other foods which can greatly modify the actual cariogenicity of a given food.

Summary

There continues to be a discussion about the nature of the relationship between sugar intake and caries and whether there is a safe level, of sugar intake, but the overall weight of the evidence is exceptionally strong and based on reviews a causal relationship between sugars and dental caries has been established. This does not mean that other carbohydrates such as starches or different combinations of sugars and starch are not cariogenic [148].

However, this relationship is much weaker than in the prefluoride era. Scientific discoveries have led to a better understanding of the caries process, the ever expanding food supply and the interaction between the two [176]. As there is evidence that frequency of sugar consumption contributes to dental caries there appears to be some justification for a guideline on sugar intake, particularly in developing countries where dental caries is still a problem, such as South Africa [134,177]. It has been found that when free sugar consumption is < 15-20kg/yr dental caries is low. In addition the frequency of consumption of foods containing free sugars should be limited to a maximum of 4 times per day [138]. Establishment of good dietary practices during infancy and childhood can minimize risk of caries development throughout life. Optimal dietary habits for oral health are consistent with dietary recommendations for systemic health, growth and development [178]. Dietary advice given should not contradict general health principles when providing practical advice to reduce caries risk [176]. However, dietary modification is notoriously difficult to achieve being incumbent upon the subject's willingness to effect a change in behaviour. Dietary advice should be formulated which is both realistic and positive. Trying to dissuade children from consuming products which they perceive as tasty and pleasurable is counter productive. Also, a fundamental shift away from the idea of "good foods versus bad foods" is required and more emphasis laid on good diets opposed to bad diets [135,179].

Future Research

There is a general agreement that diet and disease patterns change over time [180], and most countries are affected by demographic transition and changing epidemiology of disease. The nutrition of children is increasingly recognized as crucial for present and future health as there is increasing evidence that childhood nutrition also influences adult health [181]. In order to prevent diseases such as dental caries and obesity and its associated maladies developing it is essential to establish the nutrient as well as the individual food item intake and change in intake over time among the same children from an early age. A key factor for future research is the recognition that continued nutritional intervention studies at different stages of life are necessary if childhood nutrition is to improve. [180]. In this way key nutrient deficiencies and poor dietary habits can be identified and this, together with the change in nutrient intake over time, can be used as a marker for identifying individuals at risk for developing diseases. Future research should concentrate on these particular deficiencies and lifestyle habits for those individuals who are at risk. Nationally this could prove a very cost effective way of combating many of the risk factors associated with disease development.

How Can this be Done?

1. Continued nutrition intervention studies to identify nutrient deficiencies and poor dietary habits and those individuals at risk
2. Nutrition education, particularly of parents, caregivers and teachers, in the correct choice of foods, theoretical and practical application of methods of cultivation of home gardens, storage, food preparation, food budgeting etc

The Future Challenges for Research

1. Increase the number of nutritional studies, particularly of a longitudinal nature, on children and adolescents to obtain a representative data base on the nutrient and food intake of children and adolescents
2. To continue evaluating the nutritional status of children and adolescents with changing circumstances in order to keep the nutrition base updated
3. With the increasing number of children developing symptoms of disease at an early age it is essential to develop new recommended intakes of nutrients appropriate for the population that do not only prevent deficiencies but are adequate to prevent disease
4. Nutrition educators face the challenge of developing and conveying educational material that is accessible and appropriate for the population concerned
5. Persuade governments that early intervention and the initial cost of nutrition surveys is a long term investment in the future health and economy of each and every country

REFERENCES

[1] Haslbeck, M. Diet and civilisation diseases – carbohydrate aspects *Wien Med Wochenschr Suppl* 1990; *106:* Suppl 7-10.

[2] *Current carbohydrate developments.* Nutrition Department South African Sugar Association, 2004.

[3] Blaak, EE; Saris, WH. Health aspects of various digestible carbohydrates. *Nutr Res* 1995; *15:* 1547-1573.

[4] FAO/WHO. *Carbohydrates in human nutrition.* Report of a joint FAO/WHO Expert Consultation. FAO Food and Nutrition Paper no. 66 Rome, 1997.

[5] Weigley, E; Mueller, D; Robinson C. Carbohydrates. in: *Robinson's basic nutrition and diet therapy.* 8th edition New Jersey; Prentice-Hall Inc. 1997.

[6] Wardlaw, GM; Insel, PM. Perspectives in Nutrition. 3rd edition Part 2. The energy yielding nutrients Chapter 3 Carbohydrates PP69. Mosby – Year Book Inc.; Missouri, USA 1996.

[7] Sanders, TA. Diet and general health: dietary counseling. *Caries Res* 2004; *28 (Suppl 1):* 3-8.

[8] Guthrie, JF; Morton, JF. Food sources of added sweeteners in the diets of Americans. *J Am Diet Assoc* 2000; *100:* 43-51.

[9] Dixon, LB; Cronin, FJ; Krebs-Smith, SM. Let the pyramid guide your food choices: capturing the total diet concept. *J Nutr* 2001; *131:* 461S-472S.

[10] Livesey, G. The impact of complex carbohydrates in energy balance. *Eur J Clin Nutr* 1995; *49 (Suppl 3):* 589-596.

[11] Hill, J; Prentice, A. Sugar and body weight regulation, *Am J Clin Nutr* 1995; *62 (Suppl 1):* 264S-274S.

[12] Mardis, AL. Current knowledge of the health effects of sugar intake. *Fam Econ Nutr Res* 2001; *13:* 87-91.

[13] Fanelli, MT; Stevenhagen, KJ. Characterising consumption patterns of food frequency methods: core foods and variety of foods in the diet of older Americans. *J Am Diet Assoc* 1985; *85:* 1570-1576.
[14] Gibney, M; Sigman-Grant, M; Stanton, JL; Keast, DR. Consumption of sugars. *Am J Clin Nutr* 1997; *65:* 1572-1574.
[15] Popkin, BM; Nielsen, SJ. The sweetening of the world's diet. *Obes Res* 2003; *11:* 1325-1332.
[16] Somerset, SM. Refined sugar intake in Australian children. *Public Health Nutr* 2003; *6:* 809-813.
[17] Hackett, AF; Rugg-Gunn, AJ; Appleton, DR; Allinson M; Eastoe, JE. Sugar eating habits of 405 11- to 14-year-old English children. *Br J Nutr* 1984; *51:* 347-356.
[18] Sigman-Grant M; Morita, J. Defining and interpreting intakes of sugars. *Am J Clin Nutr* 2005; *78:* 815S-826S.
[19] Edgar, WM. Extrinsic and intrinsic sugars: a review of recent UK recommendations o diet and caries. *Caries Res* 1993; *27 (Suppl 1):* 64-67.
[20] Kleemola-Kujala, E; Rasanen, L. Dietary patterns of Finnish children with low high caries experience. *Community Dent Oral Epidemiol* 1979; *7:* 199-205..
[21] Moshfegh, A; Miekle, S; Borrud, L *et al.* Dietary intake of children in America: beverage choices (abstract). *FASEB J* 2000; *14:* A533.
[22] Cavadini, C; Siega-Riz, AM; Popkin, BM. US adolescent food intake trends from 1965 to 1996. *Arch Dis Child* 2000; *83:* 18-24.
[23] Nielsen, SJ; Siega-Riz, AM; Popkin, BM. Trends in energy in US between 1977 and 1996: similar shifts seen across age groups. *Obes Res* 2002; *10:* 370-378 Cavadini, C; Siega-Riz, AM; Popkin, BM. US adolescent food intake trends from 1965 to 1996. *Arch Dis Child* 2000; *83:* 18-24.
[24] Soft drinks top Americans food choices. *New Food News* 1998; *3:* 5-6.
[25] Lytle, L; Seifer, S; Greenstein, J; McGovern P. How do children's eating patterns food choices change over time? Results from a cohort study. *Am J Health Promot* 2000; *14:* 222-228.
[26] Morton, JF; Guthrie, JF. Changes in children's total fat intake and their food group sources of fat. *Fam Econ Nutr Rev* 1998; *11:* 44-57.
[27] Chanmugam, P; Morton, JF; Guthrie JF. Reported changes in energy and fat intakes in adults and their food group sources (abstract). *FASEB J* 1996; *12:* A844..
[28] French, SA; Lin, BH; Guthrie, JF. National trends in soft drink consumption among children and adolescents 6 to 17 years: prevalence amounts and sources 1977/1978 to 1994/1998. *J Am Diet Assoc* 2003; *103:* 1326-1331.
[29] Morgan, KJ; Zabik, ME. Amount and food sources of total sugar intake by children ages 5 to 12 years. *Am J Clin Nutr* 1981; *34:* 404-413.
[30] Linseisen, J; Gedrich, K; Karg, G; Wolfram, G. Sucrose in Germany. *Z Ernahrungswiss* 1998; *37:* 303-314.
[31] Prynne, CJ; Paul, AA; Price, GM; Day, KC; Hilder, WS; Wadsworth, ME. Food and nutrient intake of a national sample of 4-year-old children in 1950. *Public Health Nutr* 1999; *2:* 537-547.
[32] de la Hunty, A; Lader, D; Clarke, PC. What British children are eating and drinking at age 12 – 18 months. *J Hum Nutr Diet* 2000; *13:* 83-86.

[33] Bellisle, F; Roland-Cachera, MF and the Kellogg Scientific Advisory Committee 'Child and Nutrition'. Three consecutive (1993, 1995, 1997) surveys of food intake, nutritional attitudes and knowledge, and lifestyle in 1000 French children aged 9 – 11 years. *J Hum Nutr Diet* 2000; *13:* 101-111.

[34] Astrom, AN; Samdal, O. Time trends in oral health behaviours among Norwegian adolescents 1985 –97. *Acta Odontol Scand* 2001; *59:* 193-200.

[35] Subar, AF; Krebs-Smith, SM; Cook, A; Kahle, LL. Dietary sources of nutrients among US children 1989 – 1991. *Pediatrics* 1998; *102:* 913-923.

[36] Krebs-Smith, SM; Cook, A; Subar, AF; Cleveland, L; Friday, J; Kahle, LL. Fruit and vegetable intakes of children and adolescents in the United States, *Arch Pediatr Adolesc Med* 1996; *150:* 81-86.

[37] Harnack, L; Walters, SA; Jacobs, DR Jr. Dietary intake and food sources of whole grains among US children and adolescents: data from the 1994 – 1996 Continuing Survey of Food Intakes by Individuals. *J Am Diet Assoc* 2003; *103:* 1015-1019.

[38] Rampersaud, GC; Bailey, LB; Kauwell, GP. National survey beverage consumption data for children and adolescents indicate the need to encourage a shift toward more nutritive beverages. *J Am Diet Assoc* 2003; *103:* 97-100.

[39] Forshee, RA; Storey, ML; The role of added sugars in the diet quality of children and adolescents. *J Am Coll Nutr* 2001; *20:* 32-43.

[40] Frary, CD; Johnson, RK; Wang, MQ. Children and adolescents' choices of foods and beverages high in added sugars are associated with intakes of key nutrients and food groups. *J Adolesc Health* 2004; *34:* 56-63.

[41] Hampl, JS; Betts, NM; Benes, BA. The 'age + 5' rule: comparisons of dietary fibre intake among 4- to 10-year-old children. *J Am Diet Assoc* 1998; *98:* 1418-1423.

[42] Alexy, U; Sichert-Hellert, W; Kersting, M. Associations between intake of added sugars and intake of nutrients and food groups in the diets of German children and adolescents. *Br J Nutr* 2003; *90:* 441-447.

[43] Harnack,L; Stang, J; Storey, M. Soft drink consumption among US children and adolescents: nutritional consequences. *J Am Diet Assoc* 1999; *99:* 436-441.

[44] Ballew, C; Kuester, S; Gillespie, C. Beverage choices affect adequacy of children's nutrient intake. *Arch Pediatr Adolesc Med* 2000; *154:* 1148-1152.

[45] Guenther, PM. Beverages in the diets of American teenagers. *J Am Diet Assoc* 1986; *86:* 493-499.

[46] Johnson, RK. Changing eating and physical activity patterns of US children. *Proc Nutr Soc* 2000; *59:* 295-301.

[47] Kant, AK. Reported consumption of low-nutrient-density foods by American children and adolescents: nutritional and health correlates, NHANES III, 1988 to 1994. *Arch Adolesc Med* 2003; *157:* 789-796.

[48] Farris, RP; Nicklas, TA; Myers, L; Berenson, GS. Nutrient intake and food group consumption of 10-year-olds by sugar intake level: the Bogalusa Heart Study. *J Am Coll Nutr* 1998; *17:* 579-585.

[49] Mattes, RD. Dietary compensation by humans food supplemental energy provided as ethanol or carbohydrates in fluids. *Physiol Behav* 1996; *59:* 179-187.

[50] MacKeown, JM; Cleaton-Jones, PE; Senekal, M. Individual food items in the diets of South African preschool children – energy, protein, carbohydrate, fibre, added sugar and fat intake. *S Afr J Food Sci Nutr* 1994: *6:* 100-104.

[51] Steyn, NP; Van Wyk Kotze, TJ; van Heerden L; Kotze, JP. Analysis of the diets of 12-year-old children in Cape Town. *S Afr Med J* 1986; *69:* 739-742.

[52] Walker, ARP, Walker, BF; Richardson, BD; Woolford, A. Appendicitis, fibre intake and bowel behaviour in ethnic groups in South Africa *Postgrad Med J* 1973; *49:* 243-249.

[53] MacKeown, JM; Cleaton-Jones, PE; Granath, L; Richardson, BD; Sinwel, RE. A study of the relative amounts of food items consumed by south African preschool children. *S Afr J Food Sci Nutr* 1989; *1:* 19-22.

[54] Faber, M; Benade, AJS. Nutritional status and dietary practices of 4-24 month old children from a rural South African community. *Public Health Nutr* 1999; *2:* 179-185.

[55] Oelefse, A; Faber, M; Benade, JG; Benade, AJS; Kenoyer, DG. The nutritional status of a rural community in KwaZulu, Natal, South Africa: the Ndunakazi Project. *Central Afr J Med* 1999; *45:* 14-19.

[56] Faber, M; Benade, AJS. Perceptions of infant cereals and dietary intakes of children aged 4-24 months in a rural South African community. *Int J Food Sci Nutr* 2001; *52:* 359-365.

[57] Faber, M; Smuts, CM; Benade, AJS. Dietary intake of primary school children in relation to food production in a rural area in KwaZulu, Natal, South Africa. *Int J Food Sci Nutr* 1999; *50:* 57-64.

[58] MacKeown, JM; Faber, M. Frequency of food items consumed by yong rural and urban children – essential knowledge to provide dietary advice in caries prevention. *Int Dent J* 2004; *54:* 284-290.

[59] MacKeown, JM; Cleaton-Jones, PE, Hargreaves, JA. Variety of individual food items consumed by 11-year-old children in KwaZulu and Namibia. *Ecology Food Nutr* 1994; *33:* 27-36.

[60] Steyn, NP; Badenhorst, CJ; Nel, JH. The meal pattern and snacking habits of school children in two rural areas of Lebowa. *S Afr J Food Sci Nutr* 1993; *5:* 5-9.

[61] Bartkiw, TP. Children's eating habits: a question of balance. *World Health Forum* 1993; *14:* 404-406.

[62] Vignarajah, S. A frequency survey of sugary foods and drink consumption in school children and adolescents in a West Indian island – Antigua. *Int Dent J* 1997; *47:* 293-297.

[63] Shapiro, LR. Streamlining and implementing nutritional assessment: the dietary approach. *J Am Diet Assoc* 1079; *75:* 230-237.

[64] Hagman, U; Bruce, A; Persson, L-A; Samuelson, G; Sjolin, S. Food habits and nutrient intake in childhood in relation to health and socio-economic conditions. A Swedish multicentre study 1980-81. *Act Paediatr Scand* 1986; *Suppl 328:* 1-56.

[65] US Department of Health and Human Services. Extracts of the Surgeon General's Report on Nutrition and Health [online]. The Surgeon General of the Public Health Services, Washington, DC 2001. Available at: http*://www.mcspotlight.org/media/reports/surgeonrep.html.*

[66] Sheiham, A. Dietary effects on dental, disease. *Public Health Nutr* 2001; *4:* 569-591.

[67] Nicklas, TA; Myers, L; O'Neil, C. Breakfast consumption with and without vitamin mineral supplementation use favourably impacts daily nutrient intake of ninth-grade students. *J Adolesc Health* 2000; *27:* 314-321.

[68] Albertson, AM. Breakfast patterns and the use of ready-to-eat cereal consumption on nutrient intakes of children 4-12-years old (abstract). *FASEB J* 2001; *15:* A983.

[69] Cho, S; Dietrich, M; Brown CJP; Clark, C; Block, G. The effects of breakfast type on total daily energy intake and body mass index: results from the Third National Health and Nutrition Examination Survey (NHANES III). *J Am Coll Nutr* 2003; *22:* 296-302.

[70] Johnson, RK; Frary, C. Choosing beverages and food to moderate your intake of sugars: the 2000 dietary guidelines for Americans – what's all the fuss about? *J Nutr* 2001; *131:* 2766S-2771S.

[71] Matthiessen, J; Fagt, S; Biltoft-Jensen, A; Beck, AM; Ovesen, L. Size makes a difference. *Public Health Nutr* 2003; *6:* 65-72.

[72] Irwin, CE Jr. Eating and physical activity during adolescence: does it make a difference in adult health status? *J Adolesc Health* 2004; *34:* 459-460.

[73] Wabitsch, M; Hauner, H; Hertrampf, M; Muche, R; Hay, B; Mayer, H; Kratzer, W; Debatin; KM; Heinze, E. Type II diabetes mellitus and impaired glucose regulation in Caucasian children and adolescents with obesity living in Germany. *Int J Obes Relat Metab Disord* 2004; *28:* 307-313.

[74] Martin-Iverson, N; Pacza, T; Phatouros, A. Tenant, M. Indigenous Australian dental health: a brief review of caries experience. *Aust Dent J* 2000; *45:* 17-20.

[75] Soxman, JA. Considerations for treating adolescent patients. *Gen Dent* 2003; *51:* 24-26.

[76] Ziegler, O; Quilliot, D; Guerci, B. Physiopathology of obesity. Dietary factors, and regulation of energy balance. *Ann Endocrinol (Paris)* 2000; *61 (Suppl 6):* 12-23.

[77] Popkin, BM; Paeratakul, S; Zhai, F; Ge K. A review of environmental correlates of obesity with emphasis on developing countries. *Obes Res* 1995; *3 (suppl 2):* 145S-153S.

[78] Martinez, JA. Obesity in young Europeans: genetic and environmental influences. *Eur J Clin Nutr* 2000; *54 (Suppl 1):* S56-S60.

[79] Keller, KB; Lemberg, L. Obesity and the metabolic syndrome. *Am J Crit Care* 2002; *12:* 167-170.

[80] *Obesity: preventing and managing the global epidemic.* Geneva: World Health Organisation, 2002.

[81] Storey, ML; Forshee, RA; Weaver, AR; Sansalone, WR. Demographic and lifestyle factors associated with body mass index among children and adolescents. *Int J Food Sci Nutr* 2003; *54:* 491-503.

[82] Tresaco, B; Bueno, G. Moreno, LA; Garagorri, JM; Bueno, M. Insulin resistance and impaired glucose tolerance in obese children and adolescents. *J Physiol Biochem* 2003; *59:* 217-223.

[83] Kruger, HS; Margetts, BM, Vorster, HH. Evidence for relatively greater subcutaneous fat deposition in stunted girls in the North West Province, South Africa, as compared with non-stunted girls. J Nutr 2004; *20:* 564-569.

[84] Nicklas, TA; Baranowski, T; Cullen, KW; Berenson, G. Eating patterns, dietary quality and obesity. *J Am Coll Nutr* 2001; *20:* 599-608.

[85] Flegal, KM; Carroll, MD, Ogden, MD; Johnson, CL. Prevalence and trends in obesity among US adults, 1999 – 2000. *JAMA* 2002; *288:* 1723-1727.

[86] Ogden, MD; Flegal, KM; Carroll, MD; Johnson, CL. Prevalence and trends in overweight among US children and adolescents, 1999 – 2000. *JAMA* 2002; *288:* 1728-1732.

[87] Ludwig, DS. Dietary glycemic index and obesity. *J Nutr* 2000; *130 (2S Suppl):* 280S-283S.

[88] Mokdad, AH; Marks, JS; Stoup, D; Gerberding JL. Actual causes of death in the United States. *JAMA* 2004; *291:* 1238-1245..

[89] Chu, NF. Prevalence and trends of obesity among school children in Taiwan – the Tapei Children Heart Study. *Int J Obes Relat Metab Disord* 2001; *25:* 170-176.

[90] Eisenmann, JC. Physical activity and cardiovascular disease risk factors in children and adolescents: an overview. *Can J Cardiol* 2004; *20:* 295-301.

[91] Dietz, W; Critical periods in childhood for the development of obesity. *Am J Clin Nutr* 1994; *59:* 955.

[92] Foundation for Child Development, FCD Index of Child Well being: March 2004 [online]. Avaiable at: http://www.ffcd.org/.

[93] Caprio, S. Insulin resistance in childhood obesity. *J Pediatr Endocrinol Metab* 2002; *15 (Suppl 1):* 487-492.

[94] Caius, N; Benefice, E. Food habits, physical activity and overweight among adolescents. *Rev Epidemiol Sante Publique* 2002; *50:* 531-542.

[95] Whitaker, RC; Wright, JA; Pepe, MS; Seidel, KD; Dietz, WH. Predicting obesity in young adulthood from childhood and parental obesity. *N Engl J Med* 1997; *337:* 869-873.

[96] Brown, JD; Witherspoon, EM. The mass media and American adolescents' health. *J Adolesc Health* 2002; *31:* 153-170.

[97] Kvaavik, E; Tell, GS; Klepp, KI. Predictors and tracking of body mass index from adolescence into adulthood: follow-up of 18 to 20 years in the Oslo Youth Study. *Arch Pediatr Adolesc Med* 2003; *157:* 1212-1218.

[98] Ebbeling, CB; Pawlak, DB; Ludwig, DS. Childhood obesity: public health crisis, common sense cure. *Lancet* 2002; *360:* 473-482.

[99] Friestad, C; Pirkis, J; Biehl, M; Irwin, CE Jr. Socioeconomic patterning of smoking, sedentary lifestyle, and overweight status among adolescents in Norway and the United States. *J Adolesc Health* 2003; *33:* 275-278.

[100] Lissau, I; Overpeck, MD; Ruan WJ; Due, P; Holstein, BE; Hediger, ML; Health Behaviour in School-aged Children Obesity Workshop Group. Body mass index and overweight in adolescents in 13 European countries, Israel and the United States. *Arch Pediatr Adolesc Med* 2004; *158:* 27-33.

[101] Popkin, BM; Richards, MK; Monteiro, CA. Stunting is associated with overweight in children of four nations that are undergoing the nutrition transition,. *J Nutr* 1996; *126:* 3009-3016.

[102] Kruger, HS; Venter, CS; Vorster, HH. Obesity in African women in the North West Province, South Africa is associated with the increased risk of non-communicable diseases: the THUSA study. Transition and Health during Urbanisation of South Africans. *Br J Nutr* 2001; *86:* 733-740.

[103] Steyn, K; Jooste, PL; Bourne, Lt *et al. et al.* Risk factors for coronary heart disease in the black population in the Cape Peninsula: the BRISK study. *S Afr Med J* 1991; *79:* 480-485.

[104] Monyeki, KD; van Lenthe F; Steyn, NP. Obesity: does it occur in African children in a rural community in South Africa? *Int J Epidemiol* 1999; *28:* 287-292.

[105] Nesamvuni, AE; Labadarios, DL; Steyn, NP; *et al.* The anthropometric status of children aged 1-9-years in South Africa: the National Food Consumption Survey (NFCS) of Children aged 1-9-years, South Africa, 1999. *S Afr J Clin Nutr* 2000; *13:* 98-104.

[106] Sawaya, AL; Dallal, G; Solymos, O *et al.* Obesity and malnutrition in the shantytown population in the city of Sao Paulo, Brazil. *Obes Res* 1995; *3 (Suppl 2):* 107S-115S.

[107] Cameron, N; Getz, B. Sex differences in the prevalence of obesity in rural African adolescents. *Int J Obes* 1997; *21:* 775-782.

[108] Mokhtar, N; Elati, J; Chabir, R *et al.*. Diet, culture and obesity in northern Africa. *J Nutr* 2001; *131:* 887S-892S.

[109] Troiano, RP; Flegal, KM. Overweight children and adolescents: description, epidemiology and demographics. *Pediatrics* 1998; *101:* 497-504.

[110] Tucker, LA; Seljaas, GT; Hager, RL. Body fat percentage of children varies according to their diet composition. *J Am Diet Assoc* 1997; *97:* 981-986.

[111] Holmboe-Ottesen, G. Global trends in food consumption and nutrition. *Tidsskr Nor Laegeforen* 2000; *120:* 78-82.

[112] Bell, SJ; Sears, B. Low-glycemic-load diets: impact on obesity and chronic diseases. *Crit Rev Food Sci Nutr* 2003; *43:* 357-377.

[113] Ball, SD; Keller, KR; Moyer-Mileur, LJ; Ding, YW; Donaldson, D; Jackson, WD. Prolongation of satiety after low versus moderately high glycemic index meals in obese adolescents. *Pediatrics* 2003; *111:* 488-494.

[114] Murtaugh, MA; Jacobs, DR Jr; Jacob, B; Steffen, LM; Marquart, L. Epidemiological support for the protection of whole grain against diabetes. *Proc Nutr Soc* 2003; *62:* 143-149.

[115] Ebbeling, CB; Leidig, MM; Sinclair, KB; Hangen, JP; Ludwig, DS. A reduced-glycemic load diet in the treatment of adolescent obesity *Arch Pediatr Adolesc Med* 2003; *157:* 773-779.

[116] Warren, JM; Henry, CJ; Simonite, V. Low glycemic index breakfast and reduced food intake in preschool children. *Pediatrics* 2003; 112: e414.

[117] Anand, RS; Basiotis, PP; Klein, BW. Profile of overweight children *Nutr Insights* 1999; *13:* A publication of the USDA Centre for Nutrition Policy and Promotion.

[118] Murphy, SP; Johnson, RK. The scientific basis of recent US guidelines on sugar intake. *Am J Clin Nutr 2003*; *78:* 827S-833S.

[119] Stubbs, J; Ferres, S; Horgen, G. Energy density foods: effects on energy intake. *Clin Rev Food Sci* 2000; *40:* 481-515.

[120] Rolls, BJ; Bell, EA. Dietary approaches to the treatment of obesity. *Med Clin North Am* 2000; *84:* 401-418.

[121] Ludwig, DS. The glycemic index: physiological mechanisms relating to obesity. *JAMA* 2002; *287:* 2414-2423.

[122] Ludwig, DS; Peterson, KE; Gortmaker, SL. Relation between consumption of sugar sweetened drinks and childhood obesity: a prospective observational analysis. *Lancet* 2001; *357:* 505-508.

[123] Mann, JL; Truswell, AS; Hendricks, D; Manning EB. Effects of serum lipids in normal men of reducing dietary sucrose or starch for five months. *Lancet* 1970; *1:* 870-872.

[124] Smith, JB; Niven, BE; Mann, JL. The effect of reduced extrinsic sucrose intake on plasma triglyceride level. *Eur J Clin Nutr* 1996; *50:* 498-504.

[125] Mrdjenovic, G; Levitsky, DA. Nutritional and energetic consequences of sweetened drink consumption in 6- to 13-year-old children. J Pediatr 2003; *142:* 604-610.

[126] Forshee, RA; Storey, ML. Total beverage consumption and beverage choice among children and adolescents. *Int J Food Sci Nutr* 2001; *54:* 297-307.

[127] Gillis, LJ; Bar-Or, O. Food away from home, sugar sweetened drink consumption and juvenile obesity. *J Am Coll Nutr* 2003; *22:* 539-545.

[128] Anderson, GH. Sugars, sweetness and food intake. *Am J Clin Nutr* 1995; *62 (1 Suppl):* 195S-201S.

[129] Bolton-Smith, C. Intake of sugars in relation to fatness and micronutrient adequacy. *Int J Obes Rel Metab Disord* 1996; *20 (Suppl 2):* S31-S33.

[130] Rodriguez-Artalejo, F; Garia, EL; Gorgojo, L *et al.* Consumption of bakery products, sweetened soft drinks and yoghurt among children ages 6-7-years: association with nutrient intake and overall diet quality. *Br J Nutr* 2003; *89;* 419-429.

[131] Margarey, AM; Daniels, LA; Bouton, TJ; Cockington, RA. Does fat intake predict adiposity in healthy children and adolescents aged 2-15-years? A longitudinal analysis. *Eur J Clin Nutr* 2001; *55:* 471-481.

[132] Ortega, RM; Lopez-Sobaler, AM; Quintas, ME *et al.* Differences in the breakfast habits of overweight/obese and normal weight school children. *Int J Vit Nutr Res* 1998; 68: 125-132.

[133] Wyatt, HR; Grunwald, GK; Mosca, CL; Klem, ML; Wing, RR; Hill, JO. Long-term weight loss and breakfast in subjects in the national weight control registry. *Obes Res* 2002; *10:* 78-82.

[134] Mann, JL. Sugar revisited –again. *Bulletin WHO* 2003; *81:* 552-553.

[135] Duggal, MS; van Loveren, C. Dental considerations for dietary counseling. *Int Dent J* 2001; *51 (6 Suppl 1):* 408-412.

[136] Marthaler, TM; O'Mullane, DM; Vrbic, V. The prevalence of dental caries in Europe 1990-1995, ORCA Saturday afternoon symposium 1995. *Caries Res* 1996; *30:* 237-255.

[137] Moynihan, P. The British Nutrition Foundation Oral Task Force report – issue relevant to dental health professionals. *Br Dent J* 2000; *188:* 308-312.

[138] Moynihan, P; Petersen, PE. Diet, nutrition and the prevention of dental disease. *Public Health Nutr* 2004; *7:* 201-226.

[139] *Department of Health Demographic and Health Survey 1998.* full report. Pretoria: Department of Health (RSA); 2002.

[140] *National Oral Health Survey. National Oral Health Survey 1988/89.* Pretoria: Department of Health; 1994.

[141] Featherstone, JD. The science and practice of caries prevention. *J Am Dent Assoc* 2000; *131:* 887-899.

[142] Gustafsson, BE; Quensel, C-E; Swenander-Lamke, L *et al.* The Vipeholm Dental Caries Study. *Acta Odontol Scand* 1954: *11:* 232-364.

[143] Sheinin, A; Makinen, KK; Ylitalo, K. Turku Sugar Studies 5. Final report on the effects of sucrose, fructose and xylitol diets on caries incidence in man. *Acta Odontol Scand* 1976; *34:* 179-216.

[144] Toverud, G. The influence of war and post-war conditions on the teeth of Norwegian school children 2. Caries in the permanent teeth of children aged 7-8 and 12-13-years. *Millbank Mem Fund* Q1957a; *35:* 127-196.

[145] Toverud, G. The influence of war and post-war conditions on the teeth of Norwegian school children 3. Discussion of food supply and dental conditions in Norway and other European countries. *Millbank Mem Fund* Q1957b; *35:* 373-459.

[146] Takeuchi, M. Epidemiological study on dental caries in Japanese children before, during and after world War II. *Int Dent J* 1961: *11:*443-457.

[147] Harris, R. Biology of children in Hopewood House, Bowral, Australia 4. Observations and dental caries experience extending over five years (1957-1961) *J Dent Res* 1963; *42:* 1387-1399.

[148] Zero, DT. Sugars – the arch criminal? *Caries Res* 2004; *38:* 277-285.

[149] Majewski, RF. Dental caries in adolescents associated with caffeinated carbonated beverages. *Pediatr Dent* 2001; *23:* 198-203.

[150] Touger-Decker, R; van Loveren, C. Sugars and dental caries. *Am J Clin Nutr* 2003; *78:* 881S-892S.

[151] Heller, KE; Burt, BA; Ekland, SA. Sugared soda consumption and dental caries in the United States. *J Dent Res* 2001; *80:* 1949-1953.

[152] Sreebny, LM. Sugar availability, sugar consumption and dental caries. *Community Dent Oral Epidemiol* 1982; *10:* 1-7.

[153] Honkala, E; Tala, H. Total sugar consumption and dental caries in Europe – an overview. *Int Dent J* 1987; *37:* 185-191.

[154] Marthaler, TM. Changes in the prevalence of dental caries. How much can be attributed to changes in diet? *Caries Res* 1990; *24 (Suppl 1):* 3-15.

[155] Burt, BA; Pai, S. Sugar consumption and caries risk: a systematic review. *J Dent Educ* 2001; *65:* 1017-1023.

[156] MacKeown, JM; Cleaton-Jones, PE; Edwards, AW. Energy and macronutrient intake in relation to dental caries incidence in urban black South African preschool children in 1991 and 1995: the Birth-to-Ten (BTT) study. *Public Health Nutr* 2000; *3:* 313-319.

[157] Mackeown, JM; Cleaton-Jones, PE. Dental caries incidence in relation to nutrient intake in urban preschool children. S Afr J Clin Nutr 2001; *14:* 132-136.

[158] MacKeown, JM; Cleaton-Jones, PE; Fatti, LP. Caries and micronutrient intake among urban South African children: a cohort study. *Community Dent Oral Epidemiol* 2003; *31:* 213-220.

[159] Newbrun, E. Sucrose, the arch criminal of dental caries. *ASDCJ Dent Child* 1969; *36:* 239-248.

[160] Konig, KG. Diet and dental health. *Int Dent J* 2000; *50:* 162-174.

[161] van Loveren, C. Diet and dental caries. *Eur J Pediatr Dent* 2000; *2:* 55-62.

[162] Marthaler, TM Epidemiological and clinical dental findings in relation to intake of carbohydrates. *Caries Res* 1967; *1:* 222-238.

[163] Bibby, BG. Cariogenicity of snack foods and confections. *J Am Dent Assoc* 1965; *90:* 121-132.

[164] Sreebny, LM. The sugar-caries axis. *Int Dent J* 1982; *32:* 1-12.

[165] Newbrun, E. Sugar and dental caries. A review of human studies. *Science* 1982; *217:* 418-423.

[166] Sheiham, A. Sugars and dental decay. Lancet 1983; 1(8319): 282-284.

[167] Shaw, JH. The role of sugar in the etiology of dental caries.6.Evidence from experimental animal research. *J Dent* 1983; *11:* 209-213.

[168] Rugg-Gunn, AJ. *Starch foods and fresh fruit: their relative importance as a source of caries in Britain.* Occasional paper No. 3. London, Health Education Council, 1986.

[169] Bowen, WH; Birkhed, D. Dental caries: dietary and microbiology factors; in: Granath, L; McHugh, WD. (eds): *Systemised prevention of oral disease; theory and practice.* Boca Raton, CRC Press, 1986, pp19-41.

[170] Walker, ARP, Cleaton-Jones, PE. Sugar intake and dental caries: where do we stand? *ASDC J Dent Child* 1989; *56:* 30-35.

[171] Rugg-Gunn, AJ. Diet and dental caries. *Dent Update* 1990; *17:* 198-201.

[172] Konig KG; Navia, JM. Nutritional role of sugars in oral health. *Am J Clin Nutr* 1995; *62:* 275S-282S.

[173] Ruxton, CH; Garceau, FJ; Cottrell, RC. Guidelines for sugar consumption in Europe: is a quantitative approach justified? *Eur J Clin Nutr* 1999; *53:* 503-513.

[174] Bowen, WH; Amsbaugh, SM; Monell-Torrens, S; Brunelle, J; Kuzmiak-Jones, H; Cole, MF. A method to assess the cariogenic potential of foodstuffs. *J Am Dent Assoc* 1980; *100:* 677-681.

[175] Edgar, WM; Predicton of the cariogenicity of various foods. *Int Dent J* 1985; *35:* 190-194.

[176] Mobley, CC. Nutrition and dental caries. *Dent Clin North Am* 2003; *47:* 319-336.

[177] Steyn, NP; Myburgh, NG; Nel, JH. Evidence to support a food based dietary guideline on sugar consumption in South Africa. *Bulletin WHO* 2003; *81:* 599-608.

[178] Marshall, TA. Caries prevention in paediatrics: dietary guidelines. *Quintessence Int* 2004; *35:* 332-335.

[179] van Loveren, C; Duggal, MS. Expert's opinion on the role of diet in caries prevention. *Caries Res* 2004; *38 (Suppl 1):* 16-23.

[180] British Nutrition Foundation. *Eating in the early 1980's: summary of the British Nutrition Foundation survey.* London: British Market Research Bureau, 1985.

[181] Tomkins, A. Vitamin and mineral nutrition for the health and development of children in Europe. *Public Health Nutr* 2001; *4:* 91-99.

In: Trends in Dietary Carbohydrates Research
Editor: M. V. Landlow, pp. 55-70
ISBN 1-59454-798-X

Chapter 3

Associations between Carbohydrate Intake and Risk for Coronary Heart Disease, Insulin Resistance and the Metabolic Syndrome

***Maria Luz Fernandez*[1*] *and Marcela Vergara-Jimenez*[2]**

[1] Department of Nutritional Sciences, University of Connecticut, Storrs, CT
[2] Facultad de Ciencias Quimico-Biologicas, Universidad Autónoma de Sinaloa, Culiacán, Sinaloa, México

Abstract

Because the incidence of obesity has increased dramatically over the past 20 years, finding the most appropriate diets for losing weight has become a major issue. It is also well established that overweight individuals have a higher risk of developing insulin resistance, coronary heart disease (CHD) and diabetes type II. The amount of carbohydrate in the diet may play a significant role in the maintenance of body weight and in reducing the risk factors for chronic disease.

Dietary carbohydrates are indeed at the core of the debate regarding healthy diets that promote weight loss and decrease biomarkers for heart disease and the metabolic syndrome. Very low, moderate or high carbohydrate diets have been studied in their effects on body weight, dyslipidemias, insulin sensitivity, plasma glucose, leptin levels, inflammatory cytokines and adhesive molecules. Very low carbohydrate diets have been reported to effectively reduce body weight and improve plasma lipids and insulin sensitivity in studies of short duration between 4 to 24 weeks. Moderate and high carbohydrate diets have also been shown to have beneficial effects on anthropometrics and other cardiovascular risk factors depending on the duration of the study and the investigated population. Overall the controversies of the findings depend on the type of study (parallel versus randomized crossover) the duration of the intervention, the assessed subjects (normal versus diabetic or hyperlipidemic) and the retention of subjects, which appeared to be poor in the majority of the cases. All these factors still continue to make it

* Corresponding author: Maria Luz Fernandez, Ph.D. University of Connecticut, Department of Nutritional Sciences, 3624 Horsebarn Rd. Ext. Storrs, CT 06269; Phone: 860-486-5547; Fax: 860-486-3674; Email: maria-luz.fernandez@uconn.edu

difficult to interpret the available data and to reach conclusive statements regarding the relationship between dietary carbohydrate and chronic disease.

It is the purpose of the following review to evaluate a variety of clinical interventions conducted in the past 5 years in which dietary carbohydrate was one of the main variables under investigation. The effects of different dietary interventions varying in the amount of dietary carbohydrate on symptoms associated with the metabolic syndrome, insulin resistance and increased risk for CHD are discussed.

Key Words: Very low carbohydrate diets, High carbohydrate diets, coronary heart disease, metabolic syndrome, insulin resistance, plasma triglycerides, LDL-C, HDL-C, waist circumference.

ABBREVIATIONS

Apo:	apolipoprotein,
BBB:	blood-brain barrier,
BMI:	body mass index,
CAM-1:	cell adhesion molecule-1,
CHD:	coronary heart disease,
CNS:	central nervous system,
CRP:	C-reactive protein,
GI:	glycemic index,
HDL-C:	high density lipoprotein cholesterol,
IL-6:	Interleukin-6,
LDL-C:	low density lipoprotein cholesterol,
MetSyn:	metabolic syndrome,
TC:	total cholesterol,
TG:	triglycerides,
VAT:	visceral adipose tissue,
SCAT:	subcutaneous adipose tissue,
(TNF)α:	tumor necrosis factor,
WC:	waist circumference,

INTRODUCTION

Current research does not support the theory that one weight loss program is successful for all populations [1,2]. The best approach on macronutrient composition, caloric restriction and levels of exercise is still disputed. Obesity is a public health challenge that claims approximately 300,000 lives a year [3] and depletes an estimated 9.4% of the health care budget [4]. Approximately 65% of the US population has a body mass index (BMI) of ≥ 25 kg/m^2 [5], which classifies them as overweight. Clinically, overweight and obese (BMI ≥ 30 kg/m^2) persons are at increased risk for coronary heart disease (CHD) and diabetes mellitus Type 2 [6,7]. Adequate diets for the management and prevention of obesity, CHD, and diabetes are needed. However, experts disagree on what is the best "heart healthy" diet [8]. There still is controversy regarding dietary modifications that will result in weight loss, while maintaining a healthy plasma lipid and lipoprotein profile [9].The maintenance of a healthy weight has been shown to be the best option to reduce the prevalence of biomarkers associated with chronic disease. Therefore, it is not surprising that food choices and selection of specific macronutrients aimed at reducing weight do play a major role in our health.

Recently, an increased interest on food choices varying in the concentration and type of macronutrients has emerged. It is mainly due to the higher prevalence of obesity, that the consumer has become more aware of the various food choices that are advertised to promote weight loss. Dietary carbohydrates appear to be the focal point of the surrounding confusion concerning a healthy weight loss. The American Public's main concern is with diets aimed at weight loss while the scientific community provides controversial or at the very least confusing information regarding the appropriate amount of carbohydrate to achieve the best results. It is well known for example that an excess intake of carbohydrate may have detrimental effects on the regulation of insulin [10] and on plasma triglyceride concentrations [11] while at the same time high carbohydrate diets are promoted for high-intensity resistance exercise [12]. Cohort studies have also shown an inverse association between complex carbohydrates and CHD [13]. However, other studies have demonstrated that carbohydrate intake is positively related to plasma TG, reduced insulin sensitivity and obesity [14]. Therefore it is vital to understand the interplay between insulin, dietary carbohydrates and potential abnormalities in metabolism, including biomarkers for CHD and diabetes type II.

It is particularly important to mention that per capita fructose consumption has increased during the past three decades within the same time frame as a marked increase in the prevalence of obesity [15,16]. Gross et al. [17] have shown that since 1963 carbohydrate intake has increased by 126 g/d with high fructose syrup providing 10% of total energy intake. In addition, the incidence of diabetes has increased by 47% suggesting that there could be a correlation between increased carbohydrate intake and higher prevalence of diabetes. Although refined carbohydrates have been linked to a wide array of chronic disease including diabetes, clear data are not readily available and controversy still remains [18]. In the past, fructose was considered to be beneficial in the dietary management of diabetes mellitus and insulin resistance because fructose ingestion resulted in smaller postprandial glycemic and insulin releases than do glucose and complex carbohydrates [19]. While high fructose corn syrup has a low GI and has been proposed as beneficial for diabetes type II [20], the concern about the effects of increasing plasma TG and decreasing HDL-C still remains [21]. Dietary fructose has been also associated with weight gain and induces insulin resistance, hyperlipidemia and hypertension in experimental animals. It is therefore possible that increased consumption of fructose could contribute to weight gain and its accompanying metabolic disturbances in humans.

Coronary Heart Disease and Dietary Carbohydrates

Numerous short-term studies have indicated that diets high in carbohydrates, particularly simple sugars (fructose and glucose) increase plasma TG concentrations and decrease HDL-C thus increasing the risk for CHD [22]. However, available epidemiological data indicate that high plasma TG could be more associated with the rate of absorption of dietary carbohydrate or glycemic index (GI) [23]. GI is defined as the increment area under the blood glucose response curve (IAUC) expressed as a percentage after the intake of a food containing 50 g carbohydrate by the same individual [24]. A randomized, parallel 10-wk study involving a high carbohydrate diet, reported a 10% decrease in LDL cholesterol (LDL-C) in subjects taking low compared to high GI foods [25]. Authors concluded that although there were no changes in body weight or appetite, the low GI diets may have a favorable effect in decreasing CHD risk. In contrast, a meta analysis of fifteen randomized clinical trials conducted by Kelly et al. [26] reported that the existing evidence regarding low GI and decrease risk for CHD is weak and that better controlled studies with longer duration are needed to reach any significant conclusions.

Dietary sucrose may increase hepatic TG synthesis and VLDL assembly and secretion and decrease the catabolism of TG-rich lipoproteins [27]. In addition, the presence of abdominal obesity appears to influence the effects of diets high in carbohydrates. This latter situation may be related to the increases in basal lipolysis observed in subjects with visceral obesity due to the higher fat depots, which results in a higher rate of fatty acids going to the liver. Reesterification of fatty acids in the liver provides a consistent substrate for increased VLDL production. In addition, the resistance of viscerally obese people to the action of insulin, may also contribute to the elevated concentrations of circulating TG [28]. In summary, dietary carbohydrate is highly associated with TG metabolism and the more pronounced response is observed in individuals with visceral obesity.

The optimal diet to reduce weight and cardiovascular risk factors cannot be generalized for all individuals. Both low carbohydrate and high carbohydrate (low fat) diets have been shown to cause beneficial effects on body weight and obesity-associated comorbidities with the low carbohydrate diet apparently having a greater beneficial effect at short term [28]. The use of low carbohydrate diets appears to have multiple beneficial effects on several risk factors associated with increased risk for CHD including regulation of dyslipidemias [29], lowering of blood pressure [30] and reduction in the production of inflammation markers such as cytokines and adhesive molecules [31]. Moderate carbohydrate diets (40% of energy) have also been proven successful in decreasing biomarkers for coronary heart disease [32]. Finally, a low caloric diet high in carbohydrate has been proven to successfully reduce LDL-C and overall improve plasma lipid levels [33].

Some dietary recommendations call for a low-fat (< 30% of energy), low saturated fat (< 7% of total energy) low cholesterol (< 300 mg/d) diet [34]. However high carbohydrate diets are controversial because they raise plasma TG and may negatively affect the composition and size of LDL, creating small dense LDL particles, and reduce HDL-C [35]. Sharman et al [36] conducted a study to analyze how healthy normolipidemic, normal weight men respond to a ketogenic diet in term of CHD biomarkers. Twelve men switched from their habitual diet (17% protein, 47% carbohydrate and 32% fat) to a ketogenic diet (30% protein, 8% carbohydrate and 61% fat). Fasting serum TG and insulin concentrations significantly decreased, small increases in total and LDL-C, moderate increase in HDL-C and significant weigh loss (-2.2 kg) were found. The latter might be the cause of HDL and TG decreases in this study [36]. The same research team compared the effects of a very low-carbohydrates and a low-fat diet on fasting blood lipids and postprandial lipemia in overweight men [39]. Serum LDL-C concentrations from the low-fat diet group was the only reduced biomarker. The very low-carbohydrates diet significantly reduced TG, the TG/HDL-C ratio and glucose. Both diets reduced postprandial lipemia, but the reduction was greater with the very low-carbohydrates diet and also LDL-C particle size was larger with the very low-carbohydrate diet. This study therefore suggested that low-fat diets are good to reduce LDL-C.

Very low carbohydrate ketogenic diets appear to be valuable in the treatment of obesity and hyperlipidemia [30]. In addition, very low carbohydrate diets have been shown to be useful as an adjuct therapy for improving the plasma lipid profile in overweight subjects undergoing a stable statin therapy [37]. Several studies have been conducted comparing the effects of low- and high-carbohydrate diet on improving lipid profile and decreasing the risk for CHD. Stern et al. [38] compared overweight, hyperlipidemic volunteers randomly assigned to either a low-carbohydrate (< 20 g of carbohydrate per day) or a low-fat diet (< 30% energy from fat) during 24 weeks. Higher reductions in plasma TG and elevations in HDL-C were observed in those individuals taking the low carbohydrate diet [38]. However, the authors do mention that one limitation to the study was the intake of nutritional supplements by the low carbohydrate group that might have interfered with some of the observed results. Longer term studies have also shown that low carbohydrate diet have more favorable outcomes on dyslipidemias compared to calorie restricted diets with < 30% energy from fat in obese adults [38]. Participants were advised to either restrict carbohydrate intake or to restrict caloric intake by 500 calories per day. The reduction in weight after one year was 5.1 kg for the low carbohydrate and 3.1 kg for the low calorie diet. In addition, after one year, there was a 28% decrease in plasma TG following the low fat diet while no significant changes in plasma TG were observed in subjects following the low calorie diet. Further, after adjustment for covariates, hemoglobin A_{1c} levels improved in the low carbohydrate group only.

Because it has been postulated that several energy-consuming pathways are up-regulated with a very low intake of carbohydrates, a study was conducted in obese postmenopausal women in which protein and energy were maintained constant and only carbohydrate and fat varied significantly [39]. After 6 months, no differences in plasma lipids, glucose or insulin were observed between dietary groups. However, the group assigned to the very low carbohydrate diet presented a trend for TG reduction and lower plasma insulin levels, a trend that could become significant after more subjects are evaluated since this preliminary report only presents the results of 4 subjects [39].

In contrast Jacobs et al. [33] reported that a low fat diet (29% energy) was more effective in reducing plasma TG in hypertriglyceridemic patients than a high fat (40% energy) diet when the baseline concentrations of plasma TG were higher than 396 mg/dL. After analyzing the results for the 17 subjects who participated in this cross over design, the authors concluded that those individuals who were slightly hypertriglyceridemic had a very significant lowering of plasma TG following the high carbohydrate diet. However, 5 of the 9 subjects who had baseline plasma TG > 396 mg/dL benefited more by the low-fat intervention period [33].

In another randomized trial conducted for one year, 63 obese men and women were assigned to either a low- or a high-carbohydrate diet [40]. Subjects following the low carbohydrate diet lost more weight at 3 and 6 months, however, no significant differences between groups were observed after 1 year. At the end of the intervention changes in total cholesterol and LDL-C did not differ among participants. In contrast reductions in plasma TG and increases in HDL-C were more prominent in subjects following the low carbohydrate diet [40]. A significant observation reported by the authors was that LDL-C tended to increase after 3 months in subjects on the low carbohydrate compared to those in the high carbohydrate group ($P < 0.05$). Nevertheless, on the long term there were no significant differences in plasma LDL-C concentrations between groups suggesting that the weight loss compensated the adverse effects associated with high saturated fat consumption. The authors also raised the concern of the interpretation of the clinical significance of decreased TG and increased HDL-C in the context of high saturated fat and low fiber intake and pointed out the need for more studies to clarify the overall relationship of type of diet, weight loss and risk for CHD.

Results from a recent study in which the effects of different diets were evaluated on cardiovascular risk factors did not find significant associations between carbohydrate intake and body weight or improved plasma lipid profiles [41]. In this single center trial, 160 participants were randomly assigned to a very low carbohydrate or Atkins diet (< 20 g/d), a diet with 40% of calories derived from carbohydrate (Zone diet), a Weight Watchers diet where the participants limited their caloric intake and a very low fat diet (< 10% energy from fat) [41]. After 1 year all participants experienced a decrease in the LDL/HDL ratio and moderate decreases in weight. The percentage of subjects who completed the study ranged from 50% for the weight watchers to 65% for the group assigned to the Zone diet. Overall adherence was low and the observed improvement in cardiovascular risk factors was not different among dietary groups. Results from this study suggest that weigh loss was the most significant parameter associated with overall health benefits [41].

Lofgren et al. [32] recruited 70 overweight/obese pre-menopausal women to participate in a weight loss study consisting on a dietary modification including caloric restriction (85% of total energy expenditure) and a moderately low carbohydrate diet (40% of energy). All participants presented a significant decrease in plasma TG, apolipoprotein (apo) B and E concentrations and significant reductions in the smaller LDL subfractions. In addition there was a significant decrease in LDL susceptibility to oxidation as assessed by an increased lag time and a decrease in conjugated diene formation. All these beneficial effects were obtained in plasma lipids only with slight reduction in dietary carbohydrates. When step wise regression analysis was conducted, the changes in dietary carbohydrate had a significant contribution in the reduction of plasma TG after controlling for weight loss. Lower plasma TG are associated with a lower distribution of LDL into the smaller subfractions [14], therefore and because the smaller LDL are known to substantially increase the risk for coronary heart disease [42] overall the beneficial effect of this moderately low carbohydrate diet translates into lower risk for CHD.

A comparative parallel randomized study tested the standard American diet, a low-fat, high carbohydrate diet and the same diet in conjunction with olestra on risk factors for CHD in obese subjects [43]. The low-fat diet containing olestra had the most significant effects on weight loss with a decrease of 6.27 kg compared to 4 and 1.79 for the American diet and the low-fat diet, respectively. In addition, the olestra group had more beneficial effects on CHD risk due to significant decreases in plasma LDL-C and TG, which were not observed in the other two groups. HDL-C was not lowered after 9 months for any of the dietary groups. Authors concluded that the beneficial effects in the olestra group were mostly explained by the weight loss [43].

A summary of the results of very low, moderate and high carbohydrate intake and the effects on distinct biomarkers for chronic disease is presented in Table 1.

Table 1. Effects of low, moderate and high carbohydrate (CHO) intake on Biomarkers for CHD, Insulin Resistance and the Metabolic Syndrome.

Study	CHO Amount	Duration	TG	LDL-C	HDL-C	LDL Size	LDL oxidation	Insulin	Glucose
Jacobs et al. [33][1]	42%	3-week	↓	↔	↔	ND	↓	ND	ND
Crossover design	52%	3 week	↓	↓	↔	ND	↓	ND	ND
Stern et al. [38]	33%	1 year	↓	↔	↓	ND	ND	↔	↓[2]
Parallel design	50%	1 year	↔	↔	↓	ND	ND	↔	↓
Yancy et al. [30]	10%	24-week	↓	↔	↑	ND	ND	ND	ND
Parallel design	~55%	24-week	↓	↔	↔	ND	ND	ND	ND
Sharman et al. [29]	47%	6-week	↔	↓	↔	↔	↔	↓	↓
Crossover design	8%	6-week	↓	↓	↔	↑	↔	↓	↔
Rodriguez-Villar [54]	50%	6-week	↔	↔	↔	↑	↔	↔	↓
Crossover design	40%	6-week	↓[3]	↔	↔	ND	↔	↔	↔
Zern et al.[4]	40%	10-week	↓	↓	↔	↑	↓	↓	↔
Foster et al. [40][5]	10%	1 year	↓	↔	↔	ND	ND	↔	↔
Parallel design	60 %	1 year	↔	↔	↑	ND	ND	↓	↔

Arrows indicate increases (↑), decreases (↓) or no changes (↔). ND = not determined

[1] More favorable for patients with TG levels > 4.5 mmol/L, [2] Only in diabetic individuals, [3] TG in VLDL

[4] Compared to baseline (average 53%), [5] Significant decrease in LDL-C after 3 months in 60% CHO group

THE METABOLIC SYNDROME, TYPE II DIABETES AND DIETARY CARBOHYDRATES

The term "metabolic syndrome (MetSyn)" is now preferable to "insulin resistance syndrome". Findings from the third National Health and Nutrition Survey demonstrated a prevalence of 25% in US individuals aged > 20 years, rising to 40% by age >60 [44]. The MetSyn is postulated to be resistance to insulin-mediated glucose disposal by muscle [45], 30% of adult males and 10-15% of postmenopausal women have this particular syndrome which is associated with an increased risk for heart disease.

The National Cholesterol Education Program (ATP III) [46] has classified individuals as having the MetSyn if three of the following characteristics are present: Plasma TG higher than 150 mg/dL, Plasma HDL-C lower than 45 mg/dL in men and 50 mg/dL in women, systolic/diastolic blood pressure > 125/80 mm of Hg, waist circumference (WC) > 88 cm in women and > 102 cm in men and fasting plasma glucose > 110 mg/dL. The prevalence of the MetSyn is high among Hispanics. In the III National Health and Nutrition Examination Survey, (NHANES III), Hispanics had the highest age-adjusted prevalence of the MetSyn, which was probably linked to the higher prevalence of obesity [47]. The presence of three or more features associated with the MetSyn, have been identified in the young Hispanic population (8-13 y old) with insulin resistance playing a major role in the observed dyslipidemias [48].

As described before, waist circumference seems to play an important role in the development of the MetSyn. While abdominal obesity is determined by the accumulation of both subcutaneous adipose tissue (SCAT) and visceral adipose tissue (VAT), some studies described that VAT appears to play a major role in the MetSyn [49]. VAT is located in the body cavity beneath the abdominal muscles, whereas SCAT is located beneath the skin and on top of the abdominal musculature, femoral and gluteal regions [50]. The "Portal Theory" suggests that insulin resistance and many of its related features could arise from VAT delivering free fatty acids in a high rate to the liver via the portal vein into which VAT directly drains. This in turn, would increase hepatic glucose production, reduce hepatic insulin clearance and finally lead to insulin resistance, hyperinsulinemia, hyperglycemia as well as non-alcoholic fatty liver disease [51].

Figure 1 illustrates the effects of a high carbohydrate diet in individuals with the MetSyn characterized for VAT accumulation. When carbohydrate is increased in the diet, higher concentrations of both glucose and fructose enter to the liver through portal circulation. Excess sugars can be readily converted into fatty acids, with fructose having a higher conversion rate duc to the bypassing of phosphofructokinase, a highly regulated enzyme. In addition the quick formation of glyceraldehyde - 3 phosphate from fructose favors the esterification of fatty acids for TG synthesis. This pathway has a minor contribution to increasing the synthesis of VLDL. In addition, the increased flux of fatty acids from VAT to the liver due to insulin resistance make a significant contribution to VLDL assembly and secretion resulting in higher levels of circulating TG.

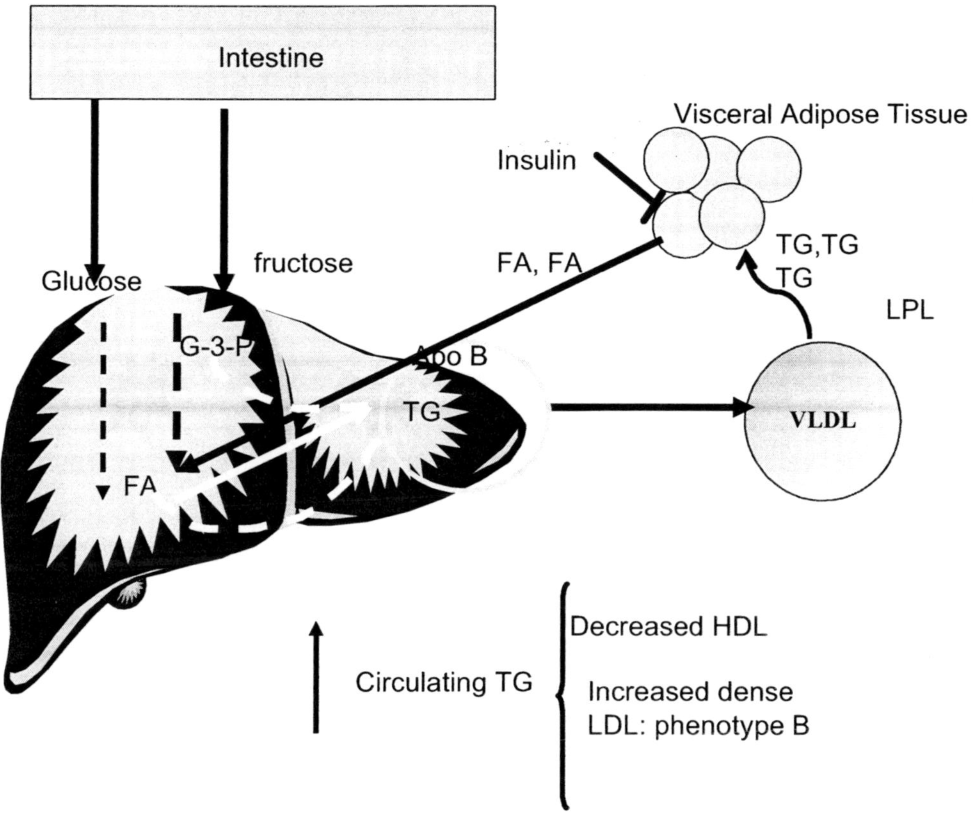

Figure 1. Increases in plasma triglycerides in subjects with the MetSyn and the consequences of a high carbohydrate diet. High carbohydrate diets promote the formation of free fatty acids. Glucose is converted to glucose 6-phospate as it enters the hepatocyte and through a series of reaction in which phsphofuctokinase, a highly regulated enzymes, the pathway progresses to lactate and then to fatty acids. In contrast, fructose bypasses this enzyme and thus it is more readily converted to fatty acids. Fatty acids are then used to form TG, which packaged with apo B result in increased secretion of VLDL. Subjects with the MetSyn because of the accumulation of visceral obesity, they develop insulin resistance and thus there is an unregulated secretion of fatty acids, which go back to the liver and are utilized for TG formation and packaging into VLDL promoting the increase of circulating TG.

Very low-carbohydrate diets seem to improve all the biomarkers associated with the MetSyn [29]. Recent studies by Volek et al [2] showed that a short-term isoenergetic very low carbohydrate diet significantly decreased fasting and postpandrial TG, increased HDL-C, decreased the total cholesterol/HDL-C ratio and did not affect CRP or TNF-α. The large increase in HDL-C could have been due to increased production by hepatocytes and the intestinal mucosa and/or increased lipoprotein-lipase (LPL), which results in disassociation of surface components that are acquired by HDL-C. Studies conducted in mice fed with a high fat diet observed a very strong correlation between increases in postheparin LPL activity and increasing HDL-C [52]. In humans, moderate to high fat diets (46 – 65% of total energy) significantly increased postheparin plasma LPL activity and skeletal muscle LPL activity [53].

The macronutrient content of the diet has been linked to the insulin resistance syndrome, for example, the effects of a high monounsaturated fat diet and a high carbohydrate diet were tested on the resistance of LDL to oxidation in Type 2 diabetic patients in an intervention, which followed a randomized crossover design [54]. In addition, high-fat, particularly high saturated fat diets, induce weight gain, insulin resistance and hyperlipidemia in humans and animals. When the acceptability of the two diets was compared at the end of 6 weeks, the high fat diet was preferred by the patients. Although no significant effects on plasma cholesterol, TG, HDL-C, parameters of LDL oxidation, body weight or glycemic control were observed between the two dietary periods, significant reductions were observed in both VLDL cholesterol and TG during the high fat period. Authors concluded that a high fat diet rich in monounsaturated fat is a good alternative for patients with type II diabetes since the diet was found to be palatable and highly accepted by the patients plus there were some additional beneficial effects on the plasma lipid profiles of these individuals [54].

Optimizing macronutrients and food preparation can have beneficial effects in individuals with visceral fat. There are some reviews that support the metabolic benefits of controlling the GI and the glycemic load (GL). In a 12-month pilot study in teens, a conventional diet was compared to the lower GI diet, which resulted in a greater total weight and fat loss without regain from months 6-12. While insulin resistance increased in the conventional diet group, the lower GI group showed no change [55]. Data from cross-sectional studies have shown that by reducing energy intake and weight loss in obese type 2 diabetic subjects, an improvement in insulin sensitivity, blood glucose levels, lipid profile and blood pressure in the short-term is observed [56]. Recently, Silvestre et al [57] showed that compared to an energy restricted low-fat diet, a short term very low-carbohydrate diet was associated with greater weight and fat loss with an apparent preferential loss of central fat. McAuley et al. [58] conducted a study in which 96 insulin resistant women were assigned either to a very low carbohydrate diet, a moderate carbohydrate diet (40% energy) or a high carbohydrate diet during 16 weeks (8 weeks of weight loss and 8 weeks of weight maintenance). When compared to the high carbohydrate diet, women on the very low and moderate carbohydrate groups had a greater reduction in waist circumference ($P < 0.01$), plasma triglycerides ($P < 0.01$) and a better effect in reducing insulin resistance. Authors concluded that the very low and the moderate carbohydrate diets are more appropriate for reducing the risk for cardiovascular disease in type 2 diabetes patients and that the high carbohydrate diet needs to include a higher amount of fiber and possible reduce saturated fat to achieve the similar effects as the lower carbohydrate groups [58].

C-reactive protein (CRP) is considered an important marker of inflammation and a risk factor for the MetSyn [59]. CRP seems to be a powerful predictor for CHD and diabetes and is positively associated with both insulin resistance and the prevalence of the MetSyn. A very low carbohydrate diet was compared to a low fat diet in a weight loss intervention to assess the effects of macronutrient intake on the inflammatory response [29]. In a crossover design, 15 overweight subjects were given either a diet with < 10% energy derived from carbohydrates or a diet with <30% energy from fat. Both diets were equally successful in decreasing tumor necrosis factor (TNF)α, Interleukin-6(IL-6), CRP and cell adhesion molecule-1 (CAM-1) indicating that weight loss is the primary driving force to reduce inflammation biomarkers. A number of studies have demonstrated the association between glycemic load and levels of CRP. O'Brien et al demonstrated a significant reduction in CRP in women after 3 months of consuming a hypocaloric-very low carbohydrate diet than after consuming a energy-matched low fat diet [60]. Weight loss could be also implicated in the reduction of CRP concentrations, thus Tchernof et al [61] suggested that a hypoenergetic very low carbohydrate or low fat diet, if used for weight loss, may lower CRP as was observed by the O'Brien study and therefore reduce the CHD and the MetSyn risk.

Dietary carbohydrates may also have influence on leptin action. Studies by Havel et al demonstrated that consumption of high-fat meals, produced smaller postprandial glucose and insulin responses than equicaloric high-carbohydrates meals, and reduced 24-h circulating leptin concentrations in humans [62]. Later on, Mueller et al associated the reductions of leptin concentrations to a decreased insulin-mediated glucose metabolism in adipose tissue [63]. Insulin and leptin function as key signals conveying information on energy intake and body fat stores to the Central Nervous System (CNS) for the long-term regulation of food intake and energy homeostasis [64]. It is possible that reduced insulin and leptin production contributes to increase energy intake, weight gain, and obesity in animals and humans consuming high-fat diets. Because fructose, unlike glucose, does not stimulate insulin secretion, Teff et al conducted a study where they hypothesized that rich fructose meals would result in lower leptin concentrations than meals containig the same amount of glucose. They fed 12 normal-weight women on 2 randomized days during which the subjects consumed three meals containing 55, 30 and 15% of total kilocalories from carbohydrates, fat, and proteins respectively, with 30% of kilocalories as either a fructose-sweetened (HFr) or glucose-sweetened (HGl) beverage. Meals were isocaloric in the two treatments. Consuming HFr beverages with meals resulted in lower circulating insulin and leptin concentrations and higer TG concentrations compared with consumption of HGl beverages [65]. Because insulin and leptin function as key signals to the CNS in the long-term regulation of energy balance, prolonged consumption of diets high in energy from fructose could lead to increased caloric intake and contribute to weigh gain and obesity. In addition, the elevation of TG concentrations after fructose consumption suggests that chronic fructose consumption, as in the case of diabetic patients, could contibute to atherogenesis, cardiovascular disease and the MetSyn. The relation between cerebrospinal fluid and serum levels of leptin in obese humans suggests that defective blood brain barrier (BBB) transport accounts for a great deal of leptin resistance in the CNS. Banks et al [66] conducted a study, where high-fat milk (98% of TG) and fat-free milk were used in vitro, in vivo and in situ in mice. They demonstrated that a high-fat diet significantly increased serum TG concentrations and that high TG levels directly inhibited the transport of leptin across the BBB and could be a major cause of leptin resistance across the CNS. Thus, authors suggested that serum TG are one of the major cause of the leptin resistance seen in both obesity and starvation [66]. This study demonstrates that just by lowering TG, it is possible to appreciate the effects of leptin on weight loss.

CONCLUSION

The review from these studies has demonstrated the importance of diet modifications in the maintenance of ideal body weight and on the reduction of biomarkers of chronic disease. It is evident that the amount of dietary carbohydrate plays a major role in determining plasma TG concentrations and other metabolic alterations associated with these plasma lipids. Elevated plasma TG are both a marker for the MetSyn and for increased risk for CHD. It is also evident from these studies that diets aimed at reducing obesity, a modifiable risk factor are beneficial independent of the amount of carbohydrates in the diet.

Although the high carbohydrate diet reduces LDL-C and with lifestyle modifications may slow the progression of atherosclerosis, evidence from the various clinical studies indicate that this diet may not be appropriate for patients who are obese (especially those with visceral obesity) or for subjects who are classified with the MetSyn. In contrast, the very low carbohydrate diet appears to be more effective for weight loss at short term and for reducing plasma TG, increasing HDL, increasing the concentration of large buoyant LDL and in some cases, reduce blood pressure and increase insulin sensitivity. However, the long-term benefits of this diet remain unconfirmed. The intake of reasonably low amounts of carbohydrate (~ 40% of total energy) could be a dietary intervention easier to follow for longer time periods and potentially become a useful alternative, specifically for those patients with hypertriglyceridemia, insulin resistance and the MetSyn.

REFERENCES

[1] Mensink RP, Zock PL, Kester ADM, Katan MB. Effects of dietary fatty acids and carbohydrates on the ration of serum total to HDL cholesterol and on serum lipids and apolipoproteins: a meta-analysis of 60 controlled trials. *Am. J. Clin. Nutr.* 2003;77: 146-1155.

[2] Volek JS, Sharman MJ, Gomez AL, Scheett TP, Kraemer WJ. An isoenergenic very low carbohydrate diet improves serum HDL cholesterol and triacylglycerol concentrations, the total cholesterol to HDL cholesterol ratio and postprandial lipemic responses compared with a low fat diet in normal weight, normolipidemic women. *J. Nutr.* 2003; 133:2756-2761.

[3] Must A, Spadano J, Coakley EH, Field AE, Colditz G, Dietz WH. The disease burden associated with overweight and obesity. *J. Am. Med. Assoc.* 1999; 282:1523-1529.

[4] Colditz G, Economic costs of obesity and inactivity. *Med Sci. Sports Exerc.* 1999;31: S663-S667.

[5] Virgin SES, JA. Metabolic syndrome. J. *Am. Assoc. Oc. Health Nurs.* 2003;51:38-37.

[6] Liu S, Willett WC, Manson JE, Hu FB, Rosner B, Colditz G. Relation between changes in intakes of dietary fiber and grain products and changes in weight and development of obesity among middle-aged women. *Am J. Clin. Nutr.* 2003;78:920-927.

[7] Lofgren IE, Herron KL, Zern TL, West KL, Patalay M, Shachter NS, Koo SI, Fernandez, ML. Waist circumference is a better predictor than body mass index of coronary heart disease risk in overweight premenopausal women. *J. Nutr.* 2004;134:1071-1076.

[8] Chahoud G, Aude YW & Methta JL. Dietary recommendations in the prevention and treatment of coronary heard disease: do we have the ideal diet yet? *Am. J. Cardiol.* 2004:94:1260-1267.

[9] Hu FB, Manson JE, Willett WC. Types of dietary fat and risk of coronary heart disease: A critical review. *J. Am. Coll. Nutr.* 2001; 20:5-19.

[10] Velasquez-Mieyer PA, Cowan PA, Arheart KL, et al. Suppression of insulin secretion is associated with weight loss and altered macronutrient intake and preference in a subset of obese adults. *Int. J. Obes.* 2003; 27:219-226.

[11] Grundy SM. Dietary influences on serum lipids and lipoproteins. *J. Lipid Res.* 1990; 31:1149-1172.

[12] Thyfault JP, Carper MJ, Richmond SR, Hulver MW, Potteiger JA. Effect of liquid carbohydrate ingestion on markers of anabolism following high-intensity resistance exercise. *J. Strenght Con. Res.* 2004; 18:174-179.

[13] Rajala, M. and P.E. Scherer, Minireview: The adipocyte - at the crossroads of energy homeostasis, inflammation and atherosclerosis. *Endocrinology*, 2003. 144:3765-3773.

[14] Dreon DM, Fernstrom HA, Williams PT, Krauss RM. LDL subclass patterns and lipoprotein response to a low-fat, high-carbohydrate diet in women. *Arterioscler. Thromb. Vasc. Biol.* 1997;17:707-714.

[15] Kuczmarski RJ, Flegal KM, Campbell SM and Johnson CL. Increasing prevalence of overweight among US adults. The National Health and Nutrition Examination Surveys, 1960 to 1991. *JAMA*. 1994;272:205-211.

[16] Putnam JJ and Allshouse JE. Food consumption, prices and expeditures, 1970-1997. Washington, DC: U.S. Deparment of Agriculture, Economic research Service.

[17] Gross LS, Li L, Ford ES and Liu S. Increased consumption of refined carbohydrates and the epidemic of type 2 diabetes in the United States: an ecological assessment. Am J. Clin. Nutr. 2004:79:774-779.

[18] Jenkins DJA, Kendalll CWC, Marchie A, Augustin LSA. Too much sugar, too much carbohydrate or just too much? *Am. J. Clin. Nutr.* 2004;79:711-712.

[19] Glinsmann WH and Bowman BA. The publica health significance of dietary fructose. *Am. J. Clin Nutr.* 1993;58(suppl):820S-823S.

[20] Osei K and Bossetti B. Dietary fructose as a natural sweetener in poorly controlled type 2 diabetes: a 12-month crossover study of effects on glucose, lipoprotein and apolipoprotein metabolism. Deabet. Med. 1989:6:506-511.

[21] Crapo PA, Koltermann OG and Henry RR. Metabolic consequence of two-week fructose feeding in diabetic subjects. Diabetes Care 1986:9:111-119.

[22] Parks EJ & Hellerstein MK. Carbohydrate-induced hypertriacylglycerolemia : historical perspective and review of biological mechanisms. *Am. J. Clin. Nutr.* 2000:71:412-413.

[23] Fried SK & Rao SP. Sugars, hyperriglyceridemia and cardiovascular disease. *Am. J. Clin. Nutr.* 2003: 78(suppl):873S-880S.

[24] Rizkalla SW, Bellisle F, Slama G. Health benefits of low glycaemic index foods, such as pulses, in diabetic patients and healthy individuals. *Br J Nutr.* 2002; 88(suppl 3):S255-S262.

[25] Sloth B, Krog-Mikkelsen I, flint A, Tetens I, Bjorck I, Vinoy S, Elmstahl H, Arstrup A, Lang V & Rabben A. No difference in body weight decrease between a low-glycemic index and high-glycemic index diet but reduced LFL cholesterol after 10-week ad libitum intake of the low-glycemic-index diet. *Am. J. Clin. Nutr.* 2004:80:337-347.

[26] Kelly S, Frost G, Whitaker V & Summerbell C. Low glycemic index diets for coronary heart disease. *Cochrane Database Syst Rev.* 2004:18:CD004467.

[27] Hellerstein MK. Carbohydrate-induced hypertriglyceridemia: modifying factors and implications for cardiovascular risk. *Curr. Op. Lipidol* 2002:13:33-40.

[28] Klein S. Clinical trial experience with fat-restricted vs carbohydrate-restricted weight-loss diets. *Obes. Res.* 2004; 12:141S-144S.

[29] Sharman MJ, Gomez AL, Kraemer WJ & Volek JS. Very low-carbohydrate and low-fat diets affect fasting lipids and postrandial lipemia differently in overweight men. *J. Nutr.* 2004;134:880-885.

[30] Yancy WS Jr, Olsen MK, Guyton JR, Bakst RP & Westman EC. A low –carbohydrate, ketogenic diet versus a low-fat diet to treat obesity and hyperlipidemia. *Annal. Int. Med.* 2004;140:769-777.

[31] Sharman MJ & Volek JS. Weight loss leads to reductions in inflammatory biomarkers after a very-low-carbohydrate diet and low-fat diet in overweight men. *Clin. Sci.* 2004;107:365-369.

[32] Lofgren IE, Zern TL, Herron KL, West KL, Sharman M, Volek JS, Shachter NS, Koo SI and Fernandez ML. Weight loss reduces the atherogenicity of LDL in premenopausal women. *Metabolism Clin. Ext.* 2005;54:133-1141.

[33] Jacobs B, De Angelis-Schierbaum G, Egert S, Assmann G & Kratz M. Individual serum triglyceride responses to high-fat and low-fat diets differ in men with modest and severe hypertriglyceridemia. *J. Nutr.* 2004;134:1400-1405.

[34] National Cholesterol Education Program Expert Panel on Detection, Evaluation and Tratment of High blood cholesterol in adults (adult treatment panel III). National Heart, lung and blood institute and national Institutes of Health, Bethesda, MD (NHI publication No. 01-3670) May 2001.

[35] Schneeman BO. Carbohydrate: friend or foe? Summary of research needs. *J. Nutr.* 2001;131:2764S-2765S.

[36] Sharman MJ, Kraemer WJ, Love DM, Avery NG, Gómez AL, Scheett TP and Volek JF. A ketogenic diet favorable affects seru biomarkers for cardiovascular disease in normal weight men. *J.Nutr.* 2002;132:1879-1885.

[37] Gann D. A low carbohydrate diet in overweight patients undergoing stable statin therapy raises high-density lipoprotein and lowers triglycerides substantially. *Clin. Cardiol.* 2004:27:563-564.

[38] Stern L, Iqbal N, Seshadri P, Chicano KL, Daily DA, McGrory J, Williams M, Gracely EJ & Samaha FF. The effects of low-carbohydrate versus conventional weight loss diets in severely obese adults: One year follow-up of a randomized trial. *Ann Intern Med* 2004;140:778-785.

[39] Segal-Isaacson CJ, Johnson S, Tomuta V, Crowell B & Stein DT. A randomized trial comparing low-fat and low carbohydrate diets matched for energy and protein. Obes. Res. 2004:12:130S-140S.

[40] Foster GD, Wyatt HR, Hill JO, McGuckin BG, Brill C, Mohammed S, Szapary PO, Rader DJ, Edman JS & Klein S. A randomized trial of low-carbohydrate diet for obesity. *New. Eng. J. Med.* 2003;328:2082-2090.

[41] Dansinger ML, Gleason JA, Griffith JL, Selker HP & Schaefer EJ. Comparison of the Atkins, Ornish,weight watchers, and zone diets for weight loss and heart disease risk reduction. A ramdomized trial. *Am. Med. Assoc.* 2005; 293: 43-53.

[42] Krauss RM. Atherogenic lipoprotein phenotype and diet-gene interactions. *J. Nutr.* 131:340S-343S.

[43] Lovejoy JC, Bray GA, Lefevre M, Smith SR, Most MM, Denkins YM, Volaufova J, Rood JC, Eldrige AL & Peters JC. Consumption of a controlled low-fat diet containing

olestra for 9 months improves health risk factors in conjuction with weight loss in obese men: the Olé study. *Int. J. Obes.* 2003;27:1242-1249.

[44] Ford ES, Giles WH, Dietz WH. Prevalence of metabolic syndrome among US adults-Finding from the Third National Health and Nutrition Examination Survey. *JAMA-J Am Med Assoc.* 2002;287:356-359.

[45] Reaven GM. Diet and syndrome X. *Curr Atheroscler. Rep.* 2000;2:503-507.

[46] Expert Panel on Detection EaToHBCiA. Executive summary of the third report of the National Cholesterol Education Program (NCEP) Expert Panel on detection, evaluation and treatment of high blood cholesterol in adults (Adult Treatment Panel III). *J. Am. Med. Assoc.* 2001;285:2486-2497.

[47] Flegal KM, Carroll MD, Ogden CL, Johnson CL. Prevalence and trends in obesity among US adults, 1999-2000. *J. Am. Med. Assoc.* 2002:288:1723-1727.

[48] Cruz ML, Weigensberg MJ, Hunag TTK, \Ball G, Shaibi GQ & Goran MI. The metabolic syndrome in overweight Hispanic youth and the role of insulin sensitivity. *J. Clin Endocrinol. Met.* 2004:89:108-113.

[49] Lamarche B. Abdominal obesity and its metabolic complications: implications for the risk of ischaemic heart disease. *Corno Artery Dis.* 1998;9:473-481.

[50] Wajchenberg BL. Subcutaneous and visceral adipose tissue: their relation to the metabolic syndrome. *Endocr Rev.* 2000;21:697-738.

[51] Bjorntorp P. "Portal" adipose tissue as a generator of risk factors for cardiovascular disease and diabetes. *Atherosclerosis.* 1990;10:493-496.

[52] Clee SM, Zhang H, Bissada N, Miao L, Ehrenborg E, Benlian P, Shen GX, Angel A, LeBoeuf, Rc and Hayden MR. Relatioship between lipoprotein lipase and high density lipoprotein cholesterol in mice: modulation by cholesteryl ester transfer protein and dietary status. *J. Lipid Res.* 1997; 38:2079-2089.

[53] Campos H, Dreon DM and Krauss RM. Association of hepatic and lipoprotein lipase activities with changes in dietary composition and low density lipoprotein subclasses. *J. Lipid Res.* 1995;36:462-472.

[54] Rodrigues-Villar C, Perez-Heras A, Mercade I, Casals E & Ros E. Comparison of a high-carbohydrate and ahihg-monounsaturated fat, olive-oil rich diet on the susceptibility of LDL to oxidative modification in subjects with Type 2 diabetes mellitus. *Diabet. UK. Diabet. Med.* 2003;21:142-149.

[55] Ebbeling CB and Ludwig DS. Treating obesity in youth: should dietary glycemic load be a consideration?. *Adv Pediatr.* 2001;48:179-217.

[56] Heilbonn LK, Noakes M and Clifton PM. Effect of energy restriction, weight loss, and diet composition on plasma lipids and glucose in patients with type 2 diabetes. *Diabetes Care.* 1999;22:889-895.

[57] Silvestre R, Sharman MJ, Gómez AL, Judelson DA, Watson G, RuffinK, Kraemer WJ and Volek JS. A very low-carbohydrate diet results in greater reductions in body weight, whole body fat, and trunk fat than a low-fat diet in overweight subjects. *In Kings-brook conference on nutritional and metabolic aspects of low carbohydrate diets. Brooklyn, University of Connecticut (Storrs).* 2004.

[58] McAuley KA, Hopkins CM, Smith KJ, McLay RT, Williams SM, Taylor RW and Mann JI. Comparison of high-fat and high-protein diets with a high carbohydrate diet in insulin-resistant obese women. Diabetologia 2004(pub med, ahead of print).

[59] Libby P, Ridker PM and MASERI a. Inflammatory bio-markers and cardiovascular risk prediction. *Circulation.* 2002;105:1135-1143.

[60] O'Brien KD, Brehm BJ, Seely RJ, Tener M, Daniels S and D Alessio D.A. Greater reduction of inflammatory markers with a low carbohydrate diet than with a carolically matched, low fat diet. *Presented at the American Heart Association,s Scientific Sessions*. 2002. November 19, Chicago IL (abs.# 117597).

[61] Tchernof A, Nolan A, Sites CK, Ades PA and Poehlman ET. Weight loss reduces C-reactive protein levels in obese postmenopausal women. *Circulation.* 2002;105:564-569.

[62] Havel PJ, Townsend r, Chaump L and teff K. High-fat meals reduce 24-h circulating leptin concentrations in women. *Diabetes.* 1999;48:334-3341.

[63] Mueller WM, Gregoire FM, stanhope KL, Mobbs CV, Mizuno TM, Warden CH, stern JS and Havel PJ. Evidence that glucose metabolism regulates leptin secretion from cultured rat adipocytes. *Endocrinology.* 1998;139:551-558.

[64] Havel PJ. Control of energy homeostasis and insulin action by adipocyte hormones: leptin, acylation stimulating protein, and adiponectin. *Curr Opin Lipidol.* 2002;13:51-59.

[65] Teff KL, Elliott SS, Tschop M, Kieffer TJ, Rader D, Heiman M, Townsend RR, Keim NL, D'alessio D and Havel PJ. Dietary fructose reduces circulating insulin and leptin, attenuates postprandial suppression of ghrelin and increases triglycerides in women.*J Clin Endocrinol Metab*. 2004;89:2963-2972.

[66] Banks WA, Coon AB, Robinson SM, Moinuddin A, Shultz JM, Nakaoke R, and Morley JE. Triglycerides induce leptin resistance at the blood-brain barrier. *Diabetes.* 2004;53:1253-1260.

In: Trends in Dietary Carbohydrates Research
Editor: M. V. Landlow, pp. 71-89
ISBN 1-59454-798-X

Chapter 4

The Effect of Carbohydrate Supplementation during the First of Two Prolonged Cycling Bouts on Immunoendocrine Responses

Tzai-Li Li[1]* and Michael Gleeson
School of Sport and Exercise Sciences, Loughborough University Loughborough, Leicestershire, United Kingdom
[1] Department of Sports and Leisure Studies, National Dong Hwa University, Hualien, Taiwan

Abstract

The purpose of this study was to examine the effect of carbohydrate feeding during the first of two 90-min cycling bouts (EX1 started at 09:00 and EX2 started at 13:30) at 60% $\dot{V}O_{2\,max}$ on leukocyte redistribution, *in vitro* lipopolysaccharide (LPS)-stimulated degranulation and phorbol-12-myristate-13-acetate (PMA)-induced oxidative burst by blood neutrophils and plasma interleukin-6 and stress hormone responses. Subjects (n = 9) consumed a 10% w/v carbohydrate (glucose) or placebo beverage during EX1: 500 mL just before exercise and 250 mL every 20 min during exercise, which were completed in a counterbalanced order and separated by at least 4 days. Venous blood samples were taken 5 min before exercise and immediately post-exercise for both trials. The main findings of the present study were that ingestion of carbohydrate compared with placebo during EX1 1) maintained higher plasma glucose concentration throughout the experimental protocol; 2) blunted the responses of plasma adrenaline, adrenocorticotrophic hormone and cortisol during EX2; 3) attenuated circulating leukocytosis and monocytosis throughout the experimental protocol, neutrophilia during the recovery interval, and lymphocytosis during EX2; 4) lessened the decline in LPS-

* Correspondence: Professor Michael Gleeson. Address: School of Sport and Exercise Sciences, Loughborough University, Loughborough, Leicestershire, LE11 3TU, United Kingdom; Telephone number: +44 1509 226345; Fax number: +44 1509 226300; Email address: m.gleeson@lboro.ac.uk

stimulated degranulation and PMA-induced oxidative burst on per neutrophil basis from 3 h post-EX1 onwards; but 5) did not affect changes in plasma interleukin-6. These findings suggest that carbohydrate ingestion during EX1 increases carbohydrate availability during both bouts of exercise; has a limited effect on immunoendocrine response during EX1 but attenuates plasma stress hormone responses during EX2; and blunts the delayed neutrophilia and concurrent decline in neutrophil functions on a per cell basis after EX1. Hence, athletes may benefit from consuming carbohydrate at the earliest opportunity when performing repeated bouts of endurance exercise in a single day.

Key Words: neutrophil degranulation, oxidative burst, interleukin-6, stress hormones

INTRODUCTION

Acute exercise alters immune cell function and modifies leukocyte trafficking between the circulation and tissue compartments and these effects may last for several hours after exercise [Gleeson and Bishop, 1999]. During this period, immunity is likely depressed and may open a window to invading pathogens, increasing opportunistic infections in stressed athletes [Pedersen, 1999]. This temporarily reversible alteration in immune function is related to elevated plasma concentrations of stress hormones [Benschop *et al.*, 1996].

Neutrophils, representing 50-60% of the total blood leukocytes, are important phagocytes in innate immunity protecting the host against various pathogenic microorganisms [Nieman, 1994]. Muns *et al.* [1994] reported that nasal neutrophil function was depressed for 3 days after prolonged running. This impairment of neutrophil microbicidal capacity may place athletes at a higher risk of infection [Fukatsu *et al.*, 1996]. Neutrophils destroy invasive microorganisms through release of degradative enzymes from preformed granule stores (degranulation) and the production of reactive oxygen species (ROS) (oxidative burst) after phagocytosis [Fukatsu *et al.*, 1996; Johnson *et al.*, 1998]. Release of elastase (one of the major lysosomal enzymes in neutrophil azurophilic granules) and luminol-enhanced chemiluminescence (CL) (mainly detecting HOCl production) are frequently used to determine neutrophil degranulation and oxidative burst activity, respectively [Elsbach, 1980; Suzuki *et al.*, 1996]. Previous studies demonstrated that the responses of neutrophil degranulation and oxidative burst activity to *in vitro* stimulants on per cell basis were depressed for several hours following intensive prolonged exercise [Pyne *et al.*, 1996; Robson *et al.*, 1999; Suzuki *et al.*, 1996; Walsh *et al.*, 2000].

Nutritional strategies are often used to manipulate exercise-induced immunoendocrine responses. Carbohydrate (CHO) supplementation during exercise is one of the most successful means to attenuate immunoendocrine responses during prolonged exercise [Gleeson *et al.*, 2001]. Ingestion of CHO compared with placebo (PLA) better maintains plasma glucose concentration, blunts hypothalamic-pituitary-adrenal axis activation [Mitchell *et al.*, 1990] and minimizes immunological perturbation to an acute single bout of non-fatiguing, fixed duration exercise [Gleeson and Bishop, 2000]. The most effective and common method applied to increase carbohydrate availability is to ingest CHO-rich drinks during prolonged exercise [Jeukendrup and Jentjens, 2000].

Training programs of endurance athletes usually involve several bouts of intensive exercise in a day. Therefore, maintenance of immune competence during repeated exercise bouts is of crucial importance to prevent athletes from immunodepression and opportunistic pathogen invasion. A few studies have examined the effect of two exercise bouts on the same day on immunoendocrine responses and have shown that the second exercise bout induces a greater hormonal response and a larger leukocyte mobilisation compared with a single identical exercise bout [Ronsen *et al.*, 2001a; Ronsen *et al.*, 2001b]. However, the limited information available is insufficient to fully evaluate the effect of repeated bouts of exercise on immune cell functions and warrants further investigation.

For various considerations, many athletes wake up in early morning and train without breakfast. However, no study has examined the effect of CHO ingestion during the first of two prolonged exercise bouts on immunoendocrine responses. Hence, the aims of this chapter were to compare the effect of CHO supplementation during the first of two prolonged cycling bouts on responses of leukocyte redistribution, lipopolysaccharide (LPS)-stimulated degranulation and phorbol-12-myristate-13-acetate (PMA)-induced oxidative burst by neutrophils, plasma stress hormones, and IL-6. We hypothesised that ingestion of CHO compared with PLA during the first exercise bout would be beneficial to attenuate the perturbation of immunoendocrine responses during the first bout, the subsequent recovery period, and second bout of exercise.

METHODS

Subjects

Nine male volunteers (age 29.7 ± 1.6 years, height 177 ± 2 cm, body mass 72.0 ± 1.6 kg, $\dot{V}O_{2\,max}$ 49.4 ± 2.0 $mL \cdot kg^{-1} \cdot min^{-1}$; means ± S.E.M.), who were recreationally active and familiar with cycling, participated in the study. After receiving written information and passing a Health Questionnaire screen, subjects signed an informed consent. Subjects were requested to complete the dietary record sheet the day prior to Trial 1 and then repeated it again before Trial 2. Subjects were also asked not to perform any strenuous exercise or consume alcohol or medication for 2 days before each trial. The protocol was approved by the Ethics Committee of Loughborough University before the study began.

Preliminary Measurements

Maximal oxygen uptake was estimated by means of a continuous incremental exercise test on a cycle ergometer (Monark 874E, Monark Exercise AB, Sweden) to volitional exhaustion. Subjects began cycling at 70 W with increments of 35 W every 3 min. The cadence was maintained at 70 $rev \cdot min^{-1}$ and heart rate was monitored using radiotelemetry. During the third minute of each work rate increment, expired gas was collected in Douglas bags. An oxygen/carbon dioxide analyser (Servomax 1400B, Crowborough, UK) was used along with a dry gas meter (Harvard Apparatus, Edenbridge, UK) for determination of $\dot{V}O_2$

and $\dot{V}CO_2$. From the $\dot{V}O_2$-work rate relationship, the work rate equivalent to 60% $\dot{V}O_{2\,max}$ was interpolated.

Experimental Procedures

The subjects completed two trials in a counterbalanced order, each separated by at least 4 days. Subjects arrived at the laboratory at 08:30 after fasting from 23:00 the previous day and were asked to empty their bladder before body mass was recorded. Subjects then performed two bouts of 90 min cycling (EX1 started at 09:00 and EX2 started at 13:30) at 60% $\dot{V}O_{2\,max}$ at 70 rev·min^{-1} on the same ergometer used to determine $\dot{V}O_{2\,max}$. Subjects were given a lemon flavoured 10% w/v CHO (glucose) or artificially sweetened placebo beverage during the first exercise bout: 500 mL just before exercise and 250 mL every 20 min during exercise. Subjects were asked to consume each drink within 3 min. Heart rate was recorded continuously during exercise by radiotelemetry. Ratings of perceived exertion were obtained at 15-min intervals using The Borg Scale of Perceived Exertion. Venous blood samples were taken 5 min before exercise and immediately post-exercise. No calories were received during the rest period between the two 90-min exercise sessions; however, water ingestion was allowed *ad libitum* during recovery interval and the second exercise bout. The laboratory temperature and relative humidity were 26.3 ± 0.2 °C and 39 ± 1%, respectively.

Blood Collection and Analysis

Venous blood samples were taken from an antecubital vein by venepuncture, and were collected into three Vacutainer tubes (Becton Dickinson, Oxford, UK). Blood samples in two K_3EDTA vacutainers (4 mL) were used for haematological analysis including hemoglobin, haematocrit, and total and differential leukocyte counts using an automated hematology analyser (A^C•T^{TM} 5diff analyser, Beckman Coulter, UK) and to determine changes in the plasma concentrations of stress hormones and interleukin-6 (IL-6). Plasma volume changes were calculated according to Dill and Costill [1974]. From blood taken into a lithium heparin vacutainer (7 mL), 1 mL was immediately added to an eppendorf tube (1.5 mL capacity) containing 50 µL of 10 mg·mL^{-1} bacterial LPS solution (Stimulant, Sigma, Poole, UK). Blood and LPS were mixed by gentle inversion and then incubated for 1 h at 37 °C, with gentle mixing every 20 min. After incubation, the mixture was centrifuged for 2 min at 15000 *g*. The supernatant was immediately stored at –80 °C prior to analysis of elastase concentration. The amount of elastase released per neutrophil in response to LPS stimulation was calculated according to Robson *et al.* [1999].

A microplate luminometer cell activation kit (Knight Scientific Limited, Plymouth, UK) was used to measure the neutrophil oxidative burst activity. Sample analysis was performed in duplicate as follows: 20 µL of K_3EDTA whole blood sample was added into a dilution tube with 2 mL of blood dilution buffer (HBSS without calcium and magnesium but with 20 mM HEPES, pH 7.4). A 20-µL aliquot of each diluted sample was then added into an opaque white microplate well. 90 µL reconstitution and assay buffer (HBSS with 20 mM HEPES, pH

7.4) was then added into each well followed by the addition of 20 μL reconstituted Adjuvant-K™ and 50 μL Pholasin® (10 μg·mL^{-1}). The microplate was placed into a luminometer (Anthos Lucy 1 Microplate Luminometer, Anthos Labtec Instrument, Austria) after adding 20 μL PMA into each well. After 1 min shaking and incubation at 37 °C, Pholasin®-enhanced chemiluminescence (CL) was measured at 1-min intervals for 30 min, and the incremental area under the curve (IAUC) was calculated. The oxidative burst activity per cell was calculated by dividing the IAUC by the numbers of neutrophils in each sample. The intra-assay coefficient of variation was 5.7% for the chemiluminescence assay.

The remaining K_3EDTA and heparinized whole blood was spun at 1500 *g* for 10 min in a refrigerated centrifuge at 4 °C within 10 min of sampling. The plasma obtained was immediately stored at −80 °C prior to analysis. Plasma aliquots were analysed to determine the concentration of glucose (GOD-PAP method, Randox, Ireland) using an automatic photometric analyser (Cobas-Mira plus, Roche). Human growth hormone (GH), cortisol (both DRG Instruments GmbH, Germany), adrenaline (IBL GmbH, Hamburg), adrenocorticotrophic hormone (ACTH) (Biomerica, Newport Beach, CA), IL-6 (Diaclone Research, France) and elastase (Merck, Lutterworth, UK) were determined using enzyme-linked immunosorbant assay (ELISA) kits. The intra-assay coefficient of variation was 1.3%, 2.4%, 6.9%, 12.7%, 5.1%, 1.6%, and 3.9% for glucose, GH, cortisol, adrenaline, ACTH, IL-6, and elastase, respectively.

Statistical Analysis

All results are presented as mean values and standard errors of the mean (± SEM). Data were checked for normality, homogeneity of variance and sphericity before statistical analysis, and where appropriate the Huynh-Feldt method was applied for adjustment of degrees of freedom for the *F*-tests. Comparisons of immunoendocrine responses were analyzed using a two-factor (trial × time) repeated measures ANOVA with *post hoc* Tukey method. Physiological variables and ratings of perceived exertion were examined using paired *t*-tests. *P*, *t*, and adjusted *F* values are presented and statistical significance was accepted at $P < 0.05$.

RESULTS

Physiological Variables and Ratings of Perceived Exertion

Exercise intensity (% $\dot{V}O_{2\,max}$), heart rate, body mass loss, water intake and the percentage change in plasma volume did not differ between trials (Table 1). The rating of perceived exertion was higher towards the end of EX2 than in EX1 ($t = 6.0$, $P < 0.001$ for CHO and $t = 7.6$, $P < 0.001$ for PLA) and higher in PLA compared with CHO in EX2 ($t = 3.5$, $P = 0.008$). There was higher heart rate response in EX2 than EX1 ($t = 3.8$, $P = 0.005$). Body mass loss and the percentage change in plasma volume in EX2 were significantly lower compared with EX1 in the CHO trial ($t = 2.9$, $P = 0.019$ and $t = 4.2$, $P = 0.003$).

Table 1. The exercise intensity and its effect on heart rate, rating of perceived exertion (RPE), body mass loss, water intake, and percentage change in plasma volume

	CHO		PLA	
	EX1	EX2	EX1	EX2
% VO_{2max}	60.7 (1.8)	59.9 (1.0)	60.9 (1.5)	59.7 (1.4)
Heart Rate (beats·min^{-1}) [a]	146 (3)	148 (3)	140 (2)	149 (2)†
RPE [a]	13.1 (0.5)	15.2 (0.4)†	13.4 (0.2)	16.8 (0.5)†¶¶
Body mass loss (kg) [b]	1.32 (0.09)	1.13 (0.09)*	1.43 (0.07)	1.24 (0.14)
Water intake (mL)	1500 (0)	768 (108)†	1500 (0)	854 (129)†
Plasma volume change (%) [c]	-7.5 (1.0)	-2.5 (0.4)†	-5.2 (0.5)	-3.7 (0.6)

Values are mean (±SEM, n = 9). Significantly different from EX1 (*$P < 0.05$, †$P < 0.01$) in same trial; significantly different from the same time point in CHO trial (¶¶ $P < 0.01$). [a] Measurements made in last 15 min of exercise. [b] After correction for water intake. [c] Immediately post-EX compared with pre-EX.

Blood Leukocyte Counts

There were significant main effects of trial ($F_{1, 8} = 26.7$, $P = 0.001$) and time ($F_{3, 24} = 48.7$, $P < 0.001$) for the circulating numbers of leukocytes (Figure 1A), with higher values in PLA than CHO. There was no effect of exercise during EX1 in CHO, but a higher value at post-EX1 compared with pre-EX1 in PLA. The blood leukocyte counts at pre-EX2 and post-EX2 were higher than pre-EX1 in both trials. There were significant main effects of trial ($F_{1, 8} = 20.8$, $P = 0.002$) and time ($F_{3, 24} = 31.4$, $P < 0.001$) and an interaction of trial and time ($F_{3, 24} = 4.0$, $P = 0.033$) for blood neutrophil counts (Figure 1B), with a higher value at pre-EX2 in PLA than CHO. No effect of exercise during EX1 in CHO was observed but a higher value at post-EX1 compared with pre-EX1 was found in PLA. The blood neutrophil counts at pre-EX2 and post-EX2 were higher than pre-EX1 in both trials. There were significant main effects of trial ($F_{1, 8} = 30.0$, $P = 0.001$) and time ($F_{3, 24} = 31.7$, $P < 0.001$) and an interaction of trial and time ($F_{3, 24} = 8.5$, $P = 0.001$) for blood lymphocyte counts (Figure 1C), with a higher value at post-EX2 compared with pre-EX1 in both trials. Furthermore, the value at post-EX2 in PLA was higher than in CHO. For blood monocyte counts (Figure 1D), there were also significant main effects of trial ($F_{1, 8} = 12.1$, $P = 0.008$) and time ($F_{3, 24} = 44.1$, $P < 0.001$) and an interaction between trial and time ($F_{3, 24} = 3.3$, $P = 0.037$), with higher values in PLA than CHO. There was no effect of exercise on monocytes during EX1 in CHO, but counts were higher at post-EX1 compared with pre-EX1 in PLA. The blood monocyte counts at pre-EX2 and post-EX2 were higher than pre-EX1 in both trials.

Plasma Stress Hormones

There were significant main effects of trial ($F_{1, 8} = 7.6$, $P = 0.025$) and time ($F_{2, 16} = 20.6$, $P = 0.001$) and an interaction of trial and time ($F_{2, 16} = 7.7$, $P = 0.009$) for plasma adrenaline (Figure 2A), which showed a higher value at post-EX2 compared with pre-EX1 in both trials and the value at post-EX2 in PLA was higher than in CHO. For plasma ACTH

(Figure 2B) and cortisol (Figure 2C), there were significant main effects of trial ($F_{1,8} = 13.7$, $P = 0.006$ and $F_{1,8} = 10.1$, $P = 0.013$) and time ($F_{3,24} = 25.9$, $P < 0.001$ and $F_{3,24} = 28.9$, $P < 0.001$) and an interaction of trial and time ($F_{3,24} = 16.5$, $P = 0.001$ and $F_{3,24} = 7.3$, $P = 0.002$), with higher values at post-EX2 in PLA compared with pre-EX1 and post-EX2 in CHO. Exercise did not affect plasma concentrations of ACTH and cortisol in CHO throughout the experimental protocol. There were significant main effects of trial ($F_{1,8} = 9.8$, $P = 0.014$) and time ($F_{3,24} = 14.7$, $P = 0.002$) and an interaction of trial and time ($F_{3,24} = 5.4$, $P = 0.009$) for plasma GH (Figure 2D), with higher values at post-EX2 compared with pre-EX1 in both trials and the value at post-EX1 in PLA was higher than in CHO.

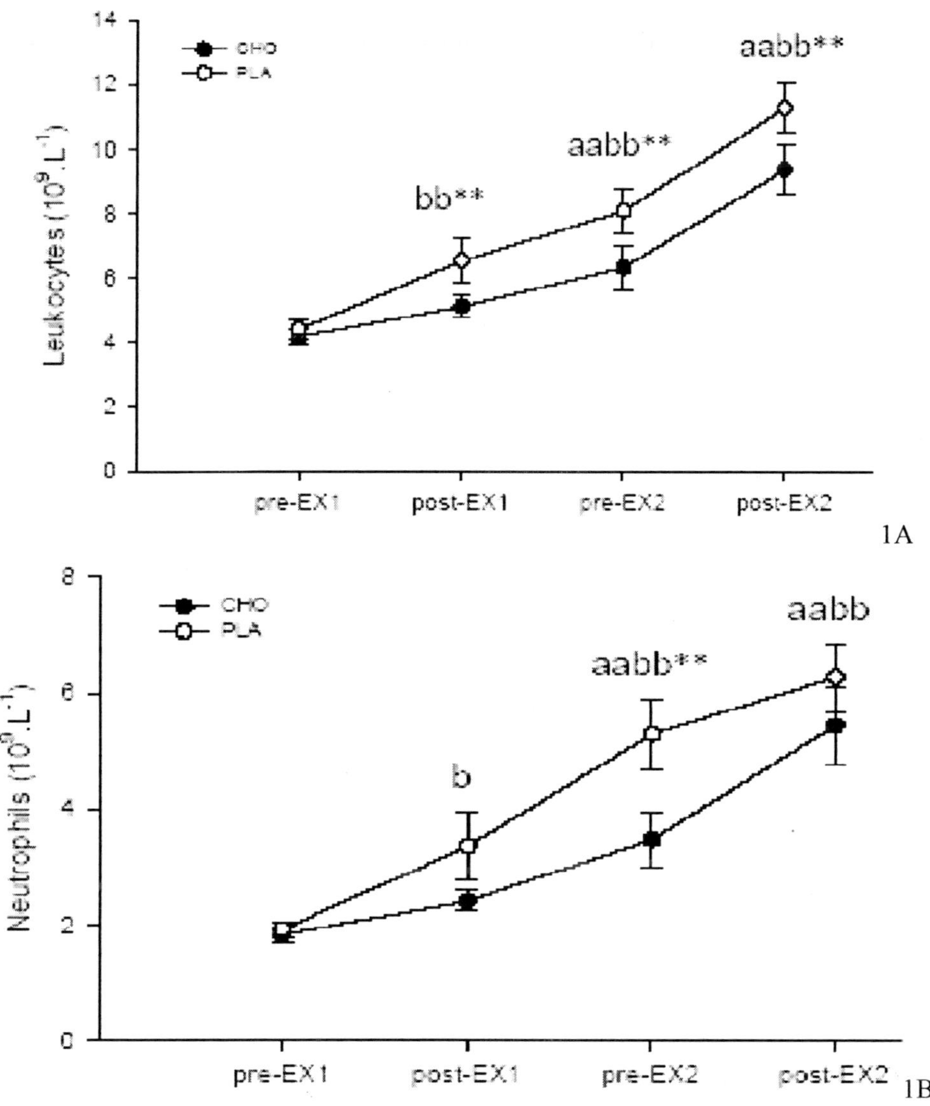

Figure 1. Continued on the next page

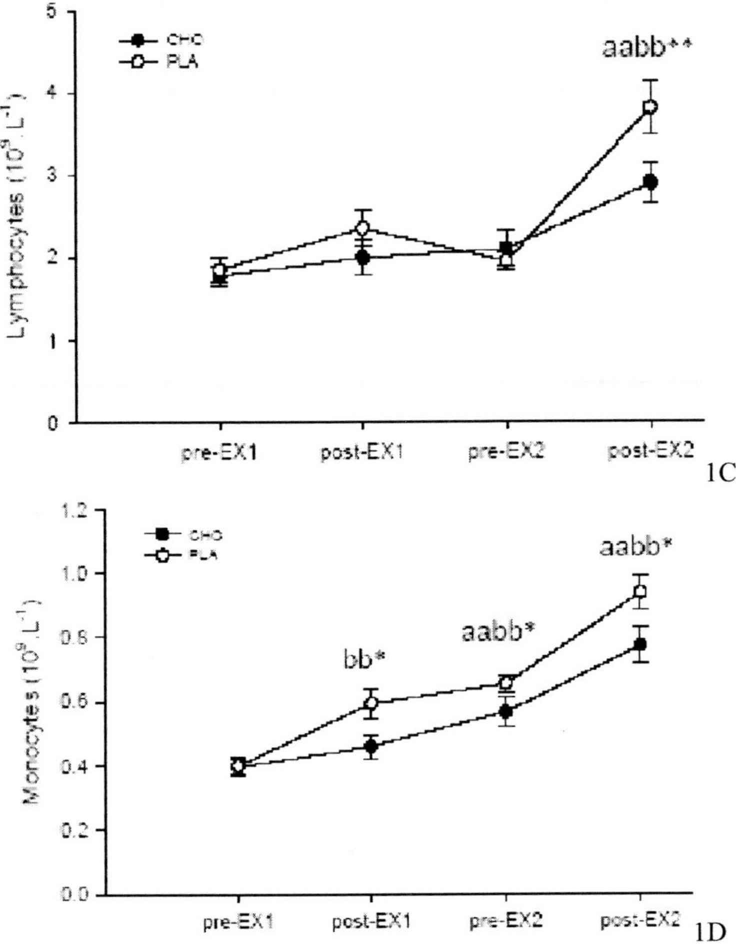

Figure 1. Changes in circulating counts of total leukocytes (1A), neutrophils (1B), lymphocytes (C), and monocytes (D). Values are means ± SEM (n = 9). Significantly different from pre-EX1 in CHO ($^{aa}P < 0.01$) and PLA ($^{b}P < 0.05$, $^{bb}P < 0.01$); significantly different between trials ($^{*}P < 0.05$, $^{**}P < 0.01$).

Plasma Glucose and IL-6

There were significant main effects of trial ($F_{1, 8} = 23.8$, $P = 0.001$) and time ($F_{3, 24} = 59.7$, $P < 0.001$) and an interaction between trial and time ($F_{3, 24} = 35.4$, $P < 0.001$) for plasma glucose concentration (Figure 3A), which showed carbohydrate feeding during EX1 significantly increased plasma glucose concentration compared with pre-EX1. However, the plasma glucose concentration was lower than pre-EX1 at pre-EX2 and post-EX2 in CHO. In PLA, the plasma glucose concentration was significantly decreased after EX1 and remained low throughout the experimental protocol. Furthermore, the plasma glucose concentrations at post-EX in CHO were significantly higher compared with the same time points in PLA. Plasma IL-6 concentrations at post-EX2 were significantly higher than pre-EX1 in both trials, but only in PLA was the IL-6 concentration higher at post-EX1 than pre-EX1 (main effect of time: $F_{3, 24} = 18.7$, $P < 0.001$, Figure 3B).

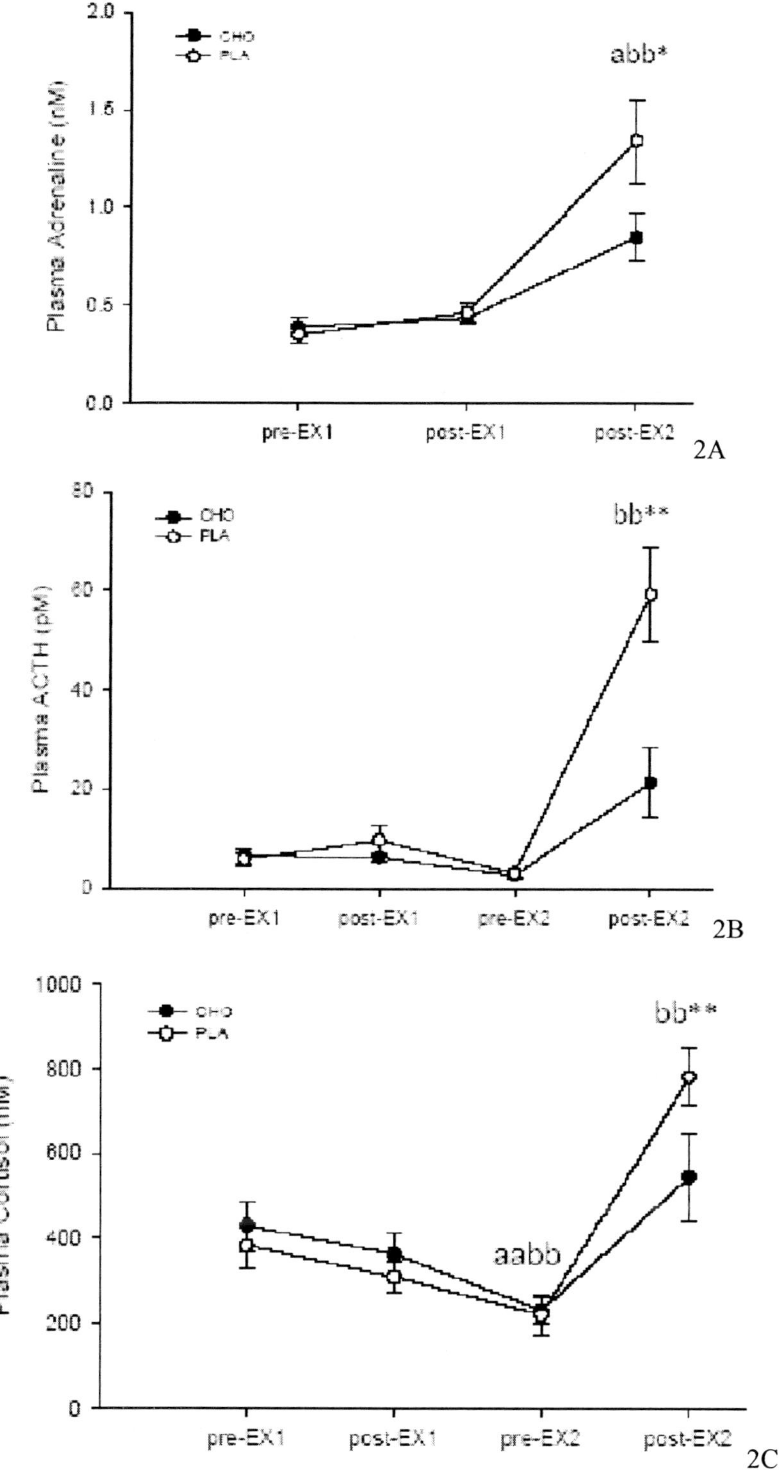

Figure 2. Continued on the next page.

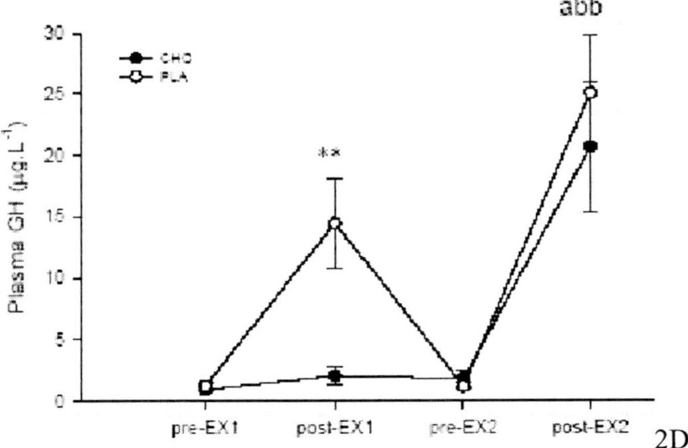

Figure 2. Changes in plasma concentrations of adrenaline (2A), adrenocorticotrophic hormone (2B), cortisol (2C), and growth hormone (2D). Values are means ± SEM (n = 9). Significantly different from pre-EX1 in CHO (^{a} $P < 0.05$, ^{aa} $P < 0.01$) and PLA (^{bb} $P < 0.01$); significantly different between trials (* $P < 0.05$, ** $P < 0.01$).

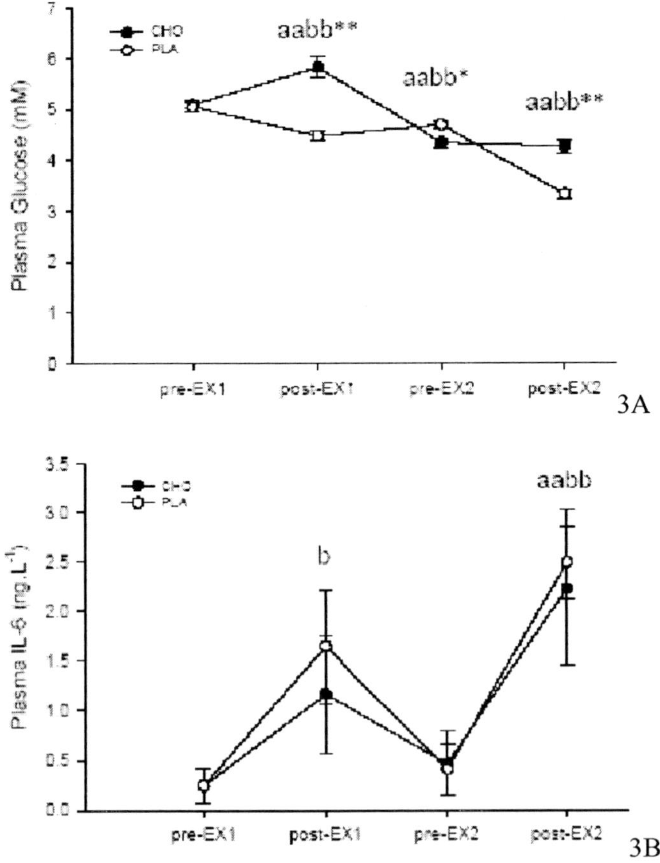

Figure 3. Changes in plasma concentrations of glucose (3A) and plasma interleukin-6 (3B). Values are means ± SEM (n = 9). Significantly different from pre-EX1 in CHO (^{aa} $P < 0.01$) and PLA (^{b} $P < 0.05$, ^{bb} $P < 0.01$); significantly different between trials (* $P < 0.05$, ** $P < 0.01$).

Neutrophil DegranulationResponse to LPS

There was a significant main effect of time ($F_{3, 24} = 25.4$, $P < 0.001$) and an interaction between trial and time ($F_{3, 24} = 4.1$, $P = 0.018$) for total LPS-stimulated elastase release, which was increased with exercise in both trials (Figure 4A). For LPS-stimulated elastase release per neutrophil, there were significant main effects of trial ($F_{1, 8} = 6.2$, $P = 0.038$) and time ($F_{3, 24} = 9.6$, $P = 0.002$), with higher values at pre-EX2 and post-EX2 in CHO compared with the same time points in PLA. In PLA, the values were lower at pre-EX2 and post-EX2 compared with pre-EX1; whereas only the value at post-EX2 was lower than pre-EX1 in CHO (Figure 4B).

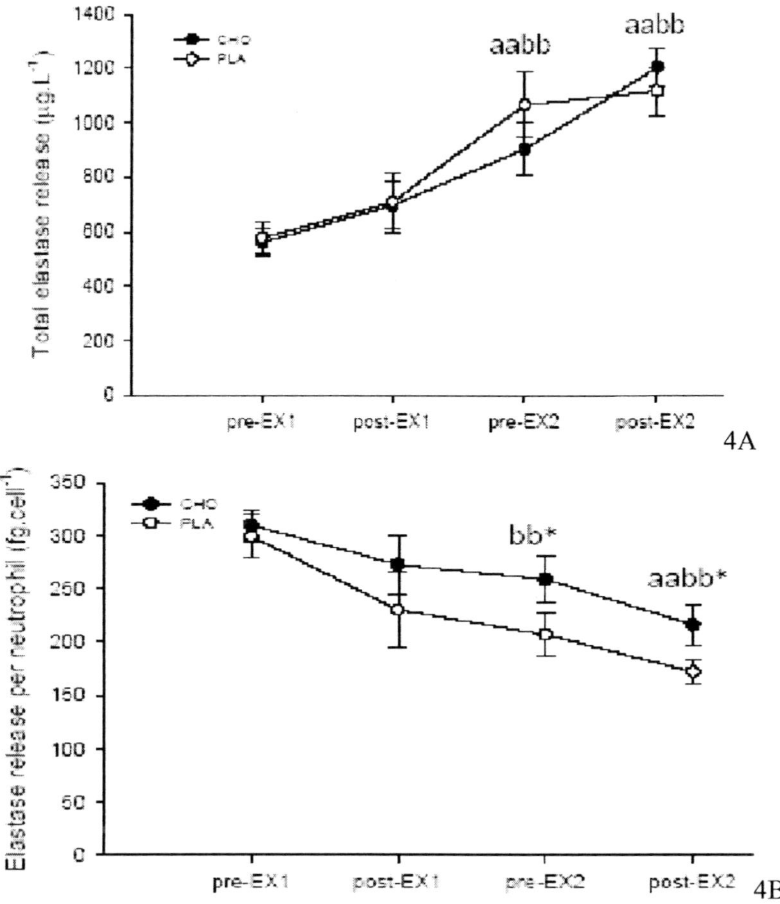

Figure 4. Changes in total LPS-stimulated elastase release (4A) and LPS-stimulated elastase release per neutrophil (4B). Values are means ± SEM (n = 9). Significantly different from pre-EX1 in CHO (^{aa} $P < 0.01$) and PLA (^{bb} $P < 0.01$); significantly different between trials (* $P < 0.05$).

Neutrophil Oxidative Burst Activity

A significant main effect of time was observed for total PMA-induced oxidative burst activity ($F_{3, 24} = 39.0$, $P < 0.001$, Figure 5A), with an increase with exercise in both trials. There were significant main effects of trial ($F_{1, 8} = 8.0$, $P = 0.022$) and time ($F_{3, 24} = 18.8$, $P < 0.001$) and an interaction between trial and time ($F_{3, 24} = 5.1$, $P = 0.007$) for PMA-induced oxidative burst activity per neutrophil (Figure 5B), which showed lower levels at pre-EX2 and post-EX2 in PLA compared with pre-EX1 and the same time points in CHO.

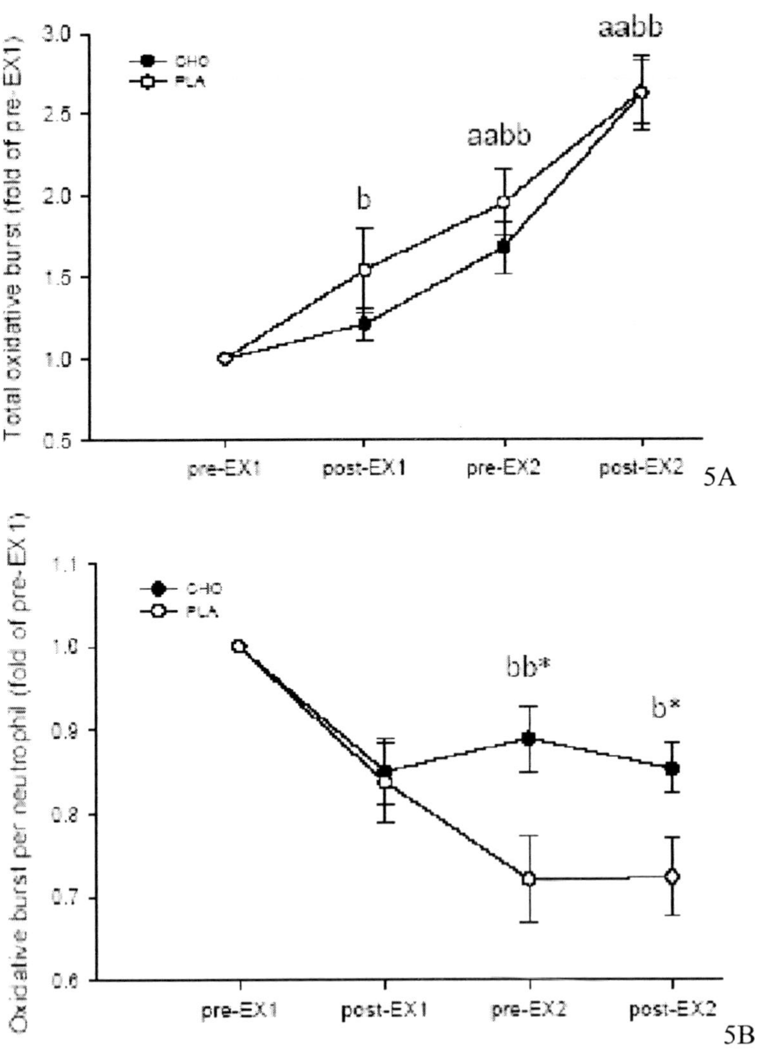

Figure 5. Changes in total PMA-induced oxidative burst (5A) and PMA-induced oxidative burst per neutrophil (5B). Values are means ± SEM (n = 9). Significantly different from pre-EX1 in CHO ($^{aa}P < 0.01$) and PLA ($^{b}P < 0.05$, $^{bb}P < 0.01$); significantly different between trials ($^{*}P < 0.05$).

DISCUSSION

The main findings of the study described in this chapter were that ingestion of CHO compared with PLA during EX1 1) maintained higher plasma glucose concentration throughout the experimental protocol; 2) blunted the responses of plasma adrenaline, ACTH and cortisol during EX2; 3) attenuated the leukocytosis and monocytosis throughout the experimental protocol, neutrophilia during the recovery interval, and lymphocytosis during EX2; 4) lessened the decline in LPS-stimulated degranulation and PMA-induced oxidative burst on per neutrophil basis from 3 h post-EX1 onwards and 5) did not affect plasma IL-6 levels.

In this chapter, ingestion of CHO compared with PLA during EX1 significantly better maintained plasma glucose concentration during EX1 and EX2. Although the amount of glucose (150g) consumed was in excess of the upper limit (~1 $g \cdot min^{-1}$) for glucose absorption during exercise [Jeukendrup and Jentjens, 2000] and might not have been completely absorbed during EX1, it helped to maintain CHO availability during EX2 since a mild hypoglycemia was only observed at post-EX2 in PLA. Plasma glucose concentration at this point was 3.3 ± 0.1 mM, reaching the threshold for evoking adrenaline (3.8 ± 0.1 mM), GH (3.7 ± 0.1 mM) and cortisol (3.2 ± 0.2 mM) secretions [Schwartz *et al.*, 1987]. Therefore, it was not surprising to find higher plasma stress hormone responses in PLA compared with CHO during EX2.

Ingesting a CHO beverage compared with PLA in this chapter attenuated the responses of plasma stress hormones and circulating leukocytes and subsets. These results were similar to previous studies, which indicated that CHO supplementation during prolonged exercise maintains euglycemia and attenuates activation of the hypothalamic-pituitary-adrenal axis, leading to a smaller perturbation of circulating leukocytes and subsets [Bishop *et al.*, 1999; Mitchell *et al.*, 1990; Nieman *et al.*, 1997]. Elevated plasma levels of catecholamines, glucocorticoids and GH during exercise are related to the redistribution (trafficking) of leukocytes [Benschop *et al.*, 1996; Cupps and Fauci, 1982; Kappel *et al.*, 1993] and alteration of neutrophil function [Liles *et al.*, 1995; Ruy *et al.*, 1997; Tintinger *et al.*, 2001]. Plasma adrenaline is likely responsible for the recruitment of lymphocytes and neutrophils into the circulation during 90 min intensive exercise, whereas the later rise of plasma cortisol seems to attenuate adrenaline-induced lymphocytosis and dominate the delayed neutrophilia and lymphopenia that develops in the first few hours after exercise cessation [Nieman, 1997]. Furthermore, GH also appears to mobilise neutrophils into the circulation [Kappel *et al.*, 1993]. The higher number of circulating monocytes after EX1 in PLA compared with CHO may be due to the effects of GH. Although there is no direct evidence to support this suggestion, we did not observe any differences between CHO and PLA in other possible candidates, such as plasma concentrations of adrenaline and cortisol or haemodynamic factors (heart rate). The higher blood counts of total leukocytes, neutrophils, lymphocytes and monocytes during EX2 and the differences between PLA and CHO are most likely attributable to the effect of elevated plasma concentrations of adrenaline and cortisol in the PLA trial.

In this chapter, the responses of LPS-stimulated elastase release per neutrophil during EX1 were similar to previous studies, which reported that during moderate duration exercise (60-90 min) CHO ingestion did not affect neutrophil degranulation on per cell basis [Bishop *et al.*, 2002; Lancaster *et al.*, 2003]. However, a significant decline in LPS-stimulated elastase release per neutrophil was found at pre-EX2 and post-EX2. A delayed blood neutrophilia induced by cortisol generally occurs after 90 min of exercise and lasts for a few hours after exercise cessation [Nieman, 1997]. Nakagawa *et al.* [1998] reported that about 10% of the circulating neutrophilia was derived from the bone marrow after infusion of the synthetic glucocorticoid dexamethasone and that these neutrophils possessed a lower content of granular digestive enzymes compared with fully mature neutrophils [Pyne, 1994]. Recent studies reported that the neutrophil degranulation response to LPS stimulation *in vitro* on per cell basis fell after 2 h cycling at 60% $\dot{V}O_{2\,max}$ [Walsh *et al.*, 2000] and following cycling to fatigue (98 ± 7 min in the CHO trial) at 75% $\dot{V}O_{2\,max}$ [Bishop *et al.*, 2001]. Accordingly, a possible explanation for why the decrease in LPS-stimulated elastase release was not observed until pre-EX2 in this chapter is that there was an influx of relatively immature and less functionally competent neutrophils from the bone marrow during the recovery period after EX1. Regarding the greater decrease in neutrophil degranulation response to LPS on per cell basis in PLA compared with CHO, this may reflect a higher number of less mature neutrophils entering the circulation from the bone marrow under the influence of higher cortisol levels in PLA.

The negative effect of exercise on PMA-induced oxidative burst activity on per neutrophil basis was blunted by CHO ingestion in the present study. Neutrophil oxidative burst is activated through receptor-dependent mechanisms, such as fMLP (N-formyl-Met-Leu-Phe), which are short-lasting (typically less than 5 min), or receptor-independent mechanisms, such as PMA, which can last for a much longer period [reviewed by Chanock *et al.*, 1994; Meenan *et al.*, 2002]. Suzuki *et al.* [1999] showed after 90 min cycling at ~53% $\dot{V}O_{2\,max}$ the PMA-induced CL response of isolated neutrophils was increased. However, a transient suppression of the oxidative burst after exercise has been also reported [Gabriel *et al.*, 1994; Pyne *et al.*, 1996]. Pyne *et al.* [1996] showed that the PMA-induced CL response of isolated neutrophils declined 41% after 40 min running at a heart rate of 140 beat·min^{-1}. However, the CL values did not change further during the 1 h recovery interval or after a second identical bout of running. The results from the PLA trial in this chapter are similar to a recent study [Morozov *et al.*, 2003], which reported that neutrophil oxidative burst activity (zymosan-induced CL) did not change until 3 h after exercise. Previous studies have shown that ingestion of CHO compared with PLA does not affect granulocyte oxidative burst activity (determined by flow cytometry) [Nieman *et al.*, 1997] or PMA-stimulated intracellular H_2O_2 production [Smith *et al.*, 1996] after a single exercise bout. However, the decrease of PMA-induced oxidative burst activity per neutrophil was blunted by CHO ingestion from 3 h after EX1 onwards in this chapter.

Many factors are associated with the regulation of neutrophil oxidative activity. However, the most important factor during exercise may be the extent of neutrophil mobilization. Berkow and Dodson [1986] reported that neutrophils in the bone marrow have lower NADPH-dependent oxidase activity and superoxide response to PMA stimulation compared to those in the circulation. Moreover, the nitro blue tetrazolium (NBT)-negative neutrophils in marginated pools produce less $O_2^{-}\cdot$ in response to *in vitro* stimulation [Suzuki *et al.*, 1996]. Therefore, the greater decline of neutrophil oxidative burst activity per cell in PLA compared with CHO in this chapter may be due to a larger influx of these two types of neutrophils into the circulation in PLA. Another possible cause is the elevated plasma adrenaline concentration, which appears to inhibit neutrophil superoxide production in a dose-related manner [Barnett *et al.*, 1997; Tintinger *et al.*, 2001]. Furthermore, neutrophil ROS producing activity is likely to decline with repeated stimulation [Prasad *et al.*, 1991]. In contrast, many studies have demonstrated that GH primes and stimulates neutrophils to produce O_2^- via Ca^{2+} signalling [Ruy *et al.*, 1997; Smith *et al.*, 1996] or protein kinase C [Fu *et al.*, 1991] pathways. However, this effect may be opposed by increased levels of other hormones that inhibit neutrophil oxidative burst activity. Laboratory techniques may also influence neutrophil oxidative responses. Many studies have measured oxidative burst activity by isolated neutrophils. However, Fukuda and Schmid-Schonbein [2002] suggested that the cell isolation procedures affect the determination of neutrophil functions. For example, neutrophil ROS production consistently increased after 1 min agitation on a test tube shaker at medium speed.

In this chapter, IL-6 levels were not affected by CHO ingestion. IL-6 is a multi-functional cytokine and mediates many physiological functions, such as maintaining glucose homeostasis, stimulating lipolysis [Gleeson, 2000] and inducing a biphasic neutrophilia [Suwa *et al.*, 2001]. However, the post-exercise plasma IL-6 concentration in this study was relatively low (2-3 $ng \cdot L^{-1}$) and may not have exerted significant metabolic effects since the threshold for initiating acute metabolic responses may be as high as 25-65 $ng \cdot L^{-1}$ [Tsigos *et al.*, 1997].

We have serially investigated the effect of CHO supplementation during different periods of two bouts of prolonged exercise in a day on immunoendocrine responses. The results showed that the ingestion of CHO compared with PLA during the recovery interval attenuates activation of the hypothalamic-pituitary-adrenal axis to the second exercise bout to a small extent [Li and Gleeson, 2004]. If CHO is supplemented during the second exercise bout, the responses of sympathetic nervous system and hypothalamic-pituitary-adrenal axis, plasma glucose, circulating leukocytosis and monocytosis during the second exercise bout are blunted compared with PLA (Li, 2004). Moreover, if CHO is ingested during the first of two bouts of prolonged exercise (as described in this chapter), the decline in neutrophil function can be prevented (compared with PLA) during the second exercise bout. It seems that when two bouts of exercise are performed on the same day, the greatest benefit in terms of circulating immunoendocrine responses is obtained by feeding CHO at the earliest opportunity.

In conclusion, ingestion of CHO compared with PLA during the first exercise bout 1) increased carbohydrate availability during both bouts of exercise; 2) had a limited effect on the immunoendocrine response during the first exercise bout, but attenuated plasma stress hormone responses during the second exercise bout and 3) blunted the delayed neutrophilia and concurrent decline in LPS-stimulated degranulation and PMA-induced oxidative burst on per neutrophil basis following the first bout of 90 min cycling at 60% $\dot{V}O_{2\,max}$. The findings of this chapter suggest that carbohydrate availability is an important determinant of immunoendocrine responses to repeated bouts of exercise. If athletes need to perform two bouts of endurance exercise in one day, the greatest benefit in terms of limiting the immunoendocrine responses appears to be obtained by regular ingestion of a CHO-rich drink providing ~ 1-2 g $CHO \cdot min^{-1}$ before and during the first exercise bout.

REFERENCES

Barnett, C. C., Moore, E. E., Partrick, D. A., & Silliman, C. C. (1997). â-Adrenergic stimulation down-regulates neutrophil priming for superoxide generation, but not elastase release. *J.Surg. Res., 70*, 166-170.

Benschop, R. J., Rodriguez-Feuerhahn, M., & Schedlowski, M. (1996). Catecholamine-induced leukocytosis: early observations, current research, and future directions. *Brain Behav. Immun., 10*, 77-91.

Berkow, R. L., & Dodson, R. W. (1986). Purification and functional evaluation of mature neutrophils from human bone marrow. *Blood, 68*(4), 853-860.

Bishop, N. C., Blannin, A. K., Walsh, N. P., & Gleeson, M. (2001). Carbohydrate beverage ingestion and neutrophil degranulation responses following cycling to fatigue at 75% VO_2 max. *Int. J. Sports Med., 22*, 226-231.

Bishop, N. C., Blannin, A. K., Walsh, N. P., Robson, P. J., & Gleeson, M. (1999). Nutritional aspects of immunosuppression in athletes. *Sports Med., 28*(3), 151-176.

Bishop, N. C., Gleeson, M., Nicholas, C. W., & Ali, A. (2002). Influence of carbohydrate supplementation on plasma cytokine and neutrophil degranulation responses to high intensity intermittent exercise. *Int. J. Sport Nutr. Exerc. Metab., 12*, 145-156.

Chanock, S. J., Nenna, J. E., Smith, R. M., & Babior, B. M. (1994). The respiratory burst oxidase. *J. Biol. Chem., 269*(40), 24519-24522.

Cupps, T. R., & Fauci, A. S. (1982). Corticosteroid-mediated immunoregulation in man. *Immunol. Rev., 65*, 133-155.

Dill, D. B., & Costill, D. L. (1974). Calculation of percentage changes in volumes of blood, plasma, and red cells in dehydration. *J. Appl. Physiol., 37*(2), 247-248.

Elsbach, P. (1980). Degradation of microorganisms by phagocytic cells. *Rev. Infect. Dis., 2*, 106-128.

Fu, Y. K., Arkins, S., Wang, B. S., & Kelley, K. W. (1991). A novel role of growth hormone and insulin-like growth factor-I. Priming neutrophils for superoxide anion secretion. *J. Immunol., 146*, 1602-1608.

Fukatsu, K., Sato, N., & Shimizu, H. (1996). 50-mile walking race suppresses neutrophil bactericidal function by inducing increases in cortisol and ketone bodies. *Life Sci., 58*(25), 2337-2343.

Fukuda, S., & Schmid-Schonbein, G. W. (2002). Centrifugation attenuates the fluid shear response of circulating leukocytes. *J. Leukoc.Biol., 72*, 133-139.

Gabriel, H., Muller, H. J., Urhausen, A., & Kindermann, W. (1994). Suppressed PMA-induced oxidative burst and unimpaired phagocytosis of circulating granulocytes one week after a long endurance exercise. *Int. J. Sports Med., 15*, 441-445.

Gleeson, M. (2000). Interleukins and exercise. *J. Physiol., 529*, 1.

Gleeson, M., & Bishop, N. C. (1999). Immunology. In R. J. Maughan (Ed.), *Basic and Applied Sciences for Sports Medicine* (pp. 199-236). Oxiford: Butterworth-Heinemann.

Gleeson, M., & Bishop, N. C. (2000). Special feature for the Olympics: effect of exercise on the immune system: modification of immune responses to exercise by carbohydrate, glutamine and anti-oxidant supplements. *Immunol. Cell Biol., 78*, 554-561.

Gleeson, M., Lancaster, G. I., & Bishop, N. C. (2001). Nutritional strategies to minimise exercise-induced immunosuppresion in athletes. *Can. J. Appl. Physiol., 26*(Suppl.), S23-S35.

Jeukendrup, A. E., & Jentjens, R. L. P. G. (2000). Oxidation of carbohydrate feedings during prolonged exercise. Current thoughts, guidelines and directions for future research. *Sports Med., 29*, 407-424.

Johnson, J. L., Moore, E. E., Tamura, D. Y., Zallen, G., Biffl, W. L., & Silliman, C. C. (1998). Interleukin-6 augments neutrophil cytotoxic potential via selective enhancement of elastase release. *J.Surg. Res., 76*, 91-94.

Kappel, M., Hansen, M. B., Diamant, M., Jorgensen, J. O. L., Gyhrs, A., & Pedersen, B. K. (1993). Effects of an acute bolus growth hormone infusion on the human immune system. *Horm. Metabol. Res., 25*, 579-585.

Lancaster, G. I., Jentjens, R. L. P. G., Moseley, L., Jeukendrup, A. E., & Gleeson, M. (2003). Effect of pre-exercise carbohydrate ingestion on plasma cytokine, stress hormone, and neutrophil degranulation responses to continuous, high intensity exercise. *Int. J. Sport Nutr. Exerc. Metab., 13*, 1-18.

Li, T.-L. (2004). The effect of repeated bouts of prolonged cycling and carbohydrate supplementation on immunoendocrine responses in man. *PhD thesis, Loughborough University.*

Li, T.-L., & Gleeson, M. (2004). The effect of carbohydrate supplementation during the recovery interval on immunoendocrine responses to a repeated bout of prolonged cycling. *Medicina Sportiva*, (Submitted).

Liles, W. C., Dale, D. C., & Klebanoff, S. J. (1995). Glucocorticoids inhibit apoptosis of human neutrophils. *Blood, 86*(8), 3181-3188.

Meenan, B. J., McConnell, J., Knight, J., Boyd, A., & Bell, A. (2002). Development of a sensitive whole blood chemiluminescence method for assessing the bioactivity of calcium phosphate powders. *Biomaterials, 23*, 2431-2445.

Mitchell, J. B., Costill, D. L., Houmard, J. A., Flynn, M. G., Fink, W. J., & Beltz, J. D. (1990). Influence of carbohydrate ingestion on counterregulatory hormones during prolonged exercise. *Int. J. Sports Med., 11*, 33-36.

Morozov, V. I., Pryatkin, S. A., Kalinski, M. I., & Rogozkin, V. A. (2003). Effect of exercise to exhaustion on myeloperoxidase and lysozyme release from blood neutrophils. *Eur. J. Appl. Physiol., 89*, 257-262.

Muns, G. (1994). Effect of long-distance running on polymorphonuclear neutrophil phagocytic function of the upper airways. *Int. J. Sports Med., 15*(2), 96-99.

Nakagawa, M., Terashima, T., D'yachkova, Y., Bondy, G. P., J.C., H., & Van Eeden, S. F. (1998). Glucocorticoid-induced granulocytosis: contribution of marrow release and demargination of intravascular granulocytes. *Circulation, 98*, 2307-2313.

Nieman, D. C. (1994). Exercise, infection, and immunity. *Int. J. Sports Med., 15*, S131-S141.

Nieman, D. C. (1997). Immune response to heavy exertion. *J. Appl. Physiol., 82*(5), 1385-1394.

Nieman, D. C., Fagoaga, O. R., Butterworth, D. E., Warren, B. J., Utter, A., Davis, J. M., Henson, D. A., & Nehlsen-Cannarelia, S. L. (1997). Carbohydrate supplementation affects blood granulocyte and monocyte trafficking but not function after 2.5 h of running. *Am. J. Clin. Nutr., 66*, 153-159.

Pedersen, B. K. (1999). Exercise and Immune Function. In M. Schedlowski & U. Tewes (Eds.), *Psychoneuroimmunology: An interdisciolinary introduction* (pp. 341-358). New York: Kluwer Academic/Plenum Publishers.

Prasad, K., Chaudhary, A. K., & Kalra, J. (1991). Oxygen-derived free radicals producing activity and survival of activated polymorphonuclear leukocytes. *Mol. Cell. Biochem., 103*(1), 51-62.

Pyne, D. B. (1994). Regulation of neutrophil function during exercise. *Sports Med., 17*(4), 245-258.

Pyne, D. B., Baker, M. S., Smith, J. A., & Telford, R. D. (1996). Exercise and the neutrophil oxidative burst: biological and experimental variability. *Eur. J. Appl. Physiol., 74*, 564-571.

Robson, P. J., Blannin, A. K., Walsh, N. P., Castell, L. M., & Gleeson, M. (1999). Effects of exercise intensity, duration and recovery on in vitro neutrophil function in male athletes. *Int. J. Sports Med., 20*, 128-135.

Ronsen, O., Haug, E., Pedersen, B. K., & Bahr, R. (2001a). Increased neuroendocrine response to a repeated bout of endurance exercise. *Med. Sci. Sports Exerc., 33*(4), 568-575.

Ronsen, O., Pedersen, B. K., Oritsland, T. R., Bahr, R., & Kjeldsen-Kragh, J. (2001b). Leukocyte counts and lymphocyte responsiveness associated with repeated bouts of strenuous endurance exercise. *J. Appl. Physiol., 91*, 425-434.

Ruy, H., Jeong, S.-M., Jun, C.-D., Lee, J.-H., Kim, J.-D., Lee, B.-S., & Chung, H.-T. (1997). Involvement of intracellular Ca2+ during growth hormone-induced priming of human neutrophils. *Brain, Behav. Immun., 11*, 39-46.

Schwartz, N. S., Clutter, W. E., Shah, S. D., & Cryer, P. E. (1987). Glycemic thresholds for activation of glucose counterregulatory systems are higher than the threshold for symptoms. *J. Clin. Invest., 79*, 777-781.

Smith, J. A., Gray, A. B., Pyne, D. B., Baker, M. S., Telford, R. D., & Weidemann, M. J. (1996). Moderate exercise triggers both priming and activation of neutrophil subpopulations. *Am. J. Physiol., 270*, R838-R845.

Suwa, T., Hogg, J. C., Klut, M. E., Hards, J., & Van Eeden, S. F. (2001). Interleukin-6 changes deformability of neutrophils and induces their sequestration in the lung. *Am. J. Respir. Crit. Care Med., 163*, 970-976.

Suzuki, K., Sato, H., Kikuchi, T., Abe, T., Nakaji, S., Sugawara, K., Totsuka, M., Sato, K., & Yamaya, K. (1996). Capacity of circulating neutrophils to produce reactive oxygen species after exhaustive exercise. *J. Appl. Physiol., 81*, 1213-1222.

Suzuki, K., Totsuka, M., Nakaji, S., Yamada, M., Kudoh, S., Liu, Q., Sugawara, K., Yamaya, K., & Sato, K. (1999). Endurance exercise causes interaction among stress hormones, cytokines, neutrophil dynamics, and muscle damage. *J. Appl. Physiol., 87*(4), 1360-1367.

Tintinger, G. R., Theron, A. J., Anderson, R., & Ker, J. A. (2001). The anti-inflammatory interactions of epinephrine with human neutrophils in vitro are acheieved by cyclic AMP-mediated accelerated resequestration of cytosolic calcium. *Biochem. Pharmacol., 61*, 1319-1328.

Tsigos, C., Papanicolaou, D. A., Kyrou, I., Defensor, R., Mitsiadis, C. S., & Chrousos, G. P. (1997). Dose-dependent effects of recombinant human interleukin-6 on glucose regulation. *J. Clin. Endocrinol. Metab., 82*(12), 4167-4170.

Walsh, N. P., Blannin, A. K., Bishop, N., Robson, P. J., & Gleeson, M. (2000). Effect of oral glutamine supplementation on human neutrophil lipopolysaccharide-stimulated degranulation following prolonged exercise. *Int. J. Sport Nutr. Exerc. Metab., 10*, 39-50.

In: Trends in Dietary Carbohydrates Research
Editor: M. V. Landlow, pp. 91-108
ISBN 1-59454-798-X

Chapter 5

PHARMACOKINETICS AND ITS RELEVANCE TO DIET

V. K. Katiyar[1] and Somna Mishra[2]

[1] Department of Mathematics, Indian Institute of Technology, Roorkee, Uttaranchal, India
[2] Department of Mathematics and Statistics,
Gurukula Kangri Vishwavidyalaya, Haridwar, Uttaranchal, India
[2]mishra_somna@yahoo.com

ABSTRACT

To understand the effect of a drug and the further response of the body, it is very important to realize what there effects can be and how they can be measured. Therefore a thorough study is usually conducted. Generally it is done by 'in vivo' experiments on animals. These drugs exert different effects and side effects on the body and are measured regularly at different time intervals. After a drug is introduced into a biological system it is subject to a number of processes whose rates control the concentration of drug in that elusive region known as the "site of action", thus affecting its onset,[1] its duration of action and intensity of biological response.

The food taken by human being is called diet. In general terms, an adequate diet is one which permits normal growth, maintenance and reproduction.

INTRODUCTION

To understand the effect of a drug and the further response of the body, it is very important to realize what there effects can be and how they can be measured. Therefore a thorough study is usually conducted. Generally it is done by 'in vivo' experiments on animals. These drugs exert different effects and side effects on the body and are measured regularly at different time intervals.

[1] Onset is defined as the amount of time required to achieving the minimum effective concentration following administration of the dosage form.

After a drug is introduced into a biological system it is subject to a number of processes whose rates control the concentration of drug in that elusive region known as the "site of action", thus affecting its onset,[2] its duration of action and intensity of biological response.

Only a drug that is completely absorbed into the blood stream will have a bio-available dose equal to that stated on the label. In the case of tablets or capsules administered orally, the bio-available dose generally be less than the administered dose. Bioavailability thus deals with the transfer of drug from the site of administration into the body itself. Since a transfer process may be characterized by both the rate of transfer and the total amount transferred. The bio-available dose refers only to the total amount transferred but the complete presentation of bioavailability of a drug must include both the rate and the amount. It can also be defined as a term used to indicate the rate and relative amount of the administered drug, which reaches the general circulation intact.

To express the drug effects more conveniently and to integrate the result obtained due to the kinetics of drug, the use of mathematical model has increased and the study of kinetics is defined as 'Pharmacokinetics'.

Some of the definitions of pharmacokinetics are as follows:

- The action of drugs in the body, including the processes of absorption, transformation, distribution to tissues, duration of action and elimination.
- Pharmacokinetics refers to the study of the metabolism and action of drugs, with particular emphasis on the time required for absorption, duration of action, distribution in body and excretion.
- The process of absorption, distribution, metabolism and excretion of a drug or vaccine.
- Process of the uptake of drugs by the body, the bio-transformation they undergo, the distribution of the drugs and their metabolites in the tissues and the elimination of the drugs and the drugs and their metabolites from the body. Both the amounts and the concentrations of the drugs and their metabolism are studied.
- Distribution of a drug in the body and the rates of biotransformation. Kinetics information includes half-life, absorption, distribution, excretion, metabolism and analysis of body fluid levels.
- This is the science, which describes quantitatively the uptake of drugs by the body, their biotransformation, their distribution, metabolism and elimination from the body.
- Study of the quantitative relationships of the rates of drug absorption, distribution, biotransformation and elimination process, data used to establish dosage and frequency of dosage for desired therapeutic response. Operationally, what the body does to drug.
- The dynamic behavior of chemicals inside biological systems, it includes the processes of uptake, distribution, metabolism and excretion.

From above definitions it is clear that the significance of pharmacokinetics in formulations, dosage form design, control release formulations deciding dosage regimen, clinical practices and therapeutic drug monitoring are of paramount importance.

---

[2] Onset is defined as the amount of time required to achieving the minimum effective concentration following administration of the dosage form.

The drug being chemical entities are handled by the biological systems and the nature and extends of activity depends on their structural features.

Pharmacokinetics is one of the various disciplines of 'Mathematical Biosciences'. It is also called the drug kinetics (or tracer kinetics or multi-compartmental analysis) deals with the distribution of drugs, chemicals, tracers or radioactive substances among the various compartments of the animal body. It is the study of the way; the body deals with the drug.

The animal body can be divided into various compartments, which are equivalent classes from the mathematical point of view. These compartments are defined from the physical properties i.e. localization, physical or electrical states, chemical states etc. these compartments may be real or fictitious spaces for drugs. The examples of the compartments are blood circulatory system, heart tissues, cells etc.

Pharmacokinetics basically deals with the rate processes of a molecule of a drug, which has to undergo on administration in biological systems. As the data of pharmacokinetics origin of bioactive molecules is quantitative in nature, it is readily adoptable to a mathematical model.

Pharmacokinetics concerns the process of the drug in the body, starting with the description of the drug administration, followed by the course of the drug concentration in the blood. Drugs often works on the receptor, so it is required to consider the effect of the drug on such a receptor. Through regular blood tests the concentration of the drug is being determined, starting just after the administration, which occurs in two possible ways: - either the drug is entered as a whole at the same time or by infusion of drug at certain intervals. The drug does not stay in the blood until its elimination. In a more realistic model the function of organs like the liver should be considered as well. Initially when the concentration of the drug in the blood is very high, a part of it is absorbed by the liver, which thus forms another important product of the process. After some time when the concentration of drug in the blood declines, the liver slowly secrets the drug it is containing into the blood until the elimination is complete and the situation of the body reaches to initial state as it was before the administration of the drug.

When a drug is absorbed from the depot, it moves directly into the blood stream. This is simplified version of the dynamic process that the drug undergoes inside the body. When the drug moves from one compartment to another compartment, there are specific rate constants with each transfer process.

Generally these rate constants follow first order kinetics in case of both the reversible and irreversible process. Exceptions will occur in cases where a capacity limited transport system or metabolic route becomes saturated and thus behaves as a zero-order rate process.

We classify the models on the basis of number of compartments:

1. Single compartment models
2. Multi-compartment models

Let us consider a simple example in pharmacology dealing with the dose-response relationship of a drug. Intravenously administered drugs distribute very rapidly throughout the body without an absorption step. For other routes of administration, absorption needs to be considered. When the drug reaches the systemic circulation, it can undergo both elimination and distribution. Elimination can be by metabolism or by excretion. Elimination processes are irreversible and responsible for the removal of the drug from the body. Each of these processes is associated with a rate constant. Rates of these processes govern the plasma drug concentration at any given time.

The rate of change in drug concentration in blood is directly proportional to the concentration remaining to undertake that process.

$$\frac{dC}{dt} = -kC. \tag{1}$$

where k is a proportionality constant known as rate constant and its value can be found experimentally. The negative sign indicates that the instantaneous rate decreases with increase in time.

Integrating equation (1), we get,

$$C(t) = C_0 e^{-kt}. \tag{2}$$

Where C_0 is the concentration when $t = 0$.

There are some other basic terms, which are of great importance in drug kinetics. These are known as pharmacokinetic parameters defined as follows: -

- *Drug Bio-transformation*: - It denotes any alterations in the chemical structure of the drug inside the body.
- *Drug Disposition*: - It is a general term that covers drug distribution, drug biotransformation and drug excretion or elimination.
- *Half-life*: - Half-life ($t_{1/2}$) of a drug is the time required to reduce the drug concentration by half. It is calculated from the equation (2) as follows:

$$C(t) = C_0 e^{-kt}.$$

In this case $C(t) = \frac{C_0}{2}$

$$\frac{C_0}{2} = C_0 e^{-kt_{1/2}}$$

$$\ln \frac{C_0}{2} = \ln C_0 - kt_{1/2}$$

$$t_{1/2} = \frac{0.693}{k}.$$

- *Clearance*: Clearance is an important pharmacokinetic parameter that describes how quickly drugs are eliminated by the body. It depends upon the intrinsic ability of the organs such as the liver and kidneys to metabolize or excrete. The elimination of a drug can be described as

$$\frac{d\chi}{dt} = -Cl.C$$

$$Cl = -\frac{\left(\frac{d\chi}{dt}\right)}{C}.$$

Here $\frac{d\chi}{dt}$ is the rate of elimination and C is the concentration of the drug remaining.

i.e. Cl = elimination rate/ C

elimination rate = $Q(C - C')$.

$$Cl = \frac{Q(C - C')}{C}.$$

Where C = Arterial blood concentration of drug

C' = Venous blood concentration of drug

Q = blood flow rate to the organ

To estimate the clearance, the drug is given intravenously. Clearance cannot be estimated after an oral dose since the total dose does not reach the systemic circulation.

- *Apparent volume of distribution*: The drug distribution is not even throughout the body at equilibrium. Some sites such as central nervous system or brain are weakly accessible to certain drug, whereas some tissues may have strong affinity for the drug. The apparent volume of distribution is not a physiological volume. It should not be regarded as a particular physiological space within the body. It would not be lower than blood or plasma volume but for some drugs it can be much larger than the body volume. The apparent volume of distribution can be defined as

V = Amount of drug in the body/concentration measured in plasma

$$V = \frac{X}{C}.$$

Immediately after the intravenous dose,

$$V = \frac{IVDose}{C(0)}.$$

The parameter V is a measure of protein binding of the drug. When drugs are highly bound to plasma proteins, V is small and results in high plasma concentrations of the drug. When drug binding to plasma proteins or tissues is negligible, V approximates the true volume of distribution, which is related to the amount of body water.

- *Area under the curve(AUC)*:- Estimation of AUC is required to determine some pharmacokinetic parameters. AUC is the area under the plot of drug concentration vs. time and is given by

$$\text{AUC} = \int_0^\infty C dt.$$

AUC can be used as a measure of drug exposure. It is derived from drug concentration and time so it gives a measure how much or how long a drug stays in a body.

- *Area under the first moment curve(AUMC)*:- AUMC is the total area under the first moment curve. First moment curve is obtained by plotting concentration-time vs. time. AUMC can be expressed as

$$\text{AUMC} = \int_0^\infty tC dt.$$

- *Compartmental Analysis*: Compartmental analysis consists of studying the exchanges of matter between the various compartments of the animal body as a function time 't'. It can be considered as a branch of internal dynamics since in compartmental analysis there is transport of matter within the animal body.
  Drugs are injected into one or more of the compartments at time t = 0 or at times t = 0,T,2T,........... or continuously. Some compartments may also be 'leaky' i.e. some part of the drug may leak from the compartment to tissues or cells outside the n-compartments.
- *Fundamental equations for 'n' compartment System*: As we have previously indicated that compartment analysis consists of studying the exchanges of matter between the compartments as a function of time 't'. So some supplementary hypothesis is required to find the mathematical equations, which quantifies the exchange of matter.
  Let there are 'n' compartments in the system, linked in both the directions. Let $\chi_i(t)$ be the amount of the drug in the ith compartment to j^{th} compartment in the time-

interval Δt. By using the concept of mass-balance we get, The change in quantity of drug in any compartment = the amount that enters the compartment – the amount that flows outside the compartment
Thus,

$$\Delta\chi_i = -\sum_{\substack{j=1\\ j\neq 1}}^{n} k_{ij}\chi_i\Delta t + \sum_{\substack{j=1\\ j\neq 1}}^{n} k_{ji}\chi_j\Delta t + o(\Delta t).$$

$$\frac{d\chi_i}{dt} = -\sum_{\substack{j=1\\ j\neq 1}}^{n} k_{ij}\chi_i + \sum_{\substack{j=1\\ j\neq 1}}^{n} k_{ji}\chi_j. \quad (i = 1,2,\ldots\ldots\ldots,n)$$

Here k_{ij} is called the transfer coefficient from i^{th} to j^{th} compartment and the zeroth compartment denotes the compartment outside the system.

Defining $$k_{ii} = -\sum_{\substack{j=1\\ j\neq 1}}^{n} k_{ij}$$

we obtain

$$\frac{d\chi_i}{dt} = \sum_{j=1}^{n} k_{ji}\chi_j. \quad (i = 1,2,\ldots\ldots,n)$$

with the initial condition $\chi_i(0) = d_i$ which is known.
It is the linear system in $\chi_i(t)$ which can be easily solved using the coefficient k_{ij} and d_i, where k_{ij} can be estimated using the experimental data.
On the other hand,
If we consider that the flow of drug from compartment i to compartment j is proportional to the product of amounts in both the compartment then we have,

$$\frac{d\chi_i}{dt} = -\sum_{\substack{i=1\\ j\neq i}}^{n} k_{ij}\chi_i\chi_j + \sum_{\substack{i=1\\ j\neq i}}^{n} k_{ji}\chi_i\chi_j. \quad (i = 1,2,\ldots\ldots\ldots,n)$$

Where $\chi_i(0) = d_i$
This is a non-linear differential system.

Single Compartment System

Intra-venous Administration

The one compartment model is the simplest and it represents the body as a single unit.

According to this model, after an IV administration the drug is eliminated by first-order kinetics. Drug concentration in blood can be expressed by equation (2). All the pharmacokinetic parameters are same as described before.

Now we consider a case where the doses of C_0 of the drug are given at equal time intervals T.

Immediately after first dose the concentration is C_0. Thus using equation (2), the concentration of drug left from the first dose after time T is $C_0 e^{-kT}$.

$$C_1 = C_0 e^{-kT} \tag{3}$$

Immediately after the second dose of C_0, the concentration will be

$$C_2 = C_0 + C_0 e^{-kT} \tag{4}$$

Immediately after third dose

$$C_3 = C_0 + \left(C_0 + C_0 e^{-kT}\right)e^{-kT} = C_0 + C_0 e^{-kT} + C_0 e^{-2kT} \tag{5}$$

Thus immediately after the nth dose,

$$C_n = C_0 + C_0 e^{-kT} + C_0 e^{-2kT} + \ldots\ldots\ldots\ldots + C_0 e^{-(n-1)kT}$$

$$= C_0\left(1 + e^{-kT} + e^{-2kT} + \ldots\ldots\ldots\ldots + e^{-(n-1)kT}\right) = C_0 \frac{1 - e^{-nkT}}{1 - e^{-kT}}.$$

When $n \longrightarrow \infty$

$$C_\infty = \frac{C_0}{1 - e^{-kt}}. \tag{6}$$

Thus it is clear that after a long run, the concentration reaches to a limiting value.

Extra-venous Administration

Administration of a drug by all routes other than IV route will involve an absorption step. When a drug is put into a depot, such as the stomach, intestines or muscle, it usually absorbed by a first-order process. The change in blood drug concentration will now be a function of both the absorption rate and elimination rate.

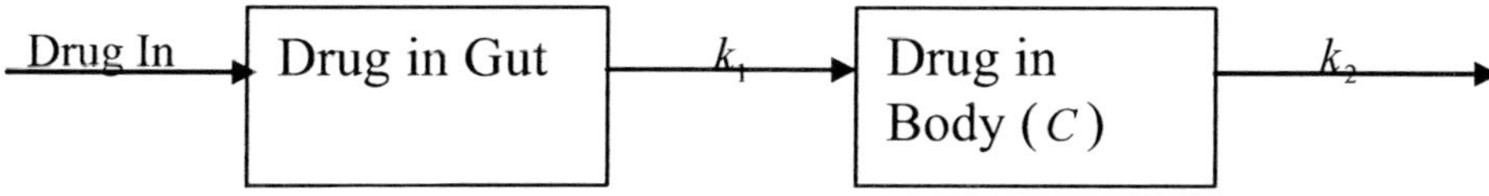

The concentration of drug in blood is given by

$$C(t) = \frac{k_1 FD\left(e^{-k_2 t} - e^{-k_1 t}\right)}{V(k_1 - k_2)}.$$

where F is the fraction of the administration dose D, which is absorbed after extra vascular administration. k_1 is the absorption rate constant and k_2 is the elimination rate constant.

METABOLISM AND EXCRETION IN ONE COMPARTMENT MODEL

Let the rate constant E_A represent the overall first-order elimination constant for loss of drug from the body by all routes i.e. if drug is eliminated by urinary excretion and metabolism, the one-compartment model become as

M $\xrightarrow{E_m}$ Blood and Tissues $\xrightarrow{E_e}$ U

Where E_m and E_e are first order rate constants for metabolism and excretion respectively.

Thus E_A can be expressed as

$$E_A = E_m + E_e$$

The individual rate constants can be calculated by knowing the fraction of dose recovered as metabolite or intact drug when the dose χ (t) becomes zero,

$$E_m = \frac{E_A M_\infty}{\chi(0)} \text{ and } E_e = \frac{E_A U_\infty}{\chi(0)}.$$

Two Compartment Model

The two Compartment model can be described as in the following figure:

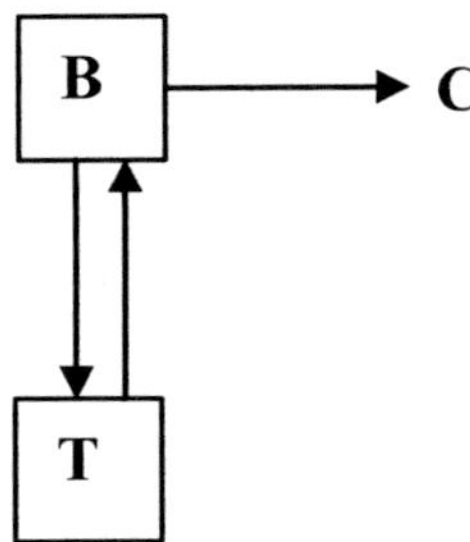

The Central Compartment, which is composed of blood and well-perfused tissue is represented by B and the tissue of the rest of the body by T. All the drug removed from the body, regardless of the route of elimination, represented by the Compartment C. The kinetics of glucose in two Compartments system can be better understand by the following example.

Mathematical Model for the Kinetics of Anti-Cancer Drugs

Cancerous tumors left unchecked, will increase in size until they ultimately kill the patient. One approach to cancer treatment is the delivery of chemotherapeutic agents designed to eradicate cancer cells. As the use of anti-cancer drugs increased rapidly over the past two decades, it became clear that a localized and quantative method of predicting drug concentrations in the various parts of the human body was necessary to provide the optimal dosing schedule for cancer chemotherapy treatment. The selection of drug doses and delivery schedules is a challenging process.

In contrast to most drugs that have high or moderate therapeutic indices, most of the antineoplastic drugs are very toxic and have a low therapeutic index, which requires that the concentrations of the drug be known accurately in both tumor and normal tissue to minimize tissue damage and maximize tumor kill. Through the use of mathematical models, a more systematic approach to drug treatment regimen development is possible.

There are two main approaches, which are used in cancer chemotherapy. The first one describes the tumor growth on macroscopic scale defining the number of cells and tumor dependent parameters.

As we know that the compartment modeling of the kinetics of a drug can be used to provide a mathematical description of the stability of drug and delivery to a specified target. For this motto a compartmental model for the anti-cancer agent topotecan (TPT) is proposed by N.D. Evans et al., which is based on underlying biological assumption and the model parameters estimated using HPLC (High Performance Liquid Chromatography) data.

The active molecule of TPT is capable of DNA binding. In aqueous media, the active form of TPT is not stable at pH and thus a reversible hydrolysis from a closed ring parent lactone form (TPT-L) to an open ringed hydroxy acid form (TPT-H). The inactivation of TPT-L and the activation of TPT-H forms the basic building block for the full cell model. The reversible hydrolysis of TPT-L can be modeled using a simple two- compartment model: -

Let $L(t)$ is the concentration of the active form of the drug (TPT-L) at time 't' after an initial dose and $H(t)$ denotes the concentration of TPT-H, which is the inactive form.

Then

$$\frac{dL(t)}{dt} = -k_0 L(t) + k_c H(t).$$

$$\frac{dH(t)}{dt} = k_0 L(t) - k_c H(t).$$

Where k_0 is the first order rate constant of inactivation of TPT-L to TPT-H and k_c is the first order rate constant by which TPT-H becomes activated to give TPT-L. The initial conditions for above two equations at time t = 0 are given by $L(0) = d$ and $H(0) = 0$, where d is the concentration of TPT administered as a single bolus input of active drug.

THREE COMPARTMENT MODEL

Consider a special case for the metabolism of glucose. There are 3 compartments in the model.

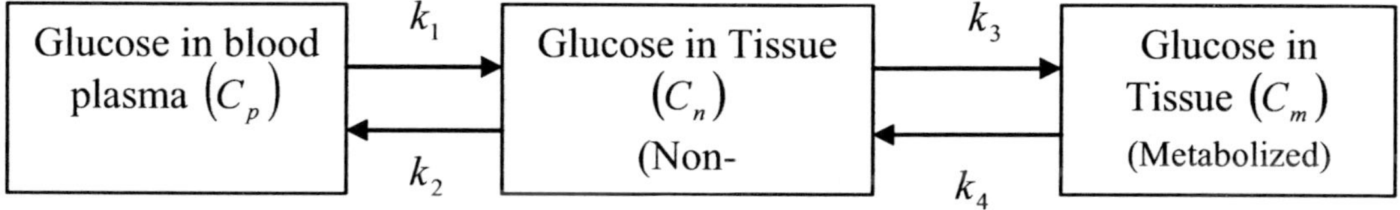

Compartment 1 is identified as blood plasma. Compartment 2 represents the organs where glucose remains un-metabolized (i.e. heart) and Compartment 3 represent the organs where glucose metabolism takes place (i.e. muscle and adipose tissues).

These 3 Compartments are referred to as 1,2 and 3 respectively and k_1 to k_4 represents the rate of movement from one Compartment to another.

Let $C_p(t)$ denotes the concentration of glucose in blood plasma, $C_n(t)$ denotes the concentration of non-metabolized glucose in tissue (i.e. the tissue of brain or nervous system that are weakly accessible to a certain drug) and $C_m(t)$ denotes the concentration of metabolized glucose in the tissues (such as the tissue of liver and intestine etc.) and $C_i(t)$ is the total concentration of glucose in tissue.

Then

$$C_i(t) = C_n(t) + C_m(t). \tag{7}$$

$$\frac{dC_i(t)}{dt} = \frac{dC_n(t)}{dt} + \frac{dC_m(t)}{dt}. \tag{8}$$

By the law of mass action, between plasma Compartment and non-metabolized Compartment and between non-metabolized Compartment and metabolized Compartment.

$$\frac{dC_n(t)}{dt} = k_1 C_p(t) - k_2 C_n(t) - k_3 C_n(t) + k_4 C_m(t).$$

$$\frac{dC_n(t)}{dt} = k_1 C_p(t) - (k_2 + k_3) C_n(t) + k_4 C_m(t). \tag{9}$$

and

$$\frac{dC_m(t)}{dt} = k_3 C_n(t) - k_4 C_m(t). \tag{10}$$

On solving these equations, we get

$$C_n(t) = \frac{k_1 C_p}{\gamma_2 - \gamma_1}\left[(k_4 - \gamma_1)e^{-\gamma_1 t} + (\gamma_2 - k_4)e^{-\gamma_2 t}\right].$$

$$C_m(t) = \frac{k_1 k_4 C_p}{\gamma_2 - \gamma_1}\left(e^{-\gamma_2 t} - e^{-\gamma_1 t}\right).$$

Where γ_1 and γ_2 are the cigen values.

DIET

The food taken by human being is called diet. In general terms, an adequate diet is one which permits normal growth, maintenance and reproduction. The following points should be taken into account while estimating adequate diet for an individual:

Essential Constituents of Diet

Normal diet must contain the following items:

(1) Proteins
(2) Fats
(3) Carbohydrates
(4) Vitamins
(5) Minerals
(6) Water and
(7) Roughage

The first three are for energy production, growth and maintenance of tissue, and the last four are essential for chemical mechanism, i.e. for the utilization of energy, synthesis of various necessary metabolites viz. enzymes, hormones etc.

Quantity of Food

Energy for physiological processes is provided by the combination of carbohydrates, fats and proteins. The daily energy requirement or the daily calorific need is the sum of the basal energy demands plus that required for the additional work of the day. The quantity of food will be proportional to the total energy requirement of the individual. The total energy requirement can be calculated from the following data:

a) *B.M.R. (basal Metabolic Rate):* B.M.R. can be determined from the surface area. On the whole, an average adult male has a surface area of 1.8 sq. meters and a B.M.R. of about 72 C per hour or 40 C per sq. meter of body surface.
b) *Nature of work done by the individual:* Work involves expenditure of energy, over and above the basal metabolic rate. The following is a rough estimate:
   i. Sedentary Work: - Without any muscular effort (such as the brain workers) : 20-25% (about 400 C)
   ii. Light work: - 30-40% (about 700 C)
   iii. Moderate Exercise: - 50-60% (about 1000 C)
   iv. Heavy work: - 100% (about 200 C)
   v. The total energy requirement will be B.M.R. plus these figures.
c) *Allowance for growth:* Infants, growing children, pregnant women, lactating mothers, athletes and convalescent patients require at least 50% more food over and above their actual B.M.R. This additional amount is necessary to provide for active growth.
d) During waking hours ingestion of food stimulates metabolism by 5-10%.

The basal calorie requirement of an individual is 40 calorie per sq. meter per hour. Thus in an average adult male, having a surface area of 1.8 sq. meter, the total energy requirement during 24 hour period may be obtained as follows:

8 hours' sleep = $(40^{*}1.8)^{*}8 = 576$ C

8 hours' awake = basal + 30% (i.e. 10% for stimulating action of food + 20% for minor activities etc.) = 576 C + 174 C = 750 C

8 hours' moderate work = basal + 1000 C = 1576 C

Total = (576+750+1576) = 2902 C $\approx$ 3000 C

To provide for the 10% loss in faulty absorption, the calorie required is about 300 C more, i.e. total 3300 C.

Thus, the average calorific requirement of a man doing light work is 3000 C net or 3300 C. The average housewife needs about 10% less (i.e. 2700 C net), lady doing more active work has the same requirement as the average male. Man doing hard work should receive up to 4000 C. The requirements of children are suggested to be as follows:

Age in Years	1-2	2-3	3-6	6-8	8-10	10-12	12-14
Calories	1000	1250	1550	1850	2150	2550	2900

Distribution of Calories in the Diet

Protein Requirement

The proteins are highly complex organic compounds made up of Carbon, Hydrogen, Oxygen and Nitrogen. A minimal amount of protein is dispensable in the diet to provide for the replacement of tissue proteins which undergo wear and tear. If the protein content of diet is in excess, the remainder is utilized to produce energy. The requirement of protein is not only quantitative but also qualitative, since metabolic aspect of protein is intimately connected with its amino acid composition. The essential amino acids must be supplied in the dietary protein, which is the basis of the qualitative aspect of protein material. For adults the adequate maintenance dose is 1 gm of protein per Kg of body weight per day. For infants and growing children 3-4 gm of proteins per Kg of body weight per day; for school boys and girls, pregnancy, lactation etc.; 2-3 gm per Kg of body weight per day.

Fat Requirement

Fats are esters of long chain fatty acids and an alcohol called glycerol. The fats are made up of the same three elements, carbon, hydrogen, and oxygen, of which the carbohydrates are made. The difference lies in the fact that fats contain less proportion of oxygen as compared to carbohydrates. Fats are esters. Every fat molecule consists of three molecules of a fatty acids and one molecule of glycerol.

$$\begin{array}{l} CH_2 \; \boxed{OH \quad H} \; OOC\text{-}F \\ | \\ CH_2 \; \boxed{OH \quad H} \; OOC\text{-}F \\ | \\ CH_2 \; \boxed{OH \quad H} \; OOC\text{-}F \end{array} \longrightarrow \begin{array}{l} CH_2OOC\text{-}F \\ | \\ CH_2OOC\text{-}F \\ | \\ CH_2OOC\text{-}F \end{array} + 3H_2O$$

Glycerol Fatty acids Mixed triglyceride

Fat produces high energy and serves as a vehicle for the fat-soluble vitamins A, D, E, and K. It also contains essential fatty acids, i.e. linoleic acid ($C_{17}H_{31}COOH$), linolenic acid ($C_{17}H_{29}COOH$). Out of the total energy requirement 20-30% should come from fats of the diet. The daily intake of fat should be between 50-100 gm per day.

Essential Fatty Acids

Our body requires a large number of fatty acids. Most of the fatty acids that are needed by our body can be prepared from carbohydrates present in our body by the body cells. Those fatty acids, which can be prepared within the body from carbohydrates, are called non-essential fatty acids. Some of the fatty acids, however, cannot be synthesized by our body cells. Those fatty acids, which cannot be synthesized within our body from carbohydrates, are called essential fatty acids. The essential fatty acids have to be supplied by the food that we eat. Essential fatty acids are present in almost all plant foods and all vegetable oils. Thus, any normal diet can provide all the essential fatty acids to our body.

Carbohydrate Requirement

Carbohydrates are the compounds made up of three elements: carbon, hydrogen and oxygen, the proportion of hydrogen and oxygen being the same as in water. Glucose ($C_6H_{12}O_6$), Sucrose ($C_{12}H_{22}O_{11}$) and Starch ($(C_6H_{10}O_5)_n$, where 'n' is a big number, are examples of Carbohydrates. Carbohydrates are the main source of energy in our body. They produce energy when they are oxidized in the body. 1 gm of Carbohydrate produces about 17 K Joules of energy and about 60-80% of the total energy contained in our diet comes from Carbohydrate present in it. For a normal person, about 400 to 500 gm of Carbohydrate required daily.

Types of Carbohydrates in food: - There are three types of carbohydrates in the foods that we eat. These are Cellulose, Starch and Sugar. Out of these cellulose is not digested by our body because our body does not have enzymes for digesting cellulose. Thus, cellulose does not provide energy to the human body and hence it is not a food. Cellulose acts as a fiber or roughage in our food. Starch and sugars are the two carbohydrates, which provide most of the energy to our body. During the process of digestion, starch and sugars get hydrolysed to glucose. Glucose so produced is absorbed by the blood and transported to various body cells. During respiration, most of the glucose is oxidized to produce energy necessary for doing work and carrying out body processes. This can be represented as:

$$C_6H_{12}O_6 + 6O_2 \longrightarrow 6CO_2 + 6H_2O + \text{Energy}$$

Glucose

Balanced Diet for Adult Man*

Dietary articles	Sedentary work		Moderate work		Heavy work	
	Vegetarian (gm)	Non-vegetarian(gm)	Vegetarian (gm)	Non-vegetarian (gm)	Vegetarian (gm)	Non-vegetarian (gm)
Cereals	400	400	475	475	650	650
Pulses	70	55	80	65	80	65
Green leafy Veg.	100	100	125	125	125	125
Other Veg.	75	75	75	75	100	100
Roots and tubers	75	75	100	100	100	100
Fruits	30	30	30	30	30	30
Milk	300	100	300	100	300	100
Sugar	30	30	40	40	55	55
Fats & oils	40	35	45	40	--	60

Balanced Diet for Adult Woman*

Dietary articles	Sedentary work		Moderate work		Heavy work		Additional allowance	
	Vegetarian (gm)	Non-vegetarian (gm)	Vegetarian (gm)	Non-vegetarian (gm)	Vegetarian (gm)	Non-vegetarian (gm)	Pregnancy (gm)	Lactation (gm)
Cereals	300	300	350	350	475	475	50	100
Pulses	60	45	70	55	70	55	--	10
Green leafy veg.	125	125	125	125	125	125	25	25
Other veg.	75	75	75	75	100	100	--	--
Roots & tubers	50	50	75	75	100	100	--	--
Fruits	30	30	30	30	30	30	--	--
Milk	200	100	200	100	200	100	125	125
Sugar	30	30	30	30	40	40	10	20
Fats & oils	35	30	40	35	50	45	--	--

Balanced Diet for Children*

Dietary articles	Pre-School children				School children			
	1-3 years		4-6 years		7-9 years		10-12 years	
	Veg.	Non-veg.	Veg.	Non-veg.	Veg.	Non-veg.	Veg.	Non-veg.
Cereals	150	150	200	200	250	250	320	320
Pulses	50	40	60	50	70	60	70	60
Green-leafy veg.	50	50	75	75	75	75	100	100
Other veg. / Roots & tubers	30	30	50	50	50	50	75	75
Fruits	50	50	50	50	60	60	60	60
Milk	500	200	400	200	500	200	400	200
Sugar	30	30	40	40	50	50	50	50
Fats & oils	20	20	25	25	30	30	35	35

Balanced Diet for Adolescent Boys and Girls*

Dietary articles	Boys				Girls	
	13-15 years		16-18 years		13-18 years	
	Veg.	Non-veg.	Veg.	Non-veg.	Veg.	Non-veg.
Cereals	430	430	450	450	350	350
Pulses	70	50	70	50	70	50
Green-leafy veg.	100	100	100	100	150	150
Other veg.	75	75	75	75	75	75
Roots & tubers	75	75	100	100	75	75
Fruits	30	30	30	30	30	30
Milk	500	200	400	150	400	150
Sugar	30	30	40	40	30	30
Fats & oils	35	40	45	50	35	40

* Adapted from Tables on Balanced diet as given the Report of the Nutrition Expert Group, Indian Council of Medical Research.

REFERENCES

[1] Neil d. Evans, R.J. Errington, M.Shelley, G.P. Feency, M.J. Chapman, K.R. Godfrey, P.J. smith, M.J. Chappell, A Mathematical Model for the in vitro kinetics of the anti-cancer agent topotecan, *Math. Biosci.* 189(2004) 185-217.

[2] Robert S. Parker, Francis J. Doyle III, Control-relevant Modelling in drug delivery, *Advanced drug delivery reviews* 48(2001) 211-228.

[3] Y. Cherruault, *Mathematical Modelling in Biomedicine*, D. Reidel Publishing Co., Holland, 1986.

[4] J.N. Kapur, *Mathematical Models in Biology and Medicine*, East-west Press, N. Delhi (2000) 316-339.

[5] C.C. Chatterjee, *Human Physiology*, Medical allied Agency, vol. 1(1994).

[6] L. Singh, M. Kaur, *Biology*, S.Chand & Co. Ltd.(1996).

[7] Vakalis I., *Pharmacokinetics: Mathematical Analysis of Drug Distribution in living organism* (2004).

[8] Haag J.D., *Time of peak response in turn over models in Pharmacokinetics and Pharmacodynamics* (2003).

In: Trends in Dietary Carbohydrates Research
Editor: M. V. Landlow, pp. 109-139
ISBN 1-59454-798-X

Chapter 6

CARBOHYDRATE EFFECTS ON THE EFFICIENCY OF UTILIZATION OF RUMINAL AMMONIA NITROGEN FOR MILK PROTEIN SYNTHESIS IN DAIRY COWS

Alexander N. Hristov•
Department of Animal and Veterinary Science, University of Idaho, Moscow, ID, USA

ABSTRACT

Ammonia is a major source of N for microbial protein synthesis in the rumen and consequently, milk protein synthesis in lactating ruminants. Effect of carbohydrate (CHO) type on ruminal fermentation, microbial protein synthesis, and the efficiency of utilization of ruminal ammonia nitrogen (N) for milk protein synthesis were studied in two in vivo experiments with lactating dairy cows. Ammonia N was labeled with ^{15}N through continuous intraruminal infusion (Exp. 1) or pulse dosing (Exp. 2) of a 20 at. % exc. $(^{15}NH_4)_2SO_4$. Recovery of ^{15}N in milk protein was determined gravimetrically. The experiments involved four ruminally and duodenally cannulated, mid- to late-lactation Holstein dairy cows. Experimental designs were cross-over (Exp. 1), or Latin square (Exp. 2). In Exp. 1 treatments were ruminally fermentable starch and sugars (RFSS; barley and molasses) vs. ruminally fermentable neutral detergent fiber (RFNDF; corn, beet pulp, and brewers grains). In Exp. 2, treatments were corn dextrose (GLU), corn starch (STA), fiber (control; NDF, white oat fiber), and a CHO mix (25% of each, apple pectin, GLU, STA, and NDF; PEC).

Ruminal ammonia concentration was lowered by RFNDF in Exp. 1. There was no effect of diet on ruminal pH, volatile fatty acid (VFA) concentrations, or microbial protein flow to the duodenum. The proportion of milk protein N originating from ruminal microbial N was greater for RFNDF than for RFSS. Cumulative recovery of ^{15}N in milk protein was 13% greater for RFNDF than for RFSS. In Exp. 2, ruminal pH was decreased by GLU, STA, and MIX compared with NDF. Concentration of ammonia in ruminal fluid and ammonia N pool size were decreased by GLU and STA. Acetate, *iso*-butyrate,

• Correspondence: A. Hristov, Department of Animal and Veterinary Science, University of Idaho, P.O. Box 442330, Moscow, ID 83844-2330 Phone: (208) 885-7204; FAX (208) 885-6420; email: ahristov@uidaho.edu

iso-valerate, and total VFA concentration in the rumen were also decreased, and butyrate was increased by GLU compared with the other CHO. Microbial N flow to the duodenum was lower for NDF than for the other CHO. Flow of microbial N formed from ammonia was greater for STA compared with GLU and NDF. The proportion of bacterial N synthesized from ammonia in the rumen was greater with STA than with NDF and MIX and was the lowest for GLU. Irreversible ammonia loss and flux were also lowered by GLU compared with STA and NDF. As percent of the dose given, cumulative secretion of ^{15}N ammonia in milk protein was greater for STA than for GLU or NDF.

Data from these two experiments indicate that diets differing in concentration of ruminally available starch and sugars and fiber produced similar level and pattern of fermentation acids and did not affect microbial protein synthesis in the rumen. Increased concentration of ruminally available starch and sugars enhanced ^{15}N-ammonia capture by ruminal bacteria, but overall transfer of ^{15}N-ammonia into milk protein was greater when cows were fed the ruminally fermentable fiber diet. The provision of readily fermentable energy as dextrose or starch in Exp. 2 decreased ammonia levels in the rumen through inhibited production of ammonia and enhanced incorporation of preformed feed amino acids, or through enhanced uptake of ammonia for microbial protein synthesis. Rapidly fermentable in the rumen energy decreases ammonia production, flux, and may decrease ammonia nitrogen cycling, but the overall efficiency of ammonia utilization for milk protein synthesis can be only increased by enhancing ruminal microbial ammonia uptake.

INTRODUCTION

The Rumen Ecosystem

The largest compartment of the complex stomach of the ruminant animal, the reticulo-rumen (the term rumen will be used in this chapter for simplicity), can be characterized as a continuous-culture fermentor designed to facilitate microbial breakdown of feed polysaccharides and the production of microbial protein and volatile fatty acids (VFA). A myriad of microorganisms inhabit the rumen and proliferate in a symbiotic relationship with the host animal. Among these microorganisms, bacteria, protozoa, and fungi are most numerous and important for the fermentation process and the host. As in any fermentor, pH, nutrients, temperature, agitation, and oxygen level are controlled to provide optimal conditions for the so-called primary reactions, i.e. the breakdown of structural and storage plant polysaccharides. Millennia of evolution have produced a unique grassing and chewing sequence designed to enhance microbial access, increase digestion surface, buffer the fermentation media, and mix substrates and microbial consortia. Plant celluloses, hemicelluloses, starches, pectins, fructosans, and other minor polysaccharides are hydrolyzed to simple sugars, which are fermented to various intermediate products and eventually to three major short-chain VFA (acetate, propionate, and butyrate), CO_2, and methane. The carbon in gasses is mostly lost to the host, but VFA are absorbed and utilized by the animal as a source for body or milk fatty acids synthesis, or as an energy source, providing up to 80% of the metabolizable energy.

Breakdown of Feed Proteins in the Rumen

Feed nitrogenous compounds undergo significant transformation in the rumen. Proteins are broken down to peptides and amino acids and amino acids are further deaminated to ammonia (NH_3) and carbon skeletons. Ammonia and pre-formed amino acids are used by the ruminal microorganisms for synthesis of cell proteins. Microbial proteins synthesized in the rumen are a major source of amino acids for synthesis of muscle and milk proteins by the host animal, contributing up to 70 to 80% of the total non-NH_3 nitrogen (N) available for absorption in the small intestine. The extensive microbial breakdown of feed proteins and deamination represent a major challenge to ruminant nutritionists; NH_3 produced in excess is absorbed through the rumen wall, mostly metabolised into urea by the liver and excreted in urine. Some of the blood plasma urea N can be recycled to the rumen through saliva and the rumen mucosa if NH_3 is needed for microbial growth and dietary N supply is low. The main form of N in urine is urea, representing from 60 to 94% of the total urinary N in cattle (Bristow et al., 1992). If mixed with feces, urea is quickly converted into NH_3 by the abundant urease activity present in fecal matter. Emitted in the atmosphere, NH_3 can be converted to ammonium aerosol and removed by dry or wet deposition. Once removed from the atmosphere, NH_3 or ammonium contribute to ecosystem fertilization, acidification, eutrophication, and can impact visibility, soil acidity, forest productivity, terrestrial ecosystem biodiversity, stream acidity, coastal productivity (Galloway and Cowling, 2002), and human health through formation of fine ($PM_{2.5}$) particulate matter (McCubbin, 2002). If not volatilized, NH_3 applied to cropland is relatively quickly oxidized to nitrate. Nitrate is completely soluble and, if in excess of crop requirements, can penetrate beyond the root zone and contaminate groundwater aquifer (Miner et al., 2000). Therefore, a better control of ruminal N, particularly NH_3, metabolism is an obvious way to achieve an improvement in the efficiency of N utilization in ruminants and to limit the excretion of nitrogenous compounds causing environmental pollution around animal production areas.

Protein Effects on Ammonia Utilization in the Rumen and Nitrogen Losses

Ammonia is a major source of N for the ruminal bacteria, particularly cellulolytics (Russell et al., 1992). Ruminal bacteria form from 38% (Table 6) to 70-80% (Mathison and Milligan, 1971; Leng and Nolan, 1984; Oldham et al., 1980; Hristov and Broderick, 1996; Koenig et al., 2000) of their N from NH_3 N and adequate NH_3 level is the first recommendation for optimization of microbial protein synthesis (MPS) in the rumen. As proportion of N intake, the irreversible loss of N from the NH_3 N pool can be as low as 23% (Table 6) or as high as 88% (Oldham et al., 1980). The relatively low efficiency of utilization of dietary N for milk protein synthesis in the dairy cow (Tamminga, 1992; MacRae et al., 1995) is due in large part to the wasteful process of intra-ruminal N cycling. Tamminga (1992) estimated that up to 50% of the dietary N is lost to the dairy cow through urinary N excretion. Of this 50%, approximately 30% is lost due to inefficient N metabolism in the rumen. Therefore, the efficiency of NH_3 utilization in the rumen is a central factor determining the economic cost and environmental impact of ruminant production. As ruminal NH_3 levels correlate positively ($r = 0.57$) with the concentration of milk urea N (MUN) in dairy cows (Broderick and Clayton, 1997) and increased NH_3 levels in the intestine have resulted in increased non-protein N content of milk (Moorby and Theobald, 1999), improving the utilization of NH_3 N in the rumen has the potential of reducing MUN content and consequently enhancing the processing quality of milk (Bachmann and Jans, 1995; Martin et al., 1997).

Ruminal NH_3 concentration is a function of both, rate of ruminal degradability and concentration of ruminally degradable dietary protein (RDP) over microbial needs and dietary energy available to the ruminal microorganisms. The effect of dietary crude protein (CP), excess RDP, and ruminally undegradable protein (RUP) supplementation on ruminal fermentation and production, particularly in dairy cows, has been covered extensively in the literature (Christensen et al., 1993; Armentano et al., 1993; Santos et al., 1998; Kebreab et al., 2001; Reynal and Broderick, 2003). Increasing CP content of the diet may result in greater milk production (Armentano et al., 1993; Tomlinson et al., 1994; Powers et al., 1995; Wu and Satter, 2000), but also leads to increased concentration of ruminal NH_3 and blood urea N and consequently greater urinary N losses (Armentano et al., 1993; Christensen et al., 1993; Metcalf et al., 1996; Castillo et al., 2001). Increasing CP concentration of the diet from 15.8 to 18.3% resulted in an increase in urinary N losses from 58 to 63% (as percentage of total losses), blood urea N (15 vs. 19 mg/100 ml), and MUN (13 vs. 16 mg/100 ml), and reduced the efficiency of utilization of ruminal NH_3 N for milk protein synthesis in dairy cows (Hristov et al., 2004a). Dietary RDP can be used for MPS provided energy is not limiting; in most feeding systems, MPS synthesis is assumed to be energy-dependent (NKJ Protein Group, 1985; Tamminga et al., 1994; NRC, 2001; GfE, 2001). If not utilized for MPS, RDP will most likely be degraded to NH_3 and detoxified in the liver (Lobley et al., 1995), although a small proportion may by-pass the rumen and contribute to the duodenal amino acid and peptide flow (Choi et al., 2002). As exemplified by Tamminga (1992), ruminal N loss is the greatest single contributor to urinary N losses, but metabolic losses, indigestible microbial N, losses in maintenance, and inefficient conversion of absorbed amino acids into milk protein comprise up to 72% of the urinary N losses in the dairy cow.

Ammonia emissions from human activities are an environmental issue of growing public concern (Cowling and Galloway, 2001) and in developed countries farm animals are the greatest contributor to these emissions (US data; Kerchner et al., 2000). Feeding, particularly dietary CP level, environment, and type of manure handling system all contribute to NH_3 losses from cattle operations. The possibility exists that reducing CP level of the diet in combination with balancing carbohydrate (CHO)/protein degradability in the rumen and accounting for the effects of manure pH and ambient temperatures can significantly reduce NH_3 losses from dairy and beef cattle operations (Külling et al., 2001; Monteny et al., 2002).

Effect of Dietary Carbohydrate Availability on Ammonia Utilization in the Rumen and Nitrogen Losses

Ammonia concentration in the rumen can vary greatly depending on diet, time of feeding, feeding frequency, animal, and other factors. This variation can result in decreased efficiency of microbial NH_3 capture and eventually, in N wastage. The extent, to which NH_3 is utilized in the rumen, depends primarily on the rate of release and the balance of CHO and N availability. Carbohydrate availability determines the rate of microbial growth in the rumen (Isaacson et al., 1975; Strobel and Russell, 1986; Hoover and Stokes, 1991) and efficiency of utilization of ruminal NH_3 (Russell et al., 1983; Newbold and Rust, 1992; Hristov et al., 1997; Heldt et al., 1999). If energy is limiting, ruminal microorganisms degrade feed proteins to NH_3, and NH_3 uptake is suppressed (Nocek and Russell, 1988; Hristov et al., 1997). Carbohydrate supplementation and source, starch degradability, and synchronization of ruminal energy and N release may be key factors in improving the efficiency of ruminal NH_3 and overall dietary N utilization in ruminants.

A survey of the literature indicated that reduction in ruminal NH_3 concentration is the most likely effect of provision of readily fermentable CHO (sugars or starch) in the rumen (Hristov and Jouany, 2005). Although more variable, MPS synthesis may increase and urinary N excretion decrease with CHO supplementation. The effect on milk N efficiency (MilkNE; N secreted with milk protein as a fraction of N intake) and MUN concentration in lactating dairy cows is less consistent. In a meta-analysis involving 846 observations (diets) from 256 feeding trials, Hristov et al. (2004b) reported that MilkNE averaged 24.7±0.14%, varying considerably between diets (min and max of 13.7 and 39.8%, respectively). This variability highlights the potential for improving the efficiency of utilization of dietary N in dairy cows and in cattle in general. Results from the Hristov et al. (2004b) analysis indicated that diets producing high MilkNE contained more corn and cereal silages and concentrate and less alfalfa forage. For example, only 29% of the diets with MilkNE greater than 30% (77 diets; average efficiency of 33%) contained alfalfa silage, compared with 50% for all diets in the dataset. Corn silage was fed with 74% of the high efficiency diets compared with 57% of all diets; average concentration of corn silage in dietary DM was similar among diets (35 and 32%, respectively). The high MilkNE diets more often contained corn grain (77%, compared with 61% for all diets) and barley grain (29 vs. 15%, respectively). Average CP concentration of the high MilkNE diets was 15.8% while the average for all diets was 17.8%. Compared with the average milk yield per cow from all diets, cows produced more milk in trials where MilkNE was high: 35.2 vs. 31.9 kg/d. Extremely high N utilization efficiencies were associated with comparatively low CP intake and very high milk yields (data by Bach et al., 2000, for example). Thus, high MilkNE was more often found with diets, in which corn silage rather than alfalfa silage was the main forage ingredient, CP concentration was low, and cows had greater milk yields. Satter et al. (2002) calculated that with diets, in which low DM alfalfa silage is the only forage, NRC (2001) predicted 20.8% dietary CP was needed to meet the requirements of a high-producing, non-pregnant dairy cow, whereas with diets, in which the forage was alfalfa hay and corn silage (1:1), the requirements of the same cow would be met at 15.8% CP. Wilkerson et al. (1997) reported proportionally greater urinary N losses and lower MilkNE with low-producing cows (<20 kg/d) than with high-producing cows (>20 kg/d milk): 37.9 vs. 34.6% and 22.0 vs. 29.7%, respectively. In general, it can be concluded that MilkNE/N losses are closely related to N intake. As demonstrated by Hof et al. (1994), below a certain level of CP in the diet, there is little that can be done to reduce N losses from dairy cows. The potential remains with diets having N content above the threshold required to maintain desired milk protein yield (16 g DVEc/MJ NELc, as expressed by Hof et al.).

A significant amount of research has been aimed at maximizing MPS through synchronizing energy and NH_3 release in the rumen. The rumen synchrony concept (Johnson, 1976) implies that MPS (and presumably NH_3 utilization) will be maximized if availabilities of energy and protein are synchronized. Synchrony can be achieved by changing the composition of the dietary CHO and N fractions, by altering the relative times of feeding of the dietary ingredients, or by a combination of both approaches (Sauvant and van Milgen,

1995; Dewhurst et al., 2000). Results suggest rapid (asynchronous) release of dietary N as the main factor in increasing ruminal NH_3 and blood urea N concentrations after feeding, irrespective of the synchrony of energy release. Sauvant and van Milgen (1995) also indicated that greater N degradation rates result in increased ruminal NH_3 levels. These authors suggested that reduction in ruminal NH_3 concentrations could be achieved either by increasing the rate of CHO degradation or decreasing the rate of N degradation. Indeed, data summarized by Hristov and Jouany (2005) support this concept. Synchronization rarely affected MPS and its efficiency in the rumen. It is likely that ruminal microorganisms have the ability to overcome periods of nutrient shortages and compensatory grow when substrate is available (Sauvant and van Milgen, 1995). Urea N recycling to the rumen is an important physiological function of the ruminant animal providing N source for the ruminal microorganisms in times when N intake/NH_3 production is low; in cattle, from 25 to 53% of the recycled urea is degraded in the rumen (Bunting et al., 1989; Huntington, 1989). Liver ureagenesis is highly and positively correlated with N intake and the body urea pool acts as a source or a sink for N, thus normalizing short-term variations in RDP supply from the diet (Huntington and Archibeque, 1999). It is also possible, as noted by Dewhurst et al. (2000), that effects attributed to synchrony may simply be effects specific to the individual CHO and protein fractions of the diet. Increasing the proportion of one fraction in the diet inevitably decreases the proportion of the other fraction(s), thus confounding attempts to determine the relative importance of the different CHO or N fractions (Armentano and Pereira, 1997).

Objectives and Hypotheses

In two metabolism trials with lactating dairy cows, we investigated the effect of dietary CHO composition or supplementation on ruminal NH_3 utilization for milk protein synthesis. We hypothesized that provision of readily fermentable in the rumen CHO (sugars, starch, or available fiber) would enhance microbial capture of ruminal NH_3 and its transfer into milk protein.

Materials and Methods

Animals and Feeding

Two experiments with lactating Holstein dairy cows were conducted (Exp. 1, Hristov and Ropp, 2003 and Exp. 2, Hristov et al., 2005). All cows were cared for according to the guidelines of the University of Idaho Animal Care and Use Committee. Cows were fitted with ruminal (Bar Diamond, Parma, ID) and simple T-type duodenal (Ankom Technology, Fairport, NY) cannulae. The duodenal cannulae were placed on the ascending duodenum anterior to the pancreatic duct. Diets were fed as total mixed rations. In Exp. 1, four multiparous, late-lactation Holstein cows (average body weight 715±33 kg; average days in milk 323±19 d) were fed two diets (Table 1) in a cross-over design. Exp. 2 involved four cows (body weight 788±31 kg; days in milk 217±35 d) subjected to four treatments (Table 2) in a 4 × 4 Latin square design.

Table 1. Composition of the diets used in Exp. 1 (% of DM) and intake of nutrients (from Hristov and Ropp, 2003)

Ingredient	Diet[1]			
	RFSS	RFNDF	SE	P
Alfalfa silage[2]	26.7	34.0		
Alfalfa hay, chopped	12.6	2.1		
Forage, % of DM	39.3	36.1		
Barley grain, rolled	38.6	-		
Corn grain, cracked	-	20.0		
Solvent soybean meal	9.7	8.2		
Brewcrs grains, dry	-	12.6		
Beet pulp, dry	-	20.7		
Molasses, dry	9.1	-		
Blood meal	0.8	-		
Mono calcium phosphate	0.5	0.4		
Sodium bicarbonate	1.4	1.4		
Mineral/vitamin mix[3]	0.6	0.6		
Composition, % of DM				
CP	19.5	19.1		
NDF	26.1	34.1		
ADF	13.5	17.7		
Starch	26.7	17.7		
Ether extract	1.6	2.5		
Lignin	1.7	2.0		
Ash	8.4	8.8		
ANDF[4]	22.0	29.2		
NSC[5]	47.8	40.3		
NSP[6]	21.2	22.6		
Intakes (kg/d)				
DM	24.2	21.5	0.72	0.12
OM	21.7	19.2	0.63	0.10
N	0.754	0.658	0.0216	0.08
NDF	6.3	7.3	0.30	0.13
ADF	3.3	3.8	0.16	0.13
Available NDF (ANDF)[7]	5.3	6.3	0.26	0.11
Fermentable ANDF	1.9	2.6	0.10	0.04
NSC[8]	11.6	8.7	0.24	0.01
Starch	5.8	3.8	0.09	0.004
Fermentable starch	4.8	2.5	0.03	0.0004
NSP[9]	5.1	4.9	0.17	0.40
Fermentable NSP	3.3	3.4	0.12	0.43
Total FCHO[10]	10.0	8.5	0.22	0.05

[1] RFSS, ruminally fermentable non-structural CHO; RFNDF, ruminally fermentable fiber.

[2] Alfalfa silage was 44%, DM.

[3] Composition: 34.5-41.4% NaCl, 26.9-33.8% ground rice hulls, 27.9% barley, 0.24% $MnSO_4$, 0.21% ZnO_3, 0.052% Cu_2SO_4, 0.0014% Fe_2CO_3, 0.0059% $CaI_2O_6.H_2O$, 0.0010% $CoCO_3$, 932 KIU/kg Vitamin A, 818 KIU/kg Vitamin D, and 15 KIU/kg Vitamin E.

[4] ANDF (available NDF); calculated as: NDF – (Lignin × 2.4) (CPM Dairy).

[5] NSC (non-structural CHO); calculated as: 100 – CP – (NDF-NDFCP) – Ash – Ether extract (CPM Dairy).

[6] NSP (non-starch polysaccharides); calculated as: NSC – starch.

[7] Available NDF was calculated as: NDF – (Lignin × 2.4).

[8] NSC (non-structural CHO) was calculated as: 100 – CP – (NDF-NDFCP) – Ash – Ether extract.

[9] NSP (non-starch polysaccharides) was calculated as: NSC – starch.

[10] Total FCHO (total fermentable CHO intake) was found as: Fermentable ANDF intake + Fermentable starch intake + Fermentable NSP intake.

Table 2. Composition of the basal diet used in Exp. 2 and intake of nutrients (from Hristov et al., 2005)

Ingredient	% of DM[1]
Alfalfa hay[2], chopped	73.2
Carbohydrate[3]	20.6
Blood meal, ring dried	3.6
Monosodium phosphate	0.4
Sodium bicarbonate	0.9
Mineral/vitamin premix[4]	1.3
Composition, % of DM	
NE_L, Mcal/kg[5]	1.37
CP	22.1
NDF	48.1
ADF	34.3

Intakes, kg/d	GLU	STA	NDF	MIX	SE	P[6]
DM	21.8	21.4	22.6	22.5	0.48	0.17
OM	19.9	19.8	20.4	20.3	0.43	0.46
N	0.634	0.630	0.662	0.651	0.0174	0.22
NDF	8.3^m	8.3^m	12.4^k	9.6^l	0.23	<0.0001

[1] With added water DM concentration of the diet was 71.6%.

[2] Alfalfa hay was 91.7% DM, 18.7% CP, and 49.7% NDF.

[3] CHO treatments were: corn dextrose, GLU; corn starch (STA); white oat fiber fiber (NDF), and a CHO mix (25% of each): apple pectin, GLU, STA, and NDF (MIX). Proportion of CHO varied between cows and treatments depending on total DMI. The average CHO proportion in dietary DM was: GLU, 20.7%; STA, 20.8%; NDF, 20.0%; MIX, 20.8%.

[4] Composition: 34.5 to 41.4% NaCl, 26.9 to 33.8% ground rice hulls, 27.9% barley, 0.24% $MnSO_4$, 0.21% ZnO_3, 0.052% Cu_2SO_4, 0.0014% Fe_2CO_3, 0.0059% $CaI_2O_6.H_2O$, 0.0010% $CoCO_3$, 932 KIU/kg Vitamin A, 174 KIU/kg Vitamin D, and 3.3 KIU/kg Vitamin E.

[5] NRC (2001) estimate.

[6] For main effect.

Diets in Exp. 1 were fed at 0600, 1400, and 2200 at 90% of ad libitum intake determined before initiation of each experimental period. Diets contained similar proportions of alfalfa forage but had either a higher concentration of ruminally fermentable non-structural CHO (NSC, as starch and sugars; diet RFSS) or ruminally fermentable fiber (diet RFNDF) provided with the non-forage components. Diets contained (DM basis; CPM Dairy, version 2.0.23, University of Pennsylvania, Kennett Square, PA, Cornell University, Ithaca, NY and William H. Miner Agricultural Research Institute, Chazy, NY): NE_L – 1.66 and 1.67 Mcal/kg; metabolizable protein – 10.6 and 10.4%; protein fractions A + B1 (non-protein N and soluble true protein) – 33 and 33% of CP; protein fractions B2 + B3 (N soluble in neutral and acid detergents) – 60 and 59% of CP; and protein fraction C (N insoluble in acid detergent) – 7 and 8% of CP (RFSS and RFNDF, respectively). Concentration of CP was similar between the two diets. Diet RFSS had 23% lower NDF content and 51% greater starch content than diet RFNDF. Concentration of available NDF (ANDF) was by 33% greater and NSC was 16% lower in RFNDF than in RFSS. Diets contained similar proportions of non-starch polysaccharides (NSP). The intake of ruminally fermentable fiber was significantly greater in the cows fed RFNDF whereas the intake of ruminally fermentable starch was greater in the cows fed the RFSS diet (Table 1). Cows fed RFSS had greater intake of NSC and total fermentable CHO than the cows fed RFNDF.

The basal diet in Exp. 2 was energy deficient for the level of milk production of the experimental cows (NRC, 2001; Table 2). Pure CHO were dosed intraruminally, at approximately 20% of total dry matter intake (DMI) twice a day before each feeding. Treatments were: control (NDF, Canadian Harvest Oat Fiber 200-150, Opta Food Ingredients, Inc., Bedford, MA); corn dextrose (GLU, Corn Products International, Bedford Park, IL); corn starch (STA, Roquette America, Inc., Keokuk, IA); and a CHO mix (25% of each): apple pectin (Amcan Industries, Inc., Elmsford, NY), GLU, STA, and NDF (MIX). Corn dextrose and STA were selected to provide rapid or slower (respectively) release of fermentable energy in the rumen. Oat fiber served as a negative control (i.e., containing no readily fermentable in the rumen energy). The combination treatment (MIX) was designed to provide a steady supply of fermentable energy throughout the feeding cycle. Cows were fed at 0600 and 1800 at 95% of ad libitum intake determined at the beginning of the experiment.

Markers and Sampling

In both experiments ruminal NH_3 N was labeled with ^{15}N. In Exp. 1, labeling was through continuous 3-d intraruminal infusion of 20 atom percent excess (APE) $(^{15}NH_4)_2SO_4$ (Cambridge Isotope Laboratories, Inc., Andover, MA) dissolved in distilled water at final concentration of 31 mg/ml and infused into the rumen through the rumen cannula via a peristaltic pump (Table 5). In Exp. 2, NH_3 N was labeled through a pulse-dose of 10 g/cow of 20 APE $(^{15}NH_4)_2SO_4$ dissolved in McDougall's buffer (McDougall, 1948). The rumens of the cows were emptied in large carts on d 15 of each period before the 0600 feeding. Contents were weighed, thoroughly mixed by hand, a background ruminal sample was collected, the isotope, CHO, and passage rate markers were added to the ruminal contents, a 0 h sample was collected following a thorough mixing, and the ruminal contents were returned to the rumen of the cows.

In Exp. 1, whole ruminal contents samples were collected before (0 h, background) and 1, 3, 5, 9, 13, 17, 21, 25, 29, 33, 37, 41, 45, 49, 53, 57, 61, 65, 69, 72, 75, 78, 84, 90, 96, 102, 108, and 114 h after initiation of the $(^{15}NH_4)_2SO_4$ infusion. In Exp. 2, samples were collected at 0 (background), 0.5, 1, 2, 4, 6, 8, 10, 14, 18, 24, and 30 h following the $(^{15}NH_4)_2SO_4$ dosing. Samples were collected from four locations in the rumen: ventral sac, reticulum, and two from the feed mat in the dorsal rumen (approximately 250 g each). The four samples were composited, squeezed through two layers of cheesecloth, and analyzed for fermentation variables (Hristov and Ropp, 2003). Ruminal NH_3 and bacterial pellets were analyzed for ^{15}N enrichment (Hristov et al., 2001). In Exp. 1, following initiation of the $(^{15}NH_4)_2SO_4$ infusion, cows were milked at 0 (background), 5, 10, 15, 20, 25, 30, 35, 40, 45, 50, 55, 60, 65, 70, 75, 80, 85, 90, 95, 100, 105, 110, 115, 125, 135, 145, and 155 h. In Exp. 2, cows were milked at 0 (background), 5, 10, 15, 20, 25, 30, 35, 40, 45, 50, 55, 60, 65, 70, 75, 80, 85, 90, 95, 105, and 120 h following the $(^{15}NH_4)_2SO_4$ dose. At each milking, milk weights were recorded and aliquot samples were analyzed for protein N and ^{15}N-enrichment. Milk protein was precipitated with 5% (w/v; final concentration) trichloroacetic acid. Protein pellets were sedimented by centrifuging at 20,000 × *g* for 15 min at 4°C, freeze-dried, and analyzed for N and ^{15}N-enrichment (Hristov et al., 2001).

Table 5. Effect of dietary carbohydrate type and fermentability on ^{15}N enrichment of various N pools and ^{15}N calculations in dairy cows, Exp. 1 (from Hristov and Ropp, 2003)

	Diet[1]			
	RFSS	**RFNDF**	**SE**	***P***
^{15}N dosed, mg	5104	5029	38.4	0.30
Ruminal NH_3-^{15}N, APE[2]	0.441	0.556	0.1434	0.62
Bacterial-^{15}N, APE	0.241	0.189	0.0015	0.01
AUC[3], bacterial N	27.5	21.3	0.36	0.006
AUC, milk protein N	7.99	9.36	0.151	0.02
Milk protein N from ruminal bacterial N[4], %	29.4	44.0	0.69	0.004
Regression analysis of cumulative milk ^{15}N excretion (estimate ± approx. SE)				
Maximum ^{15}N excreted[6],				
% of infused	12.7±0.36	14.4±0.59	0.01	
Rate related parameter	0.045±0.0017	0.043±0.0023	0.79	
Comparison of excretion lines			0.04	

[1] RFSS, ruminally fermentable non-structural CHO; RFNDF, ruminally fermentable fiber.
[2] Atom percent excess.
[3] Area under the ^{15}N curve, APE × h.
[4] Calculated as: $(AUC_{\text{milk protein}} \div AUC_{\text{rumen bacteria}}) \times 100$.
[5] Nitrogen-15 secretion in milk (mg) is expressed as percentage of ^{15}N infused in the rumen (mg). Data were fitted to a logistic model.
[6] Theoretical maximum.

Calculations

In Exp.1, milk and ruminal bacteria ^{15}N-enrichment (APE) curves were plotted vs. time and fitted to the multicompartmental model of Dhanoa et al. (1985), restricted to two compartments and to a five-parameter modified Gaussian model [f=y0+a*exp(-0.5*abs((x-x0)/b)^c] (SigmaPlot, SPSS Inc., Chicago, IL), respectively. Criteria for best fit were: R^2 (the coefficient of determination), the ANOVA *P* value for the regression (describing the association between the dependent and independent variables), the Predicted Residual Error Sum of Squares (PRESS, an indicator of how well a regression model predicts new data), the Normality test (indicating the normality of distribution of source population around the regression), and the residuals distribution around the 0 line. Ammonia concentration in the rumen of the cows varied greatly in Exp. 1. As a result, regression models were not created for ^{15}N enrichment of ruminal NH_3 N and consequently, proportions of bacterial and milk protein N originating from NH_3 N were not calculated. In Exp. 2, ruminal NH_3, bacteria, and milk protein ^{15}N-enrichment curves were fitted to a three-parameter single exponential decay model [$f=y_0+a*exp(-b*x)$], a four-parameter double exponential decay model [$f=y_0+a*exp(-b*x)+c*exp(-d*x)$], or the double exponential model of Dhanoa et al. (1985; PROC NLIN, SAS Inst. Inc., Cary, NC), respectively. Criteria for best fit were as for Exp. 1, or the proportion of the variance explained by the model in the case of milk protein. Areas under the predicted milk protein, bacterial, and NH_3 ^{15}N curves (AUC, ^{15}N atom % excess × h) were computed using the trapezoidal rule (AREA.XFM transform, SigmaPlot). Proportions of milk protein N originating from ruminal bacterial (Exp. 1) and NH_3 N and the proportion of bacterial N originating from ruminal NH_3 N were derived based on the respective AUC (Nolan and Leng, 1974). In Exp. 2, the total flux, irreversible loss, and recycling rate of ruminal NH_3 N were calculated from NH_3 ^{15}N-enrichment data, the NH_3 ^{15}N AUC, and by the difference according to Nolan and Leng (1974). The microbial N leaving the rumen that originated from ruminal NH_3 N was calculated as: microbial N flow × proportion of bacterial N originating from NH_3 N. The proportion of the irreversible NH_3 N loss incorporated into microbial protein leaving the rumen was calculated as: [(microbial N flow × proportion of bacterial N derived from NH_3 N) ÷ irreversible loss of NH_3 N] × 100. The cumulative amounts of ^{15}N secreted in milk protein (as percentage of the ^{15}N infused in the rumen of each individual cow) was calculated as milk output for each milking interval was multiplied by the trichloroacetic acid-precipitable N concentration in milk and by its ^{15}N-enrichment. In Exp. 1, data were fitted to a logistic model:

$$y = m \div (1 + \exp(-k(x-L)) \qquad (1)$$

In Exp. 2, cumulative milk ^{15}N secretion data were fitted to a single rectangular two-parameter hyperbola model of the type:

$$y = m \times x \div (b + x) \qquad (2)$$

In both models y represented the cumulative ^{15}N secretion in milk protein as percentage of the ^{15}N infused/dosed in the rumen at time x and m represented the theoretical maximum for y.These models were fitted to each treatment within each experiment and each model was assessed for adequate fit. The estimated models were compared using the dummy variable regression technique (Bates and Watts, 1988).

All data were analyzed by analysis of variance assuming cross-over or Latin square designs (PROC GLM or PROC MIXED, Exp. 1 and Exp. 2, respectively; SAS, 1999; SAS Inst., Inc., Cary, NC).

RESULTS

Ruminal pH and concentration of reducing sugars in ruminal fluid were not different (P = 0.90 and 0.50) between the two diets (Table 3) in Exp. 1. Ammonia concentration was lowered (P = 0.04) by RFNDF compared to RFSS. Polysaccharide-degrading activities in the rumen were not affected (P = 0.20 to 0.89) by treatment. There were no differences (P = 0.18 to 0.73) in total or individual VFA concentrations or acetate to propionate ratio between the diets, except diet RFSS produced greater concentrations of propionate and butyrate (P = 0.08 and 0.07, respectively). Fractional outflow rate of the fluid phase of the rumen contents did not differ (P = 0.43) between diets. Microbial nitrogen flow to the small intestine (P = 0.40), daily excretion of urinary allantoin ($P = 0.57$), or the efficiency of microbial CP synthesis in the rumen ($P = 26$) were not different between the diets.

Table 3. Effect of dietary carbohydrate type and fermentability on ruminal fermentation and microbial protein synthesis in dairy cows, Exp. 1 (from Hristov and Ropp, 2003)

Parameter	Diet[1]			
	RFSS	RFNDF	SE	*P*
pH	6.01	6.02	0.045	0.90
Ammonia, m*M*	11.4	9.8	0.24	0.04
Reducing sugars, m*M*	2.57	2.17	0.152	0.50
Volatile Fatty Acids, m*M*				
Acetate	77.4	75.5	1.48	0.46
Propionate	26.5	25.9	0.13	0.08
iso-Butyrate	1.56	1.48	0.074	0.51
Butyrate	19.3	17.0	0.48	0.07
iso-Valerate	2.09	2.00	0.147	0.73
Valerate	2.60	2.68	0.144	0.72
Total VFA	129.5	124.6	1.76	0.18
Acetate/Propionate	2.99	2.95	0.031	0.49
Polysaccharide-degrading activities[2]				
CMCase	49.4	44.3	2.10	0.22
Xylanase	189.8	184.9	22.94	0.89
Amylase	86.0	72.6	4.96	0.20
Liquid phase FOR[3], %/h	15.0	18.0	0.01	0.43
MN[4] flow, g/d	340	321	12.8	0.40
MN, g/kg OMTDR[5]	25	30	2.1	0.26
Urinary allantoin, g/d	81.7	83.3	1.68	0.57

[1] RFSS, ruminally fermentable non-structural CHO; RFNDF, ruminally fermentable fiber.
[2] Expressed as nmol of RS as glucose released per ml of ruminal fluid per minute; CMCase, carboxymethylcellulase.
[3] FOR, fractional outflow rate.
[4] MN, microbial nitrogen.
[5] OMTDR, organic matter truly digested in the rumen.

In Exp. 2, the two CHO containing glucose, GLU and MIX, produced the lowest (throughout the course of sampling; $P = 0.02$ to 0.0002) ruminal pH (Table 4). Average pH was also lower ($P = 0.005$) for STA compared with NDF. The GLU treatment (and to a lesser extent MIX) resulted in a noticeable decline in pH immediately after CHO dosing; STA decreased pH in a similar pattern, but the lowest pH occurred between 2 and 4 h post-dose. There was a significant interaction ($P < 0.001$) between CHO source and time of sampling. Ruminal pH was lower ($P < 0.001$) for GLU compared with all other CHO at 0 (except MIX), 0.5, and 1 h and compared with NDF at 2 h after feeding/CHO dosing. Similarly, pH was lower ($P < 0.001$) for MIX compared with NDF at 0, 0.5, 1, and 2 h and compared with STA at 0, 0.5, and 1 h. Ruminal pH was lower ($P = 0.06$) for STA compared with NDF at 1 h, compared with MIX and NDF at 2 h ($P = 0.01$ and $P < 0.001$, respectively), and compared with all CHO at 4 h ($P = 0.02$ to $P < 0.001$). The MIX treatment had lower ($P = 0.03$ to $P = 0.004$) pH than all other CHO at 8 h after feeding. At 14 h (or 2 h after the 1800 feeding), pH of ruminal fluid was greater ($P = 0.01$ to $P < 0.001$) for NDF compared with all other CHO. The lowest overall NH_3 concentration was associated with GLU and STA, MIX was intermediate, and NDF had the greatest NH_3 levels in the rumen ($P < 0.001$; interaction between CHO and time of sampling was not significant for this variable; $P = 0.33$). Treatments GLU and STA maintained the lowest post-feeding NH_3 concentrations ($P = 0.02$ to 0.002 vs. NDF and MIX). In accordance, NDF and MIX had larger NH_3 N pools than GLU and STA ($P = 0.01$ compared with GLU; $P = 0.06$ and 0.09 compared with STA, respectively). Concentration of reducing sugars was greater for GLU compared with STA ($P < 0.001$), NDF ($P < 0.001$), and MIX ($P < 0.001$). The STA and MIX treatments had greater reducing sugars concentration than NDF ($P < 0.001$). Protozoal counts were not affected by treatment ($P = 0.20$). The GLU treatment had the lowest total VFA concentration compared with all other CHO ($P = 0.02$ to 0.009), which was primarily due to low acetate concentration ($P = 0.001$ to < 0.001). Propionate was not affected by treatment ($P = 76$), but butyrate concentration was greater for GLU, followed by STA and MIX, and NDF ($P = 0.002$). Concentrations of *iso*-butyrate and *iso*-valerate were dramatically decreased by GLU compared with the other CHO ($P = 0.002$ to < 0.001 for *iso*-butyrate and $P = 0.01$ to < 0.001 for *iso*-valerate). *Iso*-butyrate concentration was also decreased by STA and MIX compared with NDF ($P = 0.04$ and 0.02, respectively). *Iso*-valerate concentration was lowered ($P = 0.04$) by MIX compared with STA. Reflecting acetate concentration, acetate: propionate ratio was on average by 19% lower ($P = 0.08$) for GLU compared with the other CHO. The CMCase activity of ruminal fluid was not affected ($P = 0.23$) by treatment. The NDF and MIX treatments resulted in greater xylanase activity of ruminal fluid than GLU ($P = 0.03$ and 0.02, respectively). Amylase activity was greater ($P = 0.08$ to 0.07) with the starch-containing CHO, STA and MIX, compared with GLU and NDF. Fractional outflow rates of ruminal fluid and solids were not affected ($P = 0.62$ and 0.37, respectively) by treatment. Before feeding, cows had similar ($P = 0.25$) amounts of microbial N in their ruminal contents, representing 50 to 60% of the total NAN in the rumen. Microbial N flow was decreased by NDF compared with the other CHO ($P = 0.04$ to 0.01). The outflow of microbial N originating from NH_3 N from the rumen was increased with STA ($P = 0.04$ and 0.03, compared with GLU and NDF, respectively). Expressed per kg of organic matter truly digested in the rumen, microbial N flow was decreased by NDF compared with the other CHO ($P = 0.06$ to 0.01). Urinary allantoin excretion did not seem to parallel the microbial N flow data and was not affected ($P = 0.28$) by treatment.

Cows received similar ($P = 0.30$) doses of ^{15}N in Exp. 1 and ^{15}N-enrichment of ruminal NH_3 N was not different ($P = 0.62$) between the two diets (Table 5). Bacterial N from RFSS cows had greater ($P = 0.01$) ^{15}N-enrichment than bacterial N from RFNDF cows. The area under the ruminal bacterial ^{15}N curve was larger ($P = 0.006$) for RFSS than for RFNDF. The area under the milk protein ^{15}N curve was larger ($P = 0.02$) for RFNDF than for RFSS (Figure 1). The estimated proportion of milk protein N originating from ruminal bacterial N was 50% greater ($P = 0.004$) when cows received the RFNDF diet compared with the RFSS

Table 4. Effect of carbohydrate source on ruminal fermentation and microbial protein synthesis in dairy cows, Exp. 2 (from Hristov et al., 2005)

Item	Treatment[1]					
	GLU	STA	NDF	MIX	SE	P[2]
pH	6.00^{m}	6.19^{l}	6.41^{k}	6.05^{m}	0.049	<0.001
Ammonia, m*M*	8.5^{m}	9.6^{m}	16.4^{k}	12.4^{l}	1.05	<0.001
Ammonia N, g[3]	5.6^{l}	7.2^{l}	12.3^{k}	11.6^{k}	1.24	0.03
Reducing sugars, m*M*	12.4^{k}	9.1^{l}	4.8^{m}	9.7^{l}	0.56	<0.001
Total protozoa[4] ($\times 10^4$ cells/mL)	20.0	18.8	28.3	36.3		
(5.26)	(5.21)	(5.42)	(5.49)	(0.133)	0.20	
Volatile Fatty Acids, m*M*						
Acetate	74.0^{l}	95.4^{k}	94.5^{k}	97.0^{k}	2.45	0.002
Propionate	22.1	23.0	23.2	24.0	1.28	0.76
iso-Butyrate	0.63^{m}	1.29^{l}	1.57^{k}	1.22^{l}	0.081	0.001
Butyrate	22.2^{k}	15.0^{m}	12.4^{n}	18.9^{l}	0.81	<0.001
iso-Valerate	0.61^{m}	1.73^{k}	1.68^{kl}	1.37^{l}	0.126	0.002
Valerate	2.84	2.67	2.61	2.74	0.108	0.42
Total VFA	122.3^{m}	139.1^{kl}	135.9^{l}	145.2^{k}	3.08	0.009
Acetate/Propionate	3.36^{l}	4.26^{k}	4.08^{k}	4.06^{k}	0.211	0.08
Polysaccharide-degrading activities[5]						
CMCase	35.8	47.9	48.6	65.8	10.02	0.23
Xylanase	65.3^{l}	103.0^{kl}	133.2^{k}	140.2^{k}	19.10	0.08
Amylase	12.4^{l}	39.4^{k}	13.5^{l}	38.9^{k}	8.71	0.11
Liquid phase FOR[6], %/h	9.0	10.4	10.5	11.1	1.13	0.62
Solid phase FOR, %/h	3.1	3.0	2.7	3.4	0.24	0.37
MN in rumen[7], g	180	143	140	198	21.4	0.25
As % of total NAN	59.3	49.7	49.7	61.0	6.34	0.49
MN flow, g/d	197^{k}	185^{k}	153^{l}	188^{k}	9.7	0.05
MN from NH_3 flow[8], g/d	75^{l}	111^{k}	74^{l}	89^{kl}	10.4	0.11
MN, g/kg OMTDR[9]	15^{k}	15^{k}	12^{l}	14^{k}	0.8	0.05
Urinary allantoin, g/d	57.1	70.4	58.6	66.6	4.96	0.28

[1] CHO treatments were: corn dextrose (GLU); corn starch (STA); fiber (NDF, white oat fiber), and a CHO mix (25% of each): apple pectin, GLU, STA, and NDF (MIX).

[2] For main effect.

[3] Ammonia N pool size (g) estimated from rumen evacuation data and NH_3 concentration in ruminal fluid.

[4] Values shown are means of actual counts. The values in parentheses are the means of $\log_{10}$ transformations of the data immediately above.

[5] Expressed as nmol of reducing sugars as glucose released per mL of ruminal fluid per minute; CMCase, carboxymethylcellulase.

[6] FOR, fractional outflow rate.

[7] MN, microbial nitrogen in rumen (g) analyzed at time 0 h (rumen evacuation) as: (^{15}N enrichment of ruminal NAN, APE $\div$ ^{15}N enrichment of bacterial NAN, APE) $\times$ NAN in rumen, g.

[8] Calculated as: MN flow $\times$ proportion of bacterial N originating from NH_3 N (AUC data).

[9] OMTDR, organic matter truly digested in the rumen.

[k,l,m,n] Within a row, means without a common superscript letter differ ($P \leq 0.11$).

diet. Between 12.7 (RFSS) and 14.4% (RFNDF) of ^{15}N infused intraruminally was recovered in milk protein N after 155 h of milking. The proportion was greater (P = 0.01) for RFNDF than for RFSS. Time to reach 50% of maximum ^{15}N recovery and rate of ^{15}N secretion in milk protein were not different (P = 0.44 and 0.79, respectively), but the overall cumulative secretion lines (Figure 2) differed between the two diets at P = 0.04.

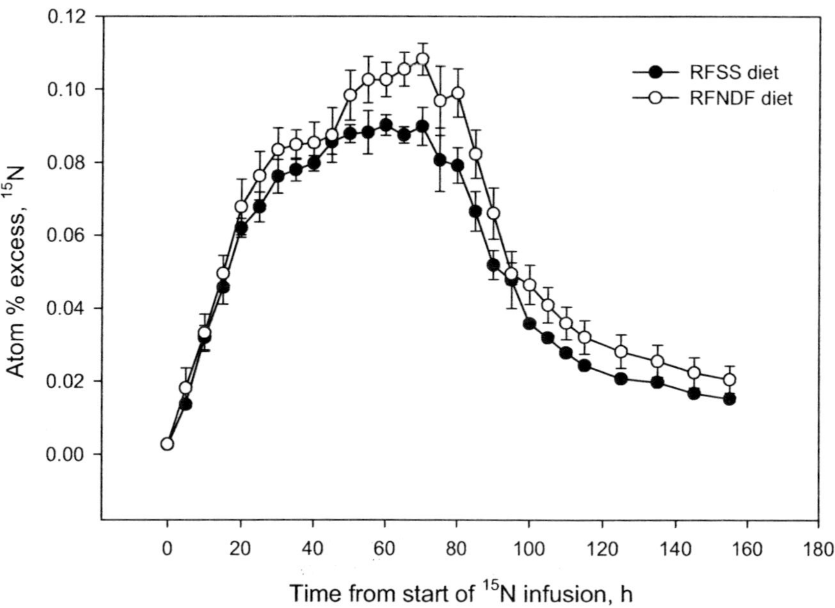

Figure 1. Effect of dietary carbohydrate type and fermentability on 15N secretion (mean ± SE) in milk protein, Exp. 1. Diet RFSS, ruminally fermentable non-structural carbohydrates; diet RFNDF, ruminally fermentable fiber (from Hristov and Ropp, 2003)

In Exp. 2, ^{15}N enrichment of ruminal NH_3 N reflected ruminal NH_3 concentrations and was greater for GLU compared with STA, NDF, and MIX (P = 0.11, 0.02, and 0.10, respectively; Table 6). Average ^{15}N enrichment of bacterial N was not different (P = 0.48) among CHO. The NH_3 ^{15}N and bacteria AUC were not affected (P = 0.15 and 51, respectively) by treatment. Enrichment of ruminal NH_3 N rapidly decreased following the ^{15}N dose and reached pre-dose levels within 5 to 6 h (Figure 3). The decline in ^{15}N enrichment of bacterial N was exponential and reached levels close to natural abundance within 30 h post-dose (Figure 4). Based on AUC data, 38 to 60% of ruminal bacterial N originated from NH_3 N, 45% of milk protein N originated from ruminal bacterial N (P = 0.65), and 17 to 28% of milk protein N originated from ruminal NH_3 N (Table 6). More bacterial N was formed from NH_3 N with STA compared with GLU, MIX, and NDF (P = 0.004, 0.04, and 0.05, respectively), which resulted in a greater proportion of milk protein N derived from NH_3 N for STA compared with the other CHO (P = 0.006, 0.08, and 0.03 compared with GLU, NDF, and MIX, respectively). The proportion of bacterial N formed from NH_3 N was greater for NDF and MIX compared with GLU (P = 0.08 and 0.11, respectively). A greater (P = 0.08) proportion of milk protein N was formed from ruminal NH_3 N with NDF than with GLU. Uptake of NH_3 ^{15}N was very rapid and within the time required to process the 0 h sample, 8.4% (SE = 1.43; P = 0.84) of bacterial N was already formed from NH_3 N. Within 30 min post-dose, 9 (GLU; P = 0.04 and 0.09 compared to NDF and MIX, respectively) to 14% (MIX; P = 0.03 compared with STA) of bacterial protein was synthesized from NH_3 N. More NH_3 N was irreversibly lost from the NH_3 N pool with STA and NDF compared with GLU (P = 0.02 and 0.05, respectively). As proportion of N intake, the irreversible loss of NH_3 N was greater for STA and NDF than for GLU (P = 0.01 and 0.07, respectively). Ruminal NH_3 N flux (absolute or as proportion of N intake) was decreased (P = 0.02 to 0.008) by GLU compared with the other CHO. Recycling of NH_3 N was not affected (P = 0.21) by treatment. The efficiency of utilization of ruminal NH_3 N for microbial protein synthesis ranged from 23 to 33% and was lower for NDF compared with the other CHO (P = 0.05 to 0.01). Average ^{15}N enrichment of milk protein N was greater for STA compared with GLU, NDF, and MIX (P = 0.11, 0.03, and 0.04, respectively). Milk protein ^{15}N AUC was not affected (P = 0.14) by treatment. Secretion of the isotope in milk was bell-shaped (Figure 5). In all treatments, peak ^{15}N concentration was measured at 15 h post-dose. Theoretical maximum cumulative secretion of the isotope in milk protein N ranged from 8.8 to 10.3% of the ruminal ^{15}N dose and was not affected by treatment (P = 0.97 to 0.48). Overall, cumulative ^{15}N secretion in milk protein (Figure 6) was greater for STA compared with GLU and NDF (P = 0.01 and P = 0.001, respectively). Secretion of the isotope for MIX was also greater (P = 0.09) compared with NDF.

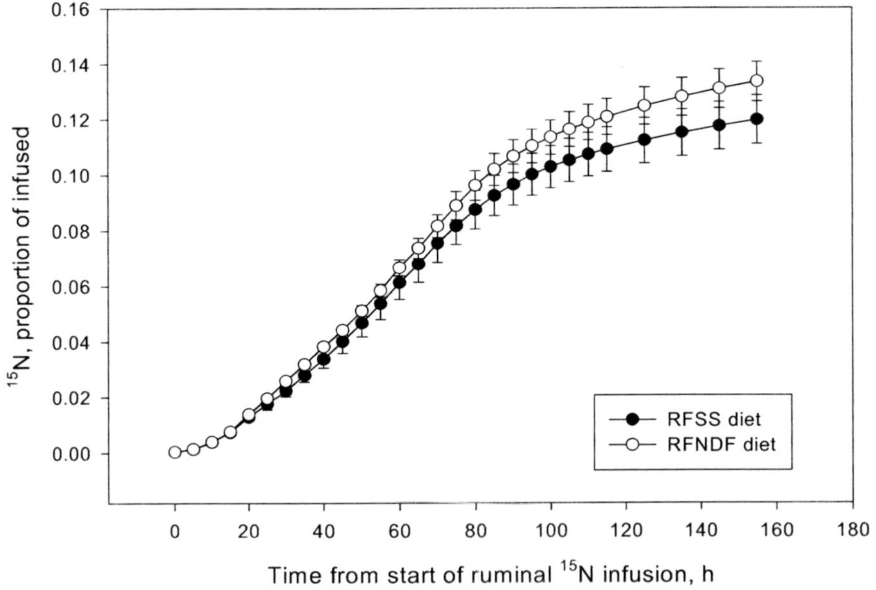

Figure 2. Effect of dietary carbohydrate type and fermentability on the cumulative secretion curves of ^{15}N in milk protein as proportion of ^{15}N infused intraruminally in Exp. 1 (predicted values; error bars represent 95% confidence intervals on the predicted values; logistic model) (from Hristov and Ropp, 2003)

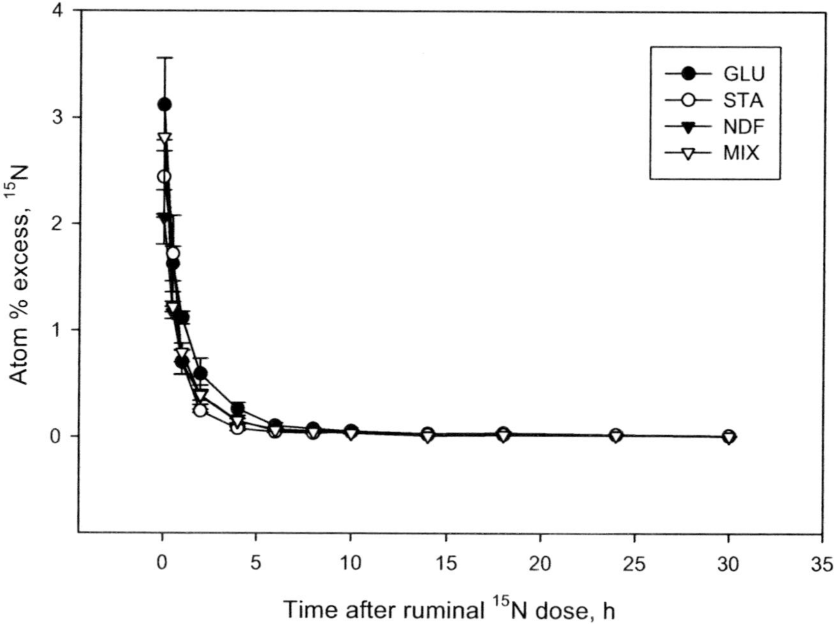

Figure 3. Effect of carbohydrate source on ^{15}N-enrichment of ruminal ammonia N in dairy cows (means ± SE), Exp. 2. Treatment GLU, corn dextrose; STA, corn starch; NDF, white oat fiber, and MIX, 25% of each, apple pectin, GLU, STA, and NDF (from Hristov et al., 2005)

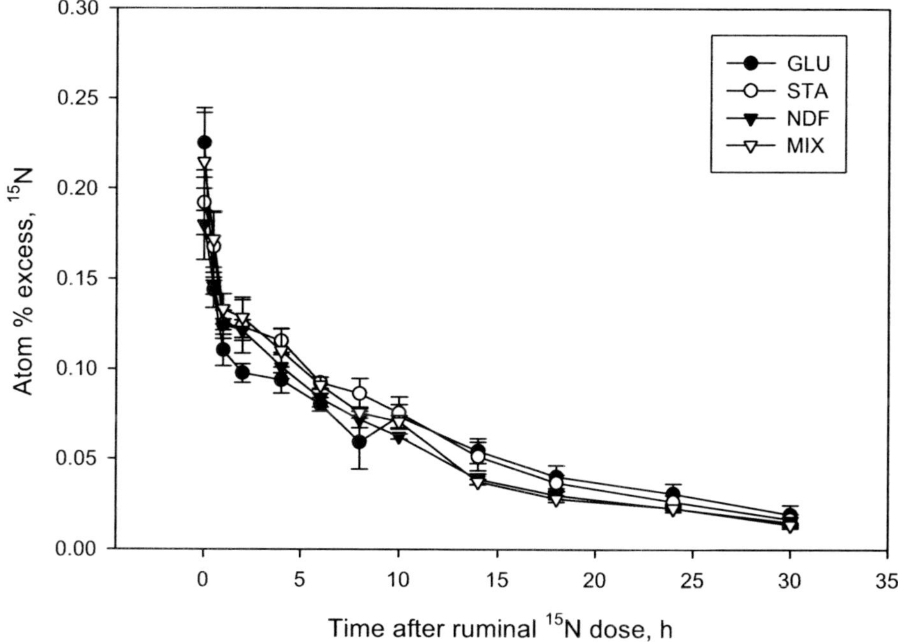

Figure 4. Effect of carbohydrate source on ^{15}N-enrichment of bacterial N in dairy cows (means ± SE), Exp. 2. Treatment GLU, corn dextrose; STA, corn starch; NDF, white oat fiber, and MIX, 25% of each, apple pectin, GLU, STA, and NDF (from Hristov et al., 2005)

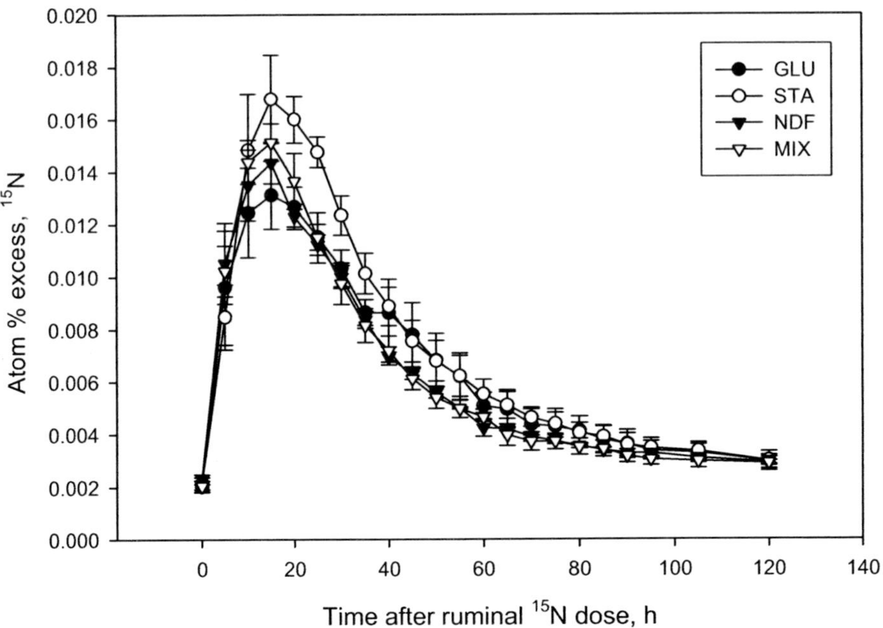

Figure 5. Effect of carbohydrate source on ^{15}N secretion (mean ± SE) in milk protein, Exp. 2. Treatment GLU, corn dextrose; STA, corn starch; NDF, white oat fiber, and MIX, 25% of each, apple pectin, GLU, STA, and NDF (from Hristov et al., 2005)

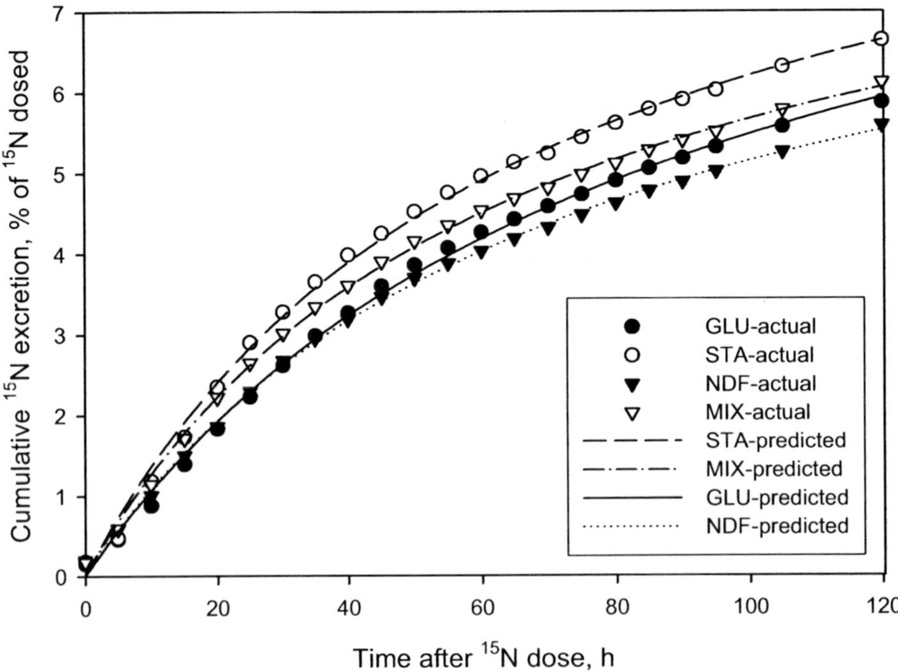

Figure 6. Effect of carbohydrate source on the cumulative secretion of ^{15}N in milk protein (as percentage of ^{15}N dosed intraruminally) in Exp. 2. Symbols are measured and lines are predicted values (single rectangular two-parameter hyperbola model). Treatment GLU, corn dextrose; STA, corn starch; NDF, white oat fiber, and MIX, 25% of each, apple pectin, GLU, STA, and NDF (from Hristov et al., 2005)

DISCUSSION

The two diets tested in Exp. 1 had similar metabolizable protein and NE_L concentrations but contrastingly different proportions of structural vs. non-structural CHO. Fiber in RFNDF had higher estimated ruminal fermentability than RFSS fiber. Beet pulp and particularly brewers grains have high concentration of ruminally fermentable NDF (Tamminga et al., 1990). The difference in NSC content was primarily from starch; NSP content was similar between the diets. Estimated starch fermentability in RFSS was also greater than fermentability of starch in RFNDF. As a result, diet RFSS provided considerably greater intakes of ruminally fermentable starch. Although, the differences in NSP content and fermentable NSP intake were not significant, the diets differed in the composition of the NSP fraction. Constituents of NSP in RFSS would include free sugars (from molasses) and β-glucans (from barley); NSP in RFNDF would originate primarily from pectins (beet pulp, Bohn et al., 1998). Thus, the main dietary factors that could have affected the results from Exp. 1 were: the greater starch content and greater starch degradation rate of barley vs. corn and presence of free sugars from molasses in RFSS and the provision of greater amount of ruminally fermentable fiber with RFNDF. These dietary differences did not affect ruminal pH, but CHO had a profound effect on this variable in Exp. 2. The effect of the rapidly fermentable CHO (from corn dextrose and starch) on ruminal fermentation was noticeable immediately after dosing. At 0.5 to 1 h, average ruminal pH was 5.3 for GLU, which was 10% lower compared with the average pH of MIX (5.9) at these sampling times. The lowest pH for STA (5.6) was similar to that for GLU but occurred between 2 and 4 h after CHO dosing. Reduction of ruminal pH in dairy cows as a result of sugar supplementation was observed by Kim et al. (1999) but not by McCormick et al. (2001) and Osborne et al. (2002).

In Exp. 1, ruminal NH_3 concentration was decreased with the RFNDF diet. The lower (-13%) intake of total dietary N, respectively ruminally degradable N in RFNDF compared with RFSS, was most likely the main reason for this effect. Structural CHO-fermenting ruminal bacteria derive their N exclusively from NH_3 (Russell et al., 1992) and it is possible that enhanced growth of fiber-degrading populations with RFNDF contributed to the reduction in NH_3 concentration with this diet. Data from Exp. 2 indicated the importance of provision of readily fermentable CHO for maximum utilization of ruminal NH_3 N. Ammonia concentration was persistently lower for GLU and STA and slightly more variable for MIX compared with the control, NDF. Apparently, this effect was a result of provision of large amounts of sugar or starch with the former treatments. However, it is possible that the mechanisms of NH_3 reduction were different between GLU and STA. Although both treatments resulted in a significant reduction in ruminal NH_3 concentration and had a similar total microbial N flow to the small intestine, a significantly larger proportion of microbial protein was synthesized from NH_3 N with STA than with GLU, which resulted in a greater flow of microbial N synthesized from NH_3. It is likely that the apparently more rapid degradation of GLU provided an immediate source of energy to the ruminal microorganisms, and feed amino acid N was rapidly utilized without passing through the NH_3 N pool. With STA, a larger proportion of alfalfa protein/amino acid N was broken down and deaminated but eventually incorporated as NH_3 N by the ruminal microorganisms. The decreased concentrations of *iso*-butyrate and *iso*-valerate and decreased irreversible NH_3 N loss and flux with GLU compared with STA support this hypothesis. In the rumen, the branched-chain

VFA (BCVFA) are derived from branched-chain amino acids (BCAA, Wolin et al., 1997). The results from Exp. 2 most likely reflect decreased BCAA concentration in the rumen with GLU compared with the other CHO due to enhanced microbial uptake and/or reduced production. Decreased NH_3 concentration in the rumen has been commonly reported in vitro when CHO are added to the incubation media (Russell et al., 1983; Hristov et al., 1997; Lee et al., 2003). Similarly, NH_3 concentration was decreased in vivo with the addition of glucose or starch (Chamberlain et al., 1985; Heldt et al., 1999; Osborne et al., 2002), sucrose or xylose (Huhtanen, 1987; Khalili and Huhtanen, 1991), and maltodextrin (Kim et al., 1999), however, in some cases sugar addition had no effect (McCormick et al., 2001; Sannes et al., 2002). In vivo studies directly comparing sugar to starch reported lower NH_3 concentration with the former CHO (Chamberlain et al., 1993; Oh et al., 1999).

Comparing diets with different rates of starch degradability in the rumen (barley vs. corn), Casper et al. (1990) found increased ruminal propionate with the barley diet. Similarly, a trend for increased propionate (and butyrate) with diet RFSS was observed in Exp. 1. No other effects on VFA concentrations were found in this experiment. Leiva et al. (2000) also reported no difference in ruminal VFA and lactate concentrations between diets containing soluble fiber (citrus pulp) and starch (corn). Diets, in which brewers grains replaced part of the forage produced greater propionate concentration in the rumen, but had no effect on total VFA concentration (Younker et al., 1998). Pereira and Armentano (2000) found no effect of the addition of non-forage NDF from wheat middlings and brewers grains on ruminal VFA concentrations. Carbohydrate source had a dramatic effect on VFA concentrations in Exp. 2. The GLU treatment drastically decreased acetate and consequently concentration of total VFA in the rumen compared with the other CHO. This reduction does not correspond well with the low pH observed for GLU. Although, lactate was not measured in this study, it seems likely that lactate production and concentration in the rumen may have been increased by GLU. Many ruminal bacteria, particularly fibrolytic species, cannot tolerate low pH (Russell et al., 1992), and the observed reduction in acetate concentration may be a result of decreased activity of structural CHO digestors. Some of the polysaccharide-degrading activities, particularly xylanase activity, were also decreased by GLU. More efficient use of ATP (Strobel and Russell, 1986; Russell, 1992) with GLU can also be partially responsible for the decreased VFA with this treatment. The increased butyrate concentration with GLU is probably indicative of stimulated growth of the major butyrate producer in the rumen, *Butyrivibrio fibrisolvens*. None of these effects were related to changes in protozoal counts. Effects of CHO on VFA concentration and ratios reported in the literature are variable. In a design similar to the present experiment, but with sheep, Chamberlain et al. (1985) found only numerical reduction in the proportion of acetate and numerical increases in the proportions of propionate and butyrate with sugar (glucose or sucrose) supplementation at 13% of DMI. In another experiment from the same study, the authors reported a significant reduction of the molar proportion of acetate and increased proportion of propionate and butyrate with sucrose supplementation. Similar effects of sugar supplementation on acetate and butyrate concentrations in vivo or in vitro were reported by others (Huhtanen, 1987; Khalili and Huhtanen, 1991; Lee et al., 2003), but in many experiments shifts in VFA proportions were not observed (McCormick et al., 2001; Osborne et al., 2002; Sannes et al., 2002).

Both CPM Dairy and NRC (2001) models predicted higher microbial protein flow at the duodenum with RFSS than with RFNDF in Exp. 1, reflecting CHO composition (CPM Dairy) or total digestible nutrients content of the diets (NRC, 2001). However, only numerical difference in the microbial protein flow between the two diets was measured in vivo. Most published work indicates microbial protein synthesis in the rumen is energy-dependent rather than N-dependent. Microbial protein produced in the rumen was found to always be greater when the diet contained greater proportion of nonstructural CHO (Hoover and Stokes, 1991; Shabi et al., 1998). Data from Exp. 2 confirmed these observations. Although GLU, STA, and MIX did not differ in their effect on microbial N outflow from the rumen, the negative control, NDF, resulted in a 23% reduction in MN flow. The flow of bacterial N formed from ruminal NH_3 N was greater (by 33%) for STA than for GLU, which, as discussed earlier, was probably due to effects on energy availability immediately after CHO dosing and deamination/uptake of alfalfa amino acids. In most published research, microbial N flow to the small intestine has been increased with addition of various sugars to the diet (Rooke et al., 1987; Khalili and Huhtanen, 1991; Kim et al., 1999). In one study (Sannes et al., 2002), microbial N flow was decreased by sucrose added at 3.2% of dietary DM, but in that study microbial N flow was determined indirectly (through urinary purine derivative excretion), and the authors had no clear explanation of the observed effect. Microbial protein synthesis in the rumen is primarily a function of availability of energy and N. The basal diet in Exp. 2 contained sufficient amounts of ruminally soluble and available N (from alfalfa hay), but was deficient in available energy (27% non-fiber CHO; NRC, 2001), and it is not surprising that addition of dextrose, starch, or a combination of ruminally available CHO enhanced microbial protein synthesis and microbial N outflow from the rumen.

Ammonia N can leave the rumen through microbial uptake or absorption; comparatively smaller amounts of NH_3 leave the rumen with the fluid digesta phase (Beever, 1996). Microbial utilization of NH_3 in the rumen is a complex process and can vary greatly, primarily depending on dietary factors. Proportions of NH_3-derived bacterial N in the rumen can be as high as 80% (Leng and Nolan, 1984; Siddons et al., 1985; Hristov and Broderick, 1996). In spite of this high affinity, microbial utilization of ruminal NH_3 can be low and variable (Exp. 2). Siddons et al. (1985) reported that 32 and 66% of the irreversible loss of ruminal NH_3 in sheep was through incorporation into microbial N (grass silage and dried grass, respectively). Thus, depending on the diet and type of animal, a significant proportion of the reduction in ruminal NH_3 is due to absorption. Our approach in estimating the proportion of NH_3-^{15}N used for milk protein synthesis was based on the assumption that most of the ruminal NH_3 that is not utilized for synthesis of microbial protein in the rumen will be detoxified in the liver and excreted as urea in the urine, and only a small proportion will be used for synthesis of non-essential amino acids, which can be used for various purposes and may or may not be eventually incorporated into milk proteins. Intravenous infusion of $^{15}NH_4Cl$ in sheep showed that less than 4% of the net ^{15}N transfer across the liver was as glutamate (Lobley et al., 1995) and 80 to 90% of the infused ^{15}N appeared in urea (Lobley et al., 1996). Therefore, absorption and incorporation into microbial protein are responsible for NH_3 N clearance from the rumen; if not captured as microbial protein, most of the NH_3 N absorbed through the ruminal wall would be used for ureagenesis by the liver.

In the two experiments reported here, transfer of NH_3 N into milk protein was measured directly; total excretion of NH_3 N tracer in milk protein was determined gravimetrically. In Exp. 1, more ^{15}N was recovered in milk protein with RFNDF than with RFSS. In agreement, the ^{15}N-AUC in milk protein was larger for RFNDF than for RFSS. The specific ^{15}N-enrichment of bacterial N and the area under the ^{15}N-bacterial N curve were larger with RFSS than with RFNDF, indicating a more intensive incorporation of ^{15}N tracer by RFSS bacteria but also a potentially smaller overall bacterial N pool with this diet compared to RFNDF. Since total milk protein yield was not different between the diets (Hristov and Ropp, 2003), the larger amount of ^{15}N recovered in milk protein from RFNDF cows could be most likely explained with a larger total flow of bacterial N to the small intestine, which in turn was used for milk protein synthesis. This hypothesis, however, was not supported by the similar microbial protein flows or urinary allantoin excretion between the two diets. Methodological problems with the procedures used in this experiment may have prevented detection of existing differences in microbial N flow from the rumen between the diets (see Perez et al., 1997 and Shingfield, 2000).

Due to the lower ruminal NH_3 N concentration and smaller pool size, average ^{15}N enrichment of NH_3 N was greater for GLU compared with some of the other CHO in Exp. 2. Bacterial N formed from NH_3 N ranged from 38 to 60%. The main difference in the proportion of bacterial N synthesized from NH_3 N was between GLU and STA. As discussed earlier, the more rapid release of ruminally fermentable energy with GLU, compared with STA, led to decreased breakdown of alfalfa amino acids and greater uptake of preformed amino acids rather than NH_3 N by the ruminal microorganisms. The more active uptake of NH_3 with STA than with NDF (or MIX) was a result of the greater availability of ruminally fermentable energy with the former treatment. The daily amount of NH_3 N leaving and not returning to the ruminal NH_3 N pool, i.e. the irreversible loss of N from this pool, would represent NH_3 leaving the rumen as microbial N, absorbed through the ruminal wall, and NH_3 outflow with digesta. Due to the decreased uptake of NH_3 N by the ruminal microorganisms, the irreversible loss was significantly lower for GLU than for STA (or NDF). Similarly, the NH_3 N flux through the ruminal NH_3 pool was significantly lower for GLU compared with all other CHO, reflecting decreased NH_3 production with the former CHO. The numerical differences between STA and the NDF-containing treatments also suggest a decreased flux of N through the NH_3 N pool with STA. Although non-significant and variable between cows, NH_3 N recycling data paralleled the trends in NH_3 flux and irreversible loss. Our data indicate that between 23 and 33% of the irreversible NH_3 N loss was with the microbial N leaving the rumen and, respectively, 77 to 67% was due to absorption or outflow with the ruminal fluid phase. Given that estimated proportions of milk protein N originating from bacterial N in Exp. 2 were similar among treatments, the proportions of milk protein N formed from ruminal NH_3 N paralleled the proportion of bacterial N synthesized from NH_3 N data. On average, 55% of milk proteins were synthesized from non-bacterial N sources (similar to the estimate for RFNDF in Exp. 1). The average NAN flow to the duodenum varied from 428 (NDF) to 536 (GLU) g/d, of which microbial N flow was 153 and 197 g/d, respectively. If NRC (2001) efficiency coefficients are used [0.64 and 0.80 for microbial and ruminally undegraded (RUP) N, respectively], these flows represent 98 and 126 g/d of metabolizable protein (MP) N from microbial and 220 and 276 g/d from non-microbial sources (NDF and GLU, respectively). The isotope data from this experiment (Table 6) indicate 42 and 43 g/d milk protein N output from microbial and 48 and 54 g/d from RUP sources for the two diets (NDF and GLU), respectively. Thus, 43 and 34% of the estimated MP flow from microbial protein and 22 and 20% from RUP (NDF and GLU, respectively) were used for synthesis of milk proteins. Milk proteins are synthesized primarily from blood free amino acids, and blood flow dictates the amount of amino acids supplied to the mammary gland (Linzell, 1974). Therefore, the above coefficients may represent the demand for amino acids by the mammary gland, respective to the stage of lactation and level of production of the experimental cows, but could also suggest differences in utilization of metabolizable protein from microbial and RUP sources as well. Raggio et al. (2003) demonstrated that the efficiency of utilization of certain amino acids for milk protein synthesis decreased linearly with increasing metabolizable protein supply. Some authors suggested lower efficiency of utilization of microbial amino acids (due to imbalanced amino acid profile) compared with casein (Cant et al., 1999). Overall, more ruminal NH_3-^{15}N was recovered in milk protein in Exp. 2 with STA than with NDF or GLU, suggesting increased efficiency of utilization of ruminal NH_3 N for milk protein synthesis with the former CHO. A variation of the technique used in this study to determine transfer of ruminal NH_3 N into milk protein was utilized in goats (Petri and Pfeffer, 1987 and Petri et al., 1988). The proportions of milk protein derived from rumen bacterial N found in these studies (from 32 to 49%) were similar to the values estimated for lactating dairy cows in Exp. 1 and 2. From the data of Petri et al. (1988), it can be calculated that, in the lactating goat, from 10 (phosphorus deficient diet) to 13-14% of the irreversible loss of ruminal NH_3 N was recovered in milk protein via microbial protein. These estimates are similar to the 13 and 14% maximum recovery of ^{15}N found in Exp. 1 and the 9 to 10% recoveries found in Exp. 2.

Analysis of a larger dataset (including Exp. 1 and 2; Hristov et al., 2003), indicated high correlation between the cumulative secretion of ^{15}N in milk, milk and milk protein yields ($r = 0.74$ and 0.75, respectively), and MilkNE ($r = 0.93$). Cumulative secretion of ^{15}N in milk protein correlated negatively with N intake and MUN concentration ($r = -0.64$, and -0.80, respectively) and with ruminal NH_3 concentration and urinary N excretion ($r = -0.50$ and -0.42, respectively), but correlation with DMI was positive ($r = 0.62$). Similar to the results from Exp. 1 and 2, this analysis showed that milk yield, protein content of milk, milk protein yield, N intake, the efficiency of utilization of dietary N for milk protein synthesis, and the rate of transfer of ruminal NH_3 N into bacterial N are significant factors influencing the efficiency of utilization of ruminal NH_3 N for milk protein synthesis in dairy cows.

CONCLUSIONS

Data from the two experiments presented here indicate that diets differing in concentration of ruminally available starch and sugars and fiber produced similar level and pattern of fermentation acids and did not affect microbial protein synthesis in the rumen. Increased concentration of ruminally available starch and sugars enhanced ^{15}N-ammonia capture by ruminal bacteria, but overall transfer of ^{15}N-ammonia into milk protein was greater when cows were fed the ruminally fermentable fiber diet. The provision of readily fermentable energy as dextrose or starch in Exp. 2, decreased ammonia levels in the rumen through inhibited production of ammonia and enhanced incorporation of preformed feed amino acids, or through enhanced uptake of ammonia for microbial protein synthesis. Rapidly fermentable in the rumen energy decreases ammonia production, flux, and may decrease ammonia nitrogen cycling, but the overall efficiency of ammonia utilization for milk protein synthesis can only be increased by enhancing ruminal microbial ammonia uptake.

Table 6. Effect of carbohydrate source on ^{15}N enrichment of various N pools and ^{15}N calculations in dairy cows, Exp. 2 (from Hristov et al., 2005)

	Treatment[1]					
Item	**GLU**	**STA**	**NDF**	**MIX**	**SE**	***P*** [2]
^{15}N enrichment of NH_3 N, APE[3]	0.601^{k}	0.468^{l}	0.383^{l}	0.465^{l}	0.0511	0.11
^{15}N enrichment of BN[4], APE	0.086	0.092	0.083	0.086	0.0041	0.48
^{15}N enrichment of MPN[5], APE	0.0068^{l}	0.0075^{k}	0.0065^{l}	0.0065^{l}	0.00035	0.10
AUC[6], NH_3 N	4.55	3.05	3.30	3.74	0.408	0.14
AUC, BN	1.73	1.82	1.57	1.67	0.115	0.51
AUC, MPN	0.77	0.83	0.73	0.72	0.041	0.14
BN from NH_3 N[7], %	38.3^{m}	60.1^{k}	48.3^{l}	47.3^{l}	3.51	0.02
0.5 h post-dose[8], %	9.0^{m}	10.3^{lm}	12.8^{kl}	14.1^{k}	1.08	0.03
MPN from BN[7], %	44.8	46.3	46.3	43.3	1.91	0.65
MPN from NH_3 N[7], %	17.1^{m}	27.7^{k}	22.4^{l}	20.8^{lm}	1.82	0.03
Irreversible loss of ruminal	230^{l}	343^{k}	320^{k}	294^{kl}	26.7	0.09
NH_3 N, g N/d						
As % of N intake	36^{l}	55^{k}	49^{k}	45^{kl}	4.0	0.08
Ruminal NH_3 N flux, g/d	350^{l}	487^{k}	533^{k}	525^{k}	39.1	0.02
As % of intake	55^{l}	77^{k}	80^{k}	80^{k}	5.9	0.04
Recycled NH_3 N, g/d	119	144	213	231	40.4	0.21
Utilization of ruminal NH_3 N for microbial protein synthesis[9], %	33^{k}	33^{k}	23^{l}	30^{k}	2.4	0.05

Regression analysis[10], cumulative milk protein ^{15}N secretion (estimate ± approx. SE)

Maximum ^{15}N secreted,

% of dosed [11] 10.2±2.23 10.3±1.81 8.8±1.55 9.2±0.36

Comparison of predicted lines (except for listed comparisons, lines did not differ among treatments, P = 0.14 to 0.60)

STA vs. GLU, $P = 0.010$

STA vs. NDF, $P = 0.001$

MIX vs. NDF, $P = 0.09$

[1] CHO treatments were: corn dextrose (GLU); corn starch (STA); fiber (NDF, white oat fiber), and a CHO mix (25% of each): apple pectin, GLU, STA, and NDF (MIX).

[2] For main effect.

[3] Atom percent excess.

[4] Bacterial N.

[5] Milk protein N.

[6] Area under the ^{15}N curve, APE × h.

[7] Calculated as: $(AUC_{\text{rumen bacteria}} \div AUC_{\text{rumen ammonia}}) \times 100$; $(AUC_{\text{milk protein}} \div AUC_{\text{rumen bacteria}}) \times 100$; or $(AUC_{\text{milk protein}} \div AUC_{\text{rumen ammonia}}) \times 100$, respectively.

[8] Based on ^{15}N enrichment (APE) of bacterial and NH_3 N at 0.5 h.

[9] Proportion of the irreversible loss of NH_3 N leaving the rumen as microbial N. Calculated as: [(MN flow × proportion of bacterial N derived from NH_3 N) ÷ irreversible loss of NH_3 N] × 100.

[10] Nitrogen-15 secretion in milk (mg) is expressed as percentage of ^{15}N infused in the rumen (mg). Data were fitted to a single rectangular two-parameter hyperbola model.

[11] Theoretical maximum; means did not differ among treatments (P = 0.48 to 0.97).

[k,l,m] Within a row, means without a common superscript letter differ ($P \leq 0.11$).

REFERENCES

[1] Armentano, L. and Pereira, M. (1997) Measuring the effectiveness of fiber by animal response trials. *Journal of Dairy Science* 80, 1416-1425.

[2] Armentano, L. E., Bertics, S. J. and Riesterer, J. (1993) Lack of response to addition of degradable protein to a low protein diet fed to midlaction dairy cows. *Journal of Dairy Science* 76, 3755-3762.

[3] Bach, A., Huntington, G. B., Calsamiglia, S. and Stern, M. D. (2000) Nitrogen metabolism of early lactation cows fed diets with two different levels of protein and different amino acid profiles. *Journal of Dairy Science* 83, 2585-2595.

[4] Bachmann, H. P. and Jans, F. (1995) Feeding can influence cheese quality. *Schweizerische Milchzeitung* 121, 3.

[5] Bates, D. M. and Watts, D. G. (1988) *Nonlinear Regression Analysis and Its Applications*. John Wiley & Sons, NY, pp. 365.

[6] Beever, D. E. (1996) Rumen function. In *Quantitative Aspects of Ruminant Digestion and Metabolism* (J. M. Forbes and France, J., Eds.). CAB International, Wallinford, U.K. pp. 515.

[7] Bohn, K., Clarke, M. A., Buchholz, K., Bliesener, K.-M., Buczys, R., Thielecke, K. and Miehe, D. (1998) Composition of sugarbeet and sugarcane and chemical behavior of constituents in processing. Page 116 in *Sugar Technology. Beet and Cane Sugar Manufacture* (P. W. van der Poel, Schiweck, H. and Schwartz, T., Eds.). Verlag Dr. Albert Bartens KG – Berlin.

[8] Bristow, A. W., Whitehead, D. C. and Cockburn, J. E. (1992) Nitrogenous constituents in the urine of cattle, sheep and goats. *Journal of the Science of Food and Agriculture* 59, 387-394.

[9] Broderick, G. A. and Clayton, M. K. (1997) A statistical evaluation of animal and nutritional factors influencing concentration of milk urea nitrogen. *Journal of Dairy Science* 80, 2964-2971.

[10] Bunting, L. D., Boling, J. A. and MacKown, C. T. (1989) Effect of dietary protein level on nitrogen metabolism in the growing bovine: I. Nitrogen recycling and intestinal protein supply in calves. *Journal of Animal Science* 67, 810-819.

[11] Cant, J. P., Qiao, F. and Toerien, C. A. (1999) Regulation of mammary metabolism. Pages 203-219 in *Protein Metabolism and Nutrition.* G. E. Lobley, White, A. and MacRae, J. C., Eds. EAAP Publication No. 96, Wageningen Press, Wageningen, The Netherlands.

[12] Casper, D. P., Schingoethe, D. J. and Eisenbeisz, W. A. (1990) Response of early lactation dairy cows fed diets varying in source of nonstructural carbohydrate and crude protein. *Journal of Dairy Science* 73, 1039-1050.

[13] Castillo, A. R., Kebreab, E. Beever,D. E., Barbi, J. H., Sutton, J. D., Kirby, H. C. and France, J. (2001) The effect of protein supplementation on nitrogen utilization in lactating dairy cows fed grass silage diets. *Journal of Animal Science* 79, 247-253.

[14] Chamberlain, D. G., Robertson, S. and Choung, J. J. (1993) Sugars versus starch as supplements to grass silage: Effects on ruminal fermentation and the supply of microbial protein to the small intestine, estimated from the urinary excretion of purine derivatives, in sheep. *Journal of the Science of Food and Agriculture* 63, 189-194.

[15] Chamberlain, D. G., Thomas, P. C., Wilson, W., Newbold, C. J. and MacDonald, J. C. (1985) The effect of carbohydrate supplements on ruminal concentrations of ammonia in animals given diets of grass silage. *Journal of Agricultural Science Cambridge* 104, 331-340.

[16] Choi, C. W., Vanhatalo, A., Ahvenjärvi, S. and Huhtanen, P. (2002) Effects of several protein supplements on flow of soluble non-ammonia nitrogen from the forestomach and milk production in dairy cows. *Animal Feed Science and Technology* 102, 15-33.

[17] Christensen, R.A., Lynch, G. L. and Clark, J. H. (1993) Influence of amount and degradability of protein on production of milk and milk components by lactating Holstein cows. *Journal of Dairy Science* 76, 3490-3496.

[18] Dewhurst, R. J., Davies, D. R. and Merry, R. J. (2000) Microbial protein supply from the rumen. *Animal Feed Science and Technology* 85, 1-21.

[19] Dhanoa, M. S., Siddons, R. C., France, J. and Gale, D. L. (1985) A multicompartmental model to describe marker excretion patterns in ruminant feces. *British Journal of Nutrition* 53, 663-671.

[20] Galloway, J. N. and E. B. Cowling. 2002. Reactive nitrogen and the world: The hundred years of change. Ambio 31:64-71.

[21] GfE (Ausschuss für Bedarfsnormen der Gesellschaft für Ernährungsphysiologie)(2001): *Empfehlungen zur Energie- und Nährstoffversorgung der Milchkühe und Aufzuchtrinder*. Energie- und Nährstoffbedarf landwirtschaftlicher Nutztiere, No. 8. DLG-Verlag, Frankfurt am Main, 135 pp.

[22] Heldt, J. S., Cochran, R. C., Mathis, C. P., Woods, B. C., Olson, K. C., Titgemeyer, E. C., Nagaraja, T. G., Vanzant, E. S. and Johnson, D. E. (1999) Effects of level and source of carbohydrate and level of degradable protein on intake and digestion of low-quality tallgrass-prairie hay by beef steers. *Journal of Animal Science* 77, 2846-2854.

[23] Hof, G., Tamminga, S. and Lenaers, P. J. (1994) Efficiency of protein utilization in dairy cows. *Livestock Production Science* 38, 169-178.

[24] Hoover, W. H. and Stokes, S. R. (1991) Balancing carbohydrates and proteins for optimum rumen microbial yield. *Journal of Dairy Science* 74, 3630-3644.

[25] Hristov, A. N. and Broderick, G. (1996) Ruminal microbial protein synthesis in cows fed alfalfa silage, alfalfa hay or corn silage and fitted with only ruminal cannulae. *Journal of Dairy Science* 79, 1627-1637.

[26] Hristov, A. N. and Jouany, J.-P. (2005) Factors affecting the efficiency of nitrogen utilization in the rumen. In: Pfeffer, E. and Hristov, A. N. (eds.) *Nitrogen and Phosphorus Nutrition of Cattle: Reducing the Environmental Impact of Cattle Operations*. CAB International, Wallingford, U.K., pp. 117-166.

[27] Hristov, A. N. and Ropp, J. K. (2003) Effect of dietary carbohydrate composition and availability on utilization of ruminal ammonia nitrogen for milk protein synthesis in dairy cows. *Journal of Dairy Science* 86, 2416-2427.

[28] Hristov, A. N., Etter, R. P., Ropp, J. K. and Grandeen, K. L. (2004a) Effect of dietary crude protein level and degradability on ruminal fermentation and nitrogen utilization in lactating dairy cows. *Journal of Animal Science* 82: 3219-3229..

[29] Hristov, A. N., Huhtanen, P., Rode, L. M., McAllister, T. A. and Acharya, S. N. (2001) Comparison of ruminal metabolism of nitrogen from ^{15}N-labeled alfalfa preserved as hay or as silage. *Journal of Dairy Science* 84, 2738-2750.

[30] Hristov, A. N., McAllister, T. A. and Cheng, K. J. (1997) Effect of carbohydrate level and ammonia availability on utilization of α-amino nitrogen by mixed ruminal microorganisms in vitro. *Proceedings, Western Section, American Society of Animal Science* 48, 186-189.

[31] Hristov, A. N., Price, W. J. and Shafii, B. (2004b) A meta-analysis examining the relationship among dietary factors, dry matter intake, and milk yield and milk protein yield in dairy cows. *Journal of Dairy Science* 87, 2184-2196.

[32] Hristov, A. N., Ropp, J. K., Grandeen, K. L., Abedi, S., Etter, R. P., Melgar, A. and Foley, A. E. (2005) Effect of carbohydrate source on ruminal fermentation and nitrogen utilization in lactating dairy cows. *Journal of Animal Science* 83:408-421.

[33] Hristov, A. N., Ropp, J. K., Grandeen, K. L., Etter, R. P., Foley, A., Melgar, A. and Price, W. (2003) Efficiency of utilization of ruminal ammonia N for milk protein synthesis in dairy cows. In *Progress in research on energy and protein metabolism*, EAAP publication No. 109, W.B. Souffrant and C.C. Metges, Eds., Wageningen Academic Publishers, pp. 601-604.

[34] Huhtanen, P. (1987) The effects of intraruminal infusions of sucrose and xylose on nitrogen and fibre digestion in the rumen intestines of cattle receiving diets of grass silage and barley. *Journal of Agricultural Science in Finland* 59, 405-424.

[35] Huntington, G. B. (1989) Hepatic urea synthesis and site and rate of urea removal from blood of beef steers fed alfalfa hay or a high concentrate diet. *Canadian Journal of Animal Science* 69, 215-223.

[36] Huntington, G. B. and Archibeque, S. L. (1999) Practical aspects of urea and ammonia metabolism in ruminants. *Proceedings of the Americal Society of Animal Science*, 1-11.

[37] Isaacson, H. R., Hinds, F. C., Bryant, M. P. and Owens, F. N. (1975) Efficiency of energy utilization by mixed rumen bacteria in continuous culture. *Journal of Dairy Science* 58, 1645-1659.

[38] Johnson, R. R. (1976) Influence of carbohydrate solubility on non-protein nitrogen utilization in the ruminant. *Journal of Animal Science* 43, 184-191.

[39] Kebreab, E., France, J., Beever, D. E. and Castillo, A. R. (2001) Nitrogen pollution by dairy cows and it's mitigation by dietary manipulation. *Nutrient Cycling in Agroecosystems* 60, 275-285.

[40] Kerchner, M., Halloran, R., Thomas, J. and Hicks, B. (2000) Airsheds and watersheds III: A shared resources workshop. The significance of ammonia to coastal and estuarine areas. Nov. 15-16, 2000. The Bay Center at Ruddertowne Dewey Beach, Delaware.

[41] Khalili, H. and Huhtanen, P. (1991) Sucrose supplement in cattle given grass silage-based diet. 1. Digestion of organic matter and nitrogen. *Animal Feed Science and Technology* 33, 247-261.

[42] Kim, K.H., Choung, J and Chamberlain, D. G. (1999) Effects of varying the degree of synchrony of energy and nitrogen release in the rumen on the synthesis of microbial protein in lactating dairy cows consuming a diet of grass silage and a cereal-based concentrate. *Journal of the Science of Food and Agriculture* 79, 1441-1447.

[43] Koenig, K. M., Newbold, C. J., McIntosh, J. F. and Rode, L. M. (2000) Effects of protozoa on bacterial nitrogen recycling in the rumen. *Journal of Animal Science* 78, 2431-2445.

[44] Külling, D. R., Menzi, H., Kröber, T. F., Neftel, A., Sutter, F., Lischer, P. and Kreuzer, M. (2001) Emissions of ammonia, nitrous oxide and methane from different types of

dairy manure during storage as affected by dietary protein content. *Journal of Agricultural Science, Cambridge* 137, 235-250.

[45] Lee, M. R. F., Merry, R. J., Davies, D. R., Moorby, J. M., Humphreys, M. O., Theodorou, M. K., Mac Rae, J. C. and Scollan, N. D. (2003) Effect on increasing availability of water-soluble carbohydrates on in vitro rumen fermentation. *Animal Feed Science and Technology* 104, 59-70.

[46] Leiva, E., Hall, M. B. and Van Horn, H. H. (2000) Performance of dairy cattle fed citrus pulp or corn products as sources of neutral detergent-soluble carbohydrates. *Journal of Dairy Science* 83, 2866-2875.

[47] Leng, R. A. and Nolan, J. V. (1984) Nitrogen metabolism in the rumen. *Journal of Dairy Science* 67, 1072-1089.

[48] Linzell, J. L. 1974. Mammary blood flow and methods of identifying and measuring precursors in milk. Pages 143-225 in *Lactation: A comprehensive Treatise.* Vol. 1. B. L. Larson and Smith, V. R., Eds. Academic Press, New York and London.

[49] Lobley, G. E., Connell, A., Lomax, M. A., Brown, D. S., Milne, E., Calder, A. G. and Farningham. D. A. H. (1995) Hepatic detoxification of ammonia in the ovine liver: possible consequences for amino acid catabolism. *British Journal of Nutrition* 73, 667-685.

[50] Lobley, G. E., Weijs, P. J. M., Connell, A., Calder, A. G., Brown, D. S. and Milne, E. (1996) The fate of absorbed and exogenous ammonia as influenced by forage or forage-concentrate diets in growing sheep. *British Journal of Nutrition* 76, 231-248.

[51] MacRae, J. C., Backwell, F. R. C., Bequette, B. J. and Lobley, G. E. (1995) Protein metabolism in specific organs. In: Nunes, A. F., Portugal, A. V., Costa, J. P. and Robeiro, J. R. (eds.) *Proceedings of the 7th EAAP Symposium on Protein Metabolism and Nutrition.* EAAP Publication No. 81, J. Vale de Santarem, Portugal: Estacao Zootechnica Nacional, p. 297.

[52] Martin, B., Coulon, J. B., Chamba, J. F. and Bugaud, C. (1997) Effect of milk urea content on characteristics of matured Reblochon cheese. *Lait* 77, 505-514.

[53] Mathison, G.W. and Milligan L.P. (1971) Nitrogen metabolism in sheep. *British Journal of Nutrition* 25, 351-366.

[54] McCormick, M. E., Redfearn, D. D., Ward, J. D. and Blouin, D. C. (2001) Effect of protein source and soluble carbohydrate addition on rumen fermentation and lactation performance of Holstein cows. *Journal of Dairy Science* 84, 1686-1697.

[55] McCubbin, D. R. 2002. Animal feeding operations, ammonia, and nitrogen particles and their effect on human health. *In* Nitrogen Losses to the Atmosphere from Livestock and Poultry Operations. 6th Discover Conference on Food Animal Agriculture, April 28 – May 1, 2002, Abe Martin Lodge, Nashville, Indiana.

[56] McDougall, E. I. (1948) The composition and output of sheep's saliva. *Biochemical Journal* 43, 99-109.

[57] Metcalf, J. A., Wray-Cahen, D., Chettle, E. E., Sutton, J. D., Beever, D. E., Crompton, L. A., MacRae, J. C., Bequette, B. J. and Backwell, F. R. C. (1996) The effect of dietary CP as protected soybean meal on mammary metabolism in the lactating dairy cow. *Journal of Dairy Science* 79, 603-611.

[58] Miner, J. R., F. J. Humenik, and M. R. Overcash. 2000. Managing Livestock Waste to Preserve Environmental Quality. Iowa State University Press, Ames, Iowa.

[59] Monteny, G. J., Smits, M. C. J., van Duinkerken, G., Mollenhorst, H and de Boer, I. J. M. (2002) Prediction of ammonia emission from dairy barns using feed characteristics part II: Relation between urinary urea concentration and ammonia emission. *Journal of Dairy Science* 85, 3389-3394.
[60] Moorby, J. M. and Theobald, V. J. (1999) Short communication: The effect of duodenal ammonia infusions on milk production and nitrogen balance of the dairy cows. *Journal of Dairy Science* 82, 2440-2442.
[61] Newbold, J. R. and Rust, S. R. (1992) Effects of asynchronous nitrogen and energy supply on growth of ruminal bacteria in batch culture. *Journal of Animal Science* 70, 538-546.
[62] NKJ Protein Group (1985) Introduction of the Nordic protein evaluation system for ruminants into practice and future research requirements. Proposals by the NKJ protein group. *Acta Agriculture Scandinavica* 25 (Suppl.), 216-220.
[63] Nocek, J. E. and Russell, J. B. (1988) Protein and energy as an integrated system. Relationship of ruminal protein and carbohydrate availability to microbial synthesis and milk production. *Journal of Dairy Science* 71, 2070-2107.
[64] Nolan, J. V. and Leng, R. A. (1974) Isotope techniques for studying the dynamics of nitrogen metabolism in ruminants. *Proceedings of the Nutrition Society* 33,1-8.
[65] NRC (2001), National Research Council. *Nutrient requirements of dairy cattle.* Seventh Revised Edition. National Academy Press, Washington, D.C.
[66] Oh, Y. G., Kim, K. H., Kim, J. H., Choung, J. J. and Chamberlain, D. G. (1999) The effect of the form of nitrogen in the diet on ruminal fermentation and the yield of microbial protein in sheep consuming diets of grass silage supplemented with starch or sucrose. *Animal Feed Science and Technology* 78, 227-237.
[67] Oldham, J. D., Bruckental, I. and Nissenbaum, A. (1980) Observations on rumen ammonia metabolism in lactating dairy cows. *Journal of Agriculture Science Cambridge* 95, 235-238.
[68] Osborne, V. R., Leslie, K. E. and McBride, B. W. (2002) Effect of supplementing glucose in drinking water on the energy and nitrogen status of the transition dairy cows. *Canadian Journal of Animal Science* 82, 427-433.
[69] Pereira, M. N. and Armentano, L. E. (2000) Partial replacement of forage with nonforage fiber sources in lactating cow diets. II. Digestion and rumen function. *Journal of airy Science* 83, 2876-2887.
[70] Perez, J. F., Balcells, J., Guada, J. A. and Castrillo, C. (1997) Contribution of dietary nitrogen and purine bases to the duodenal digesta – comparison of duodenal and polyester-bag measurements. *Animal Science* 65, 237-245.
[71] Petri, A. and Pfeffer, E. (1987) Changes of ^{15}N enrichment in N of rumen ammonia, rumen bacteria and milk protein during and following continuous intraruminal infusion of $^{15}NH_4Cl$ to goats. *Journal of Animal Physiology and Animal Nutrition* 57, 75-82.
[72] Petri, A., Müschen, H., Breves, G., Richter, O. and Pfeffer, E. (1988) Response of lactating goats to low phosphorus intake 2. Nitrogen transfer from the rumen ammonia to rumen microbes and proportion of milk protein derived from microbial amino acids. *Journal of Agricultural Science (Cambridge)* 111, 265-271.
[73] Powers, W. J., Van Horn, H. H., Harris, Jr., B. and Wilcox, C. J. (1995) Effects of variable sources of distillers dried grains plus solubles on milk yield and composition. *Journal of Dairy Science* 78, 388-396.

[74] Raggio, G., Lobley, G. E., Pacheco, D., Pellerin, D., Allard, G., Berthiaume, R., Dubreuil, P. and Lapierre, H. (2003) Effect of different levels of metabolizable protein on splanchnic fluxes of amino acids in lactating cows. Pages 223-226 In *Progress in Research on Energy and Protein Metabolism.* W. B. Souffrant and Metges, C. C., Eds. EAAP Publication No. 109, Wageningen Press, Wageningen, The Netherlands.

[75] Reynal, S.M. and Broderick, G. A. (2003) Effects of feeding dairy cows protein supplements of varying ruminal degradability. *Journal of Dairy Science* 86, 835-843.

[76] Rooke, J. A.,Lee, N. H. and Armstrong, D. G. (1987) The effects of intraruminal infusion of urea, casein, glucose syrup and a mixture of casein and glucose syrup on nitrogen digestion in the rumen of cattle receiving grass-silage diets. *British Journal of Nutrition* 57, 89-98.

[77] Russell, J. B. (1992) Glucose toxicity and the inability of *Bacteroides ruminicola* to regulate glucose transport and utilization. *Applied and Environmental Microbiology* 58, 2040-2045.

[78] Russell, J. B., O'Connor, J. D., Fox, D. G., Van Soest, P. J. and Sniffen, C. J. (1992) A net carbohydrate and protein system for evaluating cattle diets: I. Ruminal fermentation. *Journal of Animal Science* 70, 3551-3561.

[79] Russell, J.B., Sniffen, C.J. and Van Soest, P.J. (1983) Effect of carbohydrate limitation on degradation and utilization of casein by mixed rumen bacteria. *Journal of Dairy Science* 66, 763-775.

[80] Sannes, R. A., Messman, M. A. and Vagnoni, D. B. (2002) Form of rumen-degradable carbohydrate and nitrogen on microbial protein synthesis and protein efficiency of dairy cows. *Journal of Dairy Science* 85, 900-908.

[81] Santos, F. A. P., Santos, J. E. P., Theurer, C. B. and Huber, J. T. (1998) Effects of rumen-undegradable protein on dairy cow performance: A 12-year literature review. *Journal of Dairy Science* 81, 3182-3213.

[82] Satter, L. D., Klopfenstein, T. J. and Erickson, G. E. (2002) The role of nutrition in reducing nutrient output from ruminants. *Journal of Animal Science* 80 (E. Suppl. 2), E143-E156.

[83] Sauvant, D. and van Milgen, J (1995) Dynamic aspects of carbohydrate and protein breakdown and the associated microbial matter synthesis. In: Engelhardt, W. v., Leonhard-Marek, S., Breves, G. and Giesecke, D. (eds.) *Ruminant Physiology: Digestion, Metabolism, Growth and Reproduction.* Ferdinand Enke Verlag, Stuttgart, Germany, pp. 71-91.

[84] Shabi, Z., Arieli, A., Bruckental, I., Aharoni, Y., Zamwel, S., Bor, A. and Tagari, H. (1998) Effects of the synchronization of the degradation of dietary crude protein and organic matter and feeding frequency on ruminal fermentation and flow of digesta in the abomasum of dairy cows. *Journal of Dairy Science* 81, 1991-2000.

[85] Shingfield, K. J. (2000) Estimation of microbial protein supply in ruminant animals based on renal and mammary purine metabolite excretion. A review. *Journal of Animal and Feed Sciences* 9, 169-212.

[86] Siddons, R. C., Nolan, J. V., Beever, D. E. and MacRae, J. C. (1985) Nitrogen digestion and metabolism in sheep consuming diets containing contrasting forms and levels of N. *British Journal of Nutrition* 54, 175-187.

[87] Strobel, H. J. and Russell, J. B. (1986) Effects of pH and energy on bacterial protein synthesis by carbohydrate-limited cultures of mixed rumen bacteria. *Journal of Dairy Science* 69, 2941-2947.

[88] Tamminga, S. (1992) Nutrition management of dairy cows as a contribution to pollution control. *Journal of Dairy Science* 75, 345-357.

[89] Tamminga, S., van Straalen, W. M., Subnel, A. P. J., Meijer, R. G. M., Steg, A., Wever, C. J. G. and Blok, M. C. (1994) The Dutch protein evaluation system: the DVE/OEB system. *Livestock Production Science* 40, 139-155.

[90] Tamminga, S., Van Vuuren, A. M., Van der Koelen, C. J., Ketelaar, R. S. and Van der Togt, P. L. (1990) Ruminal behavior of structural carbohydrates, non-structural carbohydrates and crude protein from concentrate ingredients in dairy cows. *Netherlands Journal of Agricultural Science* 38, 513-526.

[91] Tomlinson, A. P., Van Horn, H. H., Wilcox, C. J. and Harris, Jr., B. (1994) Effects of undegradable protein and supplemental fat on milk yield and composition and physiological responses of cows. *Journal of Dairy Science* 77, 145-156.

[92] Wilkerson, V. A., Mertens, D. R. and Caster, D. P. (1997) Prediction of excretion of manure and nitrogen by Holstein dairy cows. *Journal of Dairy Science* 80, 3193-3204.

[93] Wolin, M. J., Mikker, T. L. and Steward, C. S. (1997) Microbe-microbe interactions. Pages 467-491 in *The Rumen Microbial Ecosystem*. P. N. Hobson and C. S. Steward, eds. Blackie Academic and Professional, London, U.K.

[94] Wu, Z. and Satter, L. D. (2000) Milk production during the complete lactation of dairy cows fed diets containing different amounts of protein. *Journal of Dairy Science* 83, 1042-1051.

[95] Younker, R. S., Winland, S. D., Firkins, J. L. and Hull, B. L. (1998) Effects of replacing forage fiber or nonfiber carbohydrates with dried brewers grains. *Journal of Dairy Science* 81, 2645-2656.

In: Trends in Dietary Carbohydrates Research
Editor: M. V. Landlow, pp. 141-177
ISBN 1-59454-798-X

Chapter 7

EFFECT OF CARBOHYDRATE SUPPLEMENTATION ON PERFORMANCE IN RATS EXPOSED TO HYPOBARIC HYPOXIA

Alka Chatterjee[1*], Shashi Bala Singh[2], and W. Selvamurthy[3]
[1]Directorate of Life Sciences, DRDO Headquarters, Chanakya Puri, New Delhi, India
[2]Defence Institute of Physiology and Allied Sciences, Timarpur, New Delhi, India
[3]Defence Research & Development Organisation Headquarters, New Delhi, India

ABSTRACT

The effect of a carbohydrate supplement, offered as a diet option, on feeding behavior, body weight gain and endurance exercise was studied in young and old rats exposed to hypobaric hypoxia. Male albino rats (n=47) were randomly divided into hypoxic supplemented and control groups; and a normoxic control group. They were trained to run in the Runimex for 5 days, and subsequently, the hypoxic groups were exposed to simulated high altitude equivalent to 6096 m for 11 days continuously. Food and water intakes, body weight and exercise performance were recorded before and during the exposure period. Blood glucose, and muscle and liver glycogen levels were assayed at the end of the exposure period. Blood samples were taken at the end of the exposure period for total cholesterol, HDL-Cholesterol, LDL-Cholesterol and triglyceride levels. Hypobaric hypoxia resulted in a significant decrease in food and water intakes, body weight, and blood glucose and a deterioration in exercise performance compared to the basal and normoxic group values. With the exception of one supplemented group that showed a significant decrease, there was no significant change in the total cholesterol during the hypoxic exposure. HDL-Cholesterol concentrations were significantly decreased by the end of the exposure period in all the hypoxic groups. The VLDL-Cholesterol + LDL-Cholesterol concentrations were significantly decreased in the older batch while it was significantly increased in the younger batch of animals. The plasma triglycerides showed a tendency to decrease in all the groups. The carbohydrate supplement did not ameliorate the hypoxia-induced loss in body weight, but however,

---

* E-mail: alka_cz@yahoo.com; Telephone: 26881095; Fax: 26889905

significantly ameliorated the decrement in performance in the supplemented rats compared to the hypoxic control group.

Key words: high altitude, feeding behavior, carbohydrate supplementation, exercise, lipids, weight loss

INTRODUCTION

The number of people traveling to the mountains for recreation and adventure has risen in the last few years. In the case of Armed Forces personnel, tenure at high altitude (HA) is a professional necessity. The inherent problems of the mountains viz; Acute Mountain Sickness (AMS) with its associated symptoms like reduced food intake, headache, nausea, dizziness, insomnia etc are also encountered by sojourners.

For the Armed Forces personnel, it is these initial days at altitude that are crucial during operations and a gradual or slow ascent (during which AMS could be avoided) is not always possible. Thus, the typical scenario existing under such conditions would be: a decreased food intake (Consolazio *et al*, 1969; Hannon *et al*, 1976; Rose *et al*, 1988); when in fact energy requirements are increased (Butterfield et al, 1992); concomitant with negative energy balance (Consolazio *et al*, 1972; Reynolds *et al*, 1992) reduced work capacity (Cymerman *et al*, 1989; Pugh *et al*; 1964,) and weight loss (Pugh, 1962; Consolazio *et al*, 1968; Boyer and Blume, 1984; Butterfield *et al*, 1992; Kayser, 1994).

The stresses of HA pose a severe problem in nutrition as evidenced by the feeding behavior of experimental animals under hypoxic stress. Under resting condition in rats, acute exposure to moderate and well tolerated, high altitude hypoxia inhibits both food and water intakes by mechanisms which are not fully understood (Schnakenberg, 1971; Singh *et al*, 1996; 1997a). This altitude-induced hypophagia (Hannon *et al*, 1976; Boyer and Blume, 1984; Rose *et al*, 1988; Guilland and Klepping, 1985; Askew 1989) and the resultant body weight loss (Butterfield *et al*, 1992; Kayser, 1994) have been the focus of many studies over the years. Food intakes are usually reduced by 10-50% during acute altitude exposure. Numerous attempts have been made to reverse this anorexia and hypophagia, but most have met with limited success. Access to desired foodstuffs in a chamber study also did not meet with success (Rose *et al*, 1988).

Anecdotal reports in literature cite the preference of carbohydrates over fats at high altitude (Gill and Pugh, 1964), and a distaste for fat (Richalet, 1983). Singh *et al*, (1996; 1997a) have also reported a preference for sweet-tasting (carbohydrate) solutions over other taste stimuli in rats subjected to hypoxic stress. They also reported similar preferences in human volunteers abruptly inducted to HA (Singh *et al*, 1997b). High-carbohydrate diets have been recommended as a 'non-pharmacological' method to reduce the symptoms associated with AMS and improve performance (Askew *et al*, 1989). High-carbohydrate diets have been shown to increase lung pulmonary diffusion capacity (Dramise *et al*, 1975), increase alveolar and arterial oxygen pressure (Hansen *et al*, 1972) and improve endurance during altitude acclimatization (Young *et al*, 1982).

At altitude, if sufficient food is consumed to cover energy needs, either by force or by strong encouragement and cafeteria-choice option, the metabolic responses of the body differ from that of an inadequately fed individual (Butterfield *et al*, 1996). The basal energy needs continue to be increased in the inadequately fed individuals, diuresis is minimized, and body weight and composition are maintained. Thus, weight loss at altitude may not be inevitable after all, and it's acceptance as such may have lead to the erroneous or misinterpretation of certain data. For e.g. The commonly accepted theory that the fuel of choice during exercise at altitude changes from carbohydrate (CHO) to fat with acclimatization (Young *et al*, 1982) is based on inferential measures of intact muscle glycogen stores and increased circulating levels of free fatty acids, glycerol and triglycerides. Similar circumstances are also encountered in starvation. Thus, Butterfield *et al*, 1996 argue that as most of the individuals previously studied were in negative energy balance, it was not unexpected that they would be utilizing body stores of fat as a predominant energy source.

In support of this, Brooks *et al*, (1991a), found that in men fed sufficient energy to cover energy needs, the primary source of energy appeared to be CHO, specifically glucose, after three weeks of acclimatization to 4,300 m. Similar results have been obtained by Roberts *et al* (1996a, b). Therefore, GE Butterfield, (1996), strongly recommended the consumption of a special high-calorie, nutrient-dense, palatable high-Carbohydrate, moderate protein and fat supplement providing 500 Kilocalories to help in ameliorating the hypophagia and meeting the increased need at altitude.

The feeding of high sugar diets promotes overeating and obesity in laboratory animals (Sclafani, 1987). When fed as a diet option, in the form of a solution, rats consume nearly 60% of their calories as sugar and increase their total calorie intake by 10-25% compared to control rats (Castonguay, 1981).

The goals of the present study were to ascertain whether a CHO supplement, offered as a diet option in addition to the normal diet would promote feeding and thus ameliorate high altitude induced body weight loss, to evaluate the ergogenic potential of the CHO supplement in physical and mental performance at high altitude, and also to evaluate the effects on lipid metabolism and hepatic function. All these responses were studied in young and old rats in a bid to compare the effects.

Materials and Methods

The experiments were carried out in two batches of rats. Male albino Sprague-Dawley rats, were obtained from the animal house of the Institute. The rats were bred and maintained at the animal house facility of the Defence Institute of Physiology and Allied Sciences, (DIPAS), Delhi. The rats were housed in polypropylene cages (30 x 22 x 14 cm), with a stainless steel grill, and paddy husk was used as bedding material. The bedding was changed on alternate days. The colony was maintained in a well-aerated room with a 12:12 hours light: dark cycle. The rats were housed singly. All the experimental procedures were carried out in accordance with the guidelines of the Ethical Committee of DIPAS.

Batch I : These animals (n=27), weight (250 ± 20 g), age (180 ± 10 days) were randomly divided into three groups viz., Normoxic Controls (NC, n=7); Hypoxic Control (HC, n=10), Hypoxic Experimental (HE, n=10). These rats comprised the old batch.

Batch II: These animals (n=20), weight (150 ± 20 g), age (90 ± 5 days) were randomly divided into two groups, viz., Hypoxic Control (HC, n=10), and Hypoxic Experimental (HE, n=10). These rats comprised the young batch.

Diet

The rat diet consisted of food pellets (Amrut Laboratory Animal Feeds, Pranav Agro Industries, Ltd). The calorific value of the feed was 3.41 Kilocalories / gram. Food and water were provided *ad libitum* except when food and water intakes were being measured. The food pellets were provided in a metal cup of 120-g capacity fitted with an anti-scatter rim to prevent spillage. The water was provided in 50-ml graduated glass bottles.

The diet consisted of the following components by weight: Crude Protein-21 %, fat - 5 %, Carbohydrate-53 %, Crude fiber- 4 %, Ash- 8 %, Calcium- 1 %, Phosphorus-0.6 %, and a complete vitamin supplement.

Diet Supplementation

Diet supplementation was done using a 32 % glucose solution in drinking water. Dextrose anhydrous, AR grade, was used to prepare the supplement and only the HE groups received the supplement. The remaining control groups (NC, HC) received the commercial chow only. The supplement was prepared fresh every second day and was administered in graduated 25-ml glass bottles.

Animal Environmental Chamber

The environmental chamber provided a means of studying the effects of chronic hypobaric hypoxia under controlled conditions of temperature and humidity and consisted of an exposure chamber, barometric pressure, temperature and humidity control unit, vacuum pumps, and a video camera and monitor screen to monitor the behaviour of the experimental animals.

Thus, HA conditions could be simulated by evacuating the chamber by means of powerful vacuum pumps and then maintaining the atmospheric pressure inside the chamber by appropriate inlet/ outlet valve manipulations. The temperature in the chamber was maintained at 32 ± 0.5 °C. The relative humidity inside the chamber was maintained at 50 % and fresh air was allowed to flow into the chamber at a rate of 5.5 L /m.

Runimex Setup

The Runimex is a circular runway, for testing rat or mouse endurance, and for performing 'one-way', two-way and 'either-way' avoidance tests. An IBM -PC/XT/AT or compatible computer is used as a controller for automatic presentation of stimuli and collection of results. Eight infrared beams spaced evenly around the perimeter of the runway detect the location of the animal. The floor consists of closely spaced rods, which are connected to an adjustable intensity shock generator. Eight lamps around the runway present visual stimulus to the animal, and a variable intensity sound source presents auditory stimulus. When used as an animal endurance tester, the animal is required to interrupt the infrared beams at a preset frequency to avoid being shocked. If the animal fails to interrupt the next beam within the required time, a sound stimulus warns the animal, and then a shock is delivered. The animal's average speed, distance traveled, time running, time resting and number of shock stimuli initiated are continuously updated on the computer display. Upto 2 hours conditioning is required to condition the animal to the equipment.

Even though active /passive avoidance tests were not carried out, the number of shock stimuli initiated per 100 cm traveled is a reliable indicator of the mental performance, particularly memory-related learning ability.

After one week of training, the basal endurance of all the rats was determined and all the rats were run at the same time of day. The hypoxic groups were then exposed to chronic hypobaric hypoxia equivalent to 6096 m (20,000 ft) in the specially designed and fabricated environmental chamber hypoxia for 10 consecutive days for 21 hrs daily (from 1200 hrs to 0900 hrs the next morning).

The animals were gradually exposed to reduced barometric pressure until the equivalent altitude of 6096 m (280 mm Hg) was achieved. The rats were brought to sea-level conditions every morning and this three hour period was used to replenish their food and water supplies and also to record the various parameters like food and water intakes, body weights, exercise endurance, and blood sample collection, as the protocol dictated. All the rats were given food and water inside the chamber during the exposure period. At the end of the exposure session each day, the hypoxic experimental group was administered the CHO supplement in their respective cages in addition to water. These supplement bottles were withdrawn just before the animals were restored to the chamber at 1200 hrs every day. The normoxic and untreated control groups were maintained at ambient pressure and altitude (220 m) in individual cages. During the exposure period, all the rats were regularly exercised for fixed time interval of 20 min/session.

Blood was withdrawn from the retro-orbital venous plexus under ether anesthesia between 0930 and 1000 hrs for blood glucose estimations. Blood was collected in heparinized tubes and then subsequently centrifuged. Aliquots of the plasma were stored at -70 °C till they were assayed for the various biochemical parameters.

At the termination of exposure, the rats were sacrificed by decapitation and muscle and liver samples were taken for glycogen estimations. The blood samples were collected before the start of hypoxic exposure (PE), during the first week of exposure (E I) and the second week of exposure (E II).

The protocol of the study is outlined in Chart 1.

Variables Studied

Food Intake

The food intake was recorded daily at the same time in the mornings. The food intake was recorded to the second decimal place. The food intakes are expressed as g intake/100 g body weight. The food intakes were then subsequently expressed as Kilocalories/100 g body weight of the animals.

Body Weight

Body weight was recorded every day. The animals were placed in a tared plastic 1000-ml beaker and their weights recorded to the second decimal place, and expressed in grams.

Chart 1: Experimental protocol for batches I and II

Days	Parameters recorded	Experimental conditions	
		HE HC	NC
(Training) 1. P E 2. R - X 3. E P 4 O 5 S 6 U 7 R E	• Food Intake • Body Weight • Plasma Glucose • Lipid Profile • Hepatic Function • Physical Performance • Mental Performance	Normoxia Temp. = 27± 0.5 °C RH = 50 %	Normoxia Temp. = 27± 0.5°C RH = 50 %
8 E 9 X 10 P 11 O 12 S 13 U 14 R E	• Food Intake • Body Weight • Plasma Glucose • Lipid Profile • Hepatic Function • Physical Performance • Mental Performance	Simulated hypoxia [Approx. 20,000 ft] Temp. = 32± 0.5°C RH = 50 %	Normoxia Temp. = 27± 0.5°C RH = 50 %
15 E 16 X 17 P 18 O S U R E	• Food Intake • Body Weight • Plasma Glucose • Lipid Profile • Hepatic Function • Physical Performance • Mental Performance	Simulated hypoxia [Approx. 20,000 ft] Temp. = 32± 0.5°C RH = 50 %	Normoxia Temp. =27± 0.5°C RH = 50 %
19 End of exposure [Animals sacrificed]	• Muscle Glycogen • Liver Glycogen	----	----

* CHO supplement administered to HE group only.

CHO Supplement Intake

The 32% CHO supplement intake was also measured daily. It was administered in graduated 25-ml glass bottles. It was prepared fresh every second day. The CHO supplement intake was expressed as ml ingested/100 g body weight and after determining the calorific value was added to the food intake to obtain the total energy intake expressed as Kilocalories/100 g body weight.

Exercise Endurance (Physical Performance) and Mental Performance

The endurance performance was evaluated using a Runimex (Columbus Instruments, USA). The animals were exercised on the Runimex using a fixed time interval of 20 minutes.

All the variables are reported as averages for one minute. The number of shock stimuli initiated per 100 cm traveled was taken as an indicator of the mental performance, particularly memory-related learning ability.

Blood Measurements

Blood Glucose

Blood glucose estimations were done by an enzymatic colorimetric method using kits obtained from Ranbaxy. The kit was based on the GOD-POD method of Trinder (1969).

Glycogen Content of Muscle and Liver

Tissue preparation and assay method: Immediately after decapitation, the muscles of the hind limb were skinned and rapidly exposed. A sample of muscle tissue was excised and immediately placed in pre-weighed tubes containing 30 % KOH chilled on ice. Following this, a midsagittal incision was made in the abdomen of the animals and a portion of the lateral lobe of the liver was excised and immediately freeze-clamped in a similar fashion. The glycogen content of the muscle and liver was determined by the method of Montgomery (1957).

Total Plasma Cholesterol

Total plasma cholesterol was estimated by the enzymatic colorimetric method using QualiTEST® assay kits (Rashmi Diagnostics Pvt. Ltd., India) as per the protocol.

Plasma HDL-Cholesterol

HDL- cholesterol levels were estimated by the enzymatic colorimetric method using QualiTEST® assay kits (Rashmi Diagnostics Pvt. Ltd., India) as per the protocol.

For calculation of LDL cholesterol Friedwald Formula was used [LDL =(TC)-(HDL)-TG/5].

Plasma LDL and VLDL-Cholesterol

Plasma LDL and VLDL-Cholesterol concentrations were calculated by the difference of Total-cholesterol and HDL- cholesterol.

Plasma Triglycerides

The plasma triglycerides were estimated by the enzymatic method using QualiTEST® assay kits (Rashmi Diagnostics Pvt. Ltd., India) as per the protocol.

Plasma ALT

The plasma alanine aminotransferase activity was estimated by the enzymatic method using QualiTEST® assay kits (Rashmi Diagnostics Pvt. Ltd., India) as per the protocol.

Plasma AST

The plasma aspartate aminotransferase activity was estimated by the enzymatic method using QualiTEST® assay kits (Rashmi Diagnostics Pvt. Ltd., India) as per the protocol.

Plasma LDH

The plasma lactate dehydrogenase activity was estimated by the enzymatic method using QualiTEST® assay kits (Rashmi Diagnostics Pvt. Ltd., India) as per the protocol.

STATISTICAL ANALYSIS

Statistical analysis was done by subjecting all the variables to 2-way ANOVA with multiple comparison testing done using the Student's Newman-Keul's test.

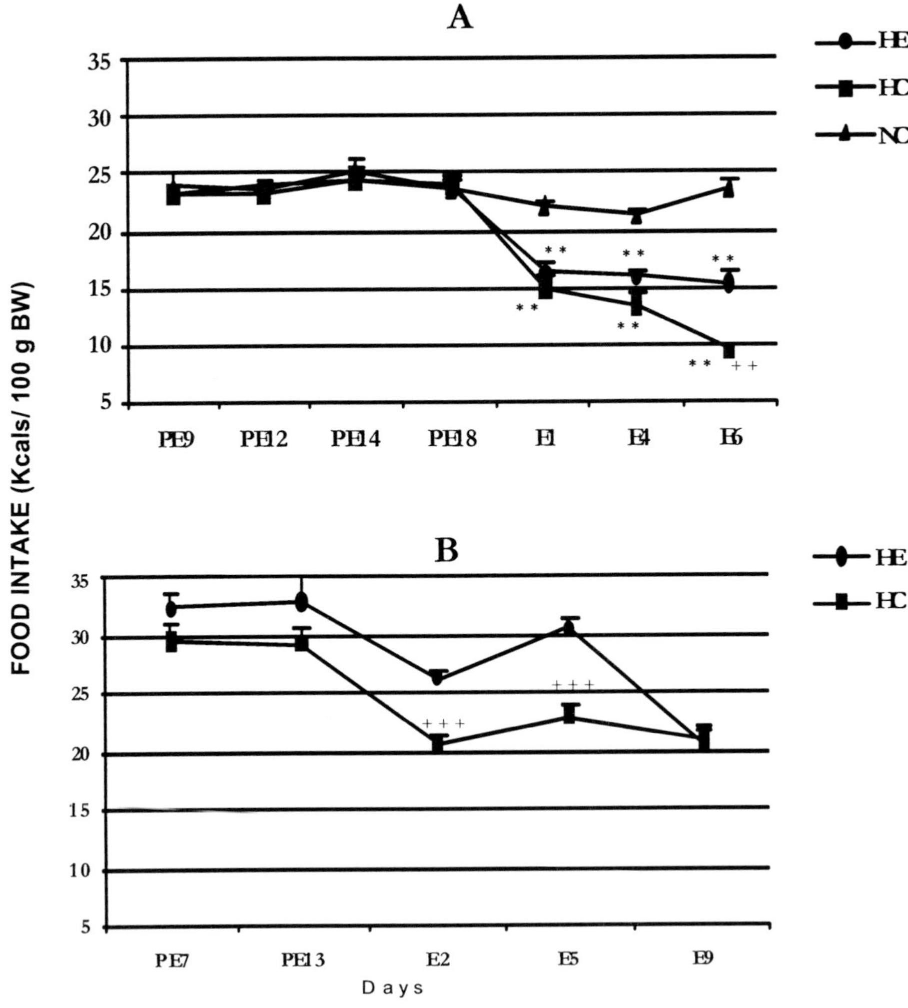

Figure 1: Effect of Hypobaric Hypoxia on food intakes of Control and CHO-supplemented rats of Batches I [A] and II [B]. ** P<0.01, significantly different compared to NC; ++ P< 0.01, significantly different compared to corresponding HE value; +++ P<0.001, significantly different compared to corresponding HE value.

RESULTS

Batch I

Food Intake

The food intake of the hypoxic (HE and HC) groups was significantly reduced ($p < 0.001$) in comparison with either their pre-exposure intakes or the intake of the normoxic group throughout the exposure period. Compared to the normoxic rats and also their pre-exposure intake, the daily food intakes of the Hypoxic Experimental rats were lower by 36.22 % and that of the Hypoxic Control group by 60.6 % by the end of the 1st week. Further, there was a significant difference in the food intakes of the Hypoxic Experimental and Hypoxic Control groups by the end of the first week [Figure 1A].

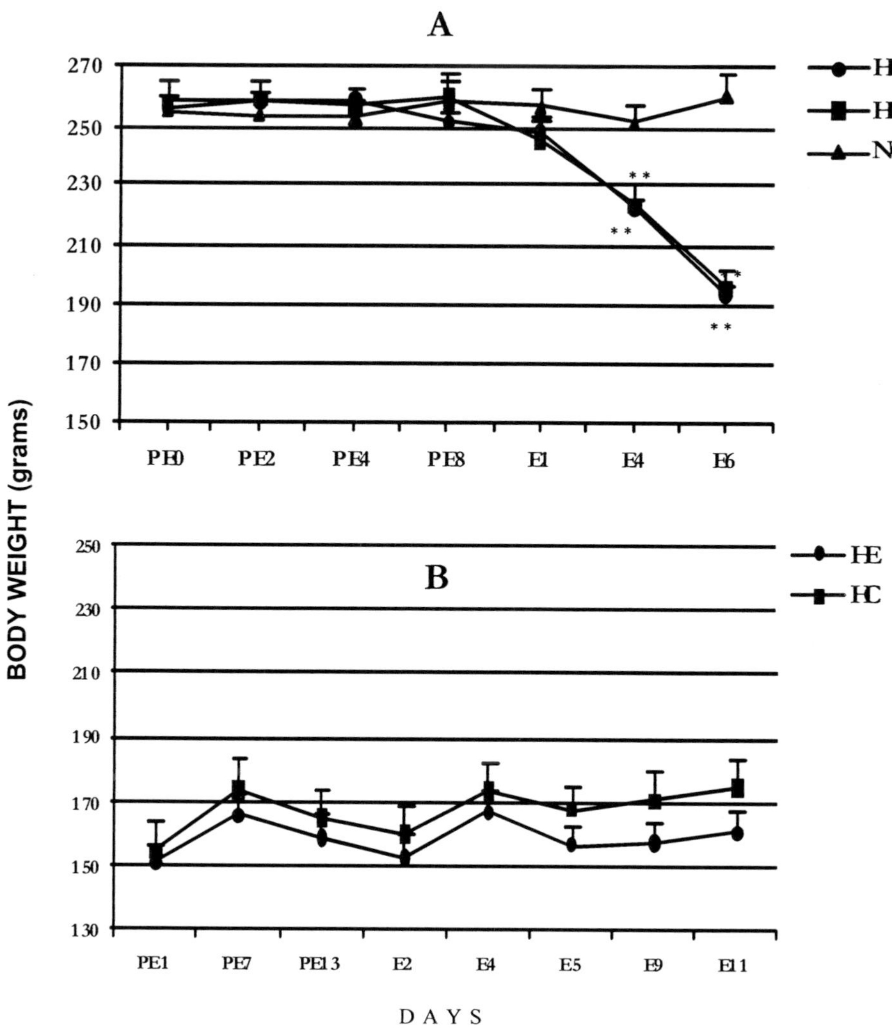

Figure 2: Effect of Hypobaric Hypoxia on Body Weight of Control and CHO-supplemented rats of Batches I [A] and II [B]. ** $P<0.01$, significantly different compared to corresponding NC value

Body Weight

The body weights of the hypoxic (HE and HC) groups during the first week of HA exposure were significantly reduced ($p < 0.001$) in comparison with their pre-exposure weights. [Figure 2]. The CHO-supplemented (HE) group had a 23 % and the Hypoxic Control group, 25 % loss of body weight by day 6 (first week) of the exposure and 29 % and 35.5 % loss respectively, by the end of the exposure period. The CHO supplement however, did not have any protective effect on the body weight as the Hypoxic Experimental group continued to lose weight in a similar fashion as the Hypoxic Control group. This was borne out by the fact that, the Hypoxic Experimental group consumed the same amount of calories as the Hypoxic Control group, by reducing the amount of chow to compensate for the CHO solution consumed. The normoxic group had a marginal and non-significant weight gain during the comparative exposure period [Figure 2 A].

Exercise Endurance Performance and Mental Performance

Hypobaric hypoxic exposure significantly reduced ($p < 0.05$) the endurance capacity of the Hypoxic Control group compared to either it's basal value (PE) or the Hypoxic Experimental and Normoxic Control groups [Table 1]. The CHO-supplemented group recorded significantly greater speed ($p < 0.05$), greater distance traveled ($p < 0.05$), longer run times ($p < 0.05$), and shorter rest times ($p < 0.05$) than the Hypoxic Control group after one week of HA exposure (E I); and greater distance traveled ($p<0.05$), longer run times ($p<0.01$), and shorter rest times ($p<0.05$) by the second week of exposure (E II) [Table 1].

Table 1: Effect of CHO supplementation during first and second weeks of exposure to hypobaric hypoxia on physical performance – batch I

Group	Endurance variables	PE	E I	E II
HE	Speed (cm/sec)	11.98 ± 1.89	11.57 ± 1.16	15.97 ± 1.87
	Distance (cm)	720.99 ± 117.2	689.38 ± 70.44	906.38 ± 148.68
	Run Time (sec)	53.41 ± 1.56	50.95 ± 2.22	51.6 ± 2.08
	Rest Time (sec)	5.51 ± 1.41	8.85 ± 2.26	6.9 ± 1.56
	Stimuli (no.)	16.39 ± 1.2	11.84 ± 0.7*	8.49 ± 1.92*
HC	Speed (cm/sec)	10.47 ± 0.8	7.03 ± 1.2**	10.61 ± 1.61
	Distance (cm)	648.72 ± 47.22	404.18 ± 69.31**	493.13 ± 75.07**
	Run Time (sec)	52.61 ± 1.41	31.02 ± 4.44**	37.68 ± 4.51**
	Rest Time (sec)	5.61 ± 0.87	24.92 ± 3.77**	17.35 ± 4.82**
	Stimuli (no.)	12.29 ± 1.16	9.1 ± 1.01	9.66 ± 0.94
NC	Speed (cm/sec)	12.37 ± 1.56	14.36 ± 1.62	14.02 ± 1.02
	Distance (cm)	727.26 ± 94.07	834.02 ± 89.66	873.2 ± 81.49
	Run Time (sec)	52.73 ± 1.42	54.98 ± 0.95	54.93 ± 1.04
	Rest Time (sec)	5.45 ± 1.27	3.85 ± 0.4	5.02 ± 1.12
	Stimuli (no.)	11.9 ± 1.14	10.45 ± 1.07	12.23 ± 1.18

Values are Means ± SEM, n=7

* Significantly different from corresponding HE values ($p<0.05$)

** Significantly different from corresponding HE and NC values ($p<0.05$)

In the case of the Hypoxic Experimental group, there was no significant difference in either the speed, distance traveled, run time, or rest time at the three different time periods viz., PE (pre-exposure), E I (during the first week of exposure), and E II (second week of exposure) [Table 2]. The number of shock stimuli avoided, however, were significantly ($p < 0.05$) increased at E I and E II in comparison to pre-exposure values.

Table 2: Effect of hypoxia on physical performance of CHO-supplemented (HE) rats of batch I

Variables	PE	E 1	E II
Speed cm/sec	12.99 ± 2.99	12.11 ± 1.71	15.97±1.87
Distance cm	784.03± 186.74	721.34± 104.17	906.38± 148.68
Run time sec	53.48 ± 2.49	51.56± 2.54	51.6± 2.08
Rest time sec	5.94± 2.29	8.16 ± 2.53	6.90 ± 1.56
Stimuli No.	16.80 ± 1.73	12.51± 1.03	9.49 ±1..92

Values are : Mean ± SEM, n = 7

Variables	Over all	PE vs E I	PE vs E II	E I vs E II
Speed cm/sec	NS	---	---	---
Distance cm	NS	---	---	---
Run time sec	NS	---	---	---
Rest time sec	NS	---	---	---
Stimuli No.	P< 0.05	NS	P< 0.05	NS

Table 3: Effect of hypoxia on physical performance of hypoxic control (HC) rats of batch I

Variables	PE	E 1	E II
Speed cm/sec	10. 55 ± 1.24	6.04 ± 1.34	10. 61 ± 1.61
Distance cm	626.37 ± 67. 36	350.15 ± 81. 98	493.13 ± 75.07
Run time sec	52.69 ± 2.41	28.34 ± 5.90	37.68 ± 4.51
Rest time sec	5.46 ± 1.39	26.54 ± 5.09	17.35 ± 4.82
Stimuli No.	12.23 ± 1.88	8.17 ± 1.54	9.66 ± 0.94

Values are : Mean ± SEM, n = 7

Variables	Over all	PE vs E I	PE vs E II	E I vs E II
Speed cm/sec	NS	---	---	---
Distance cm	NS	---	---	---
Run time sec	P< 0.05	P< 0.05	P< 0.05	NS
Rest time sec	P< 0.05	P< 0.05	NS	NS
Stimuli No.	NS	NS	---	---

When the performance of the Hypoxic Control group was compared between the different time periods viz., pre-exposure, during the first week (E I), and second week of HA exposure (E II), a significant deterioration in performance was observed with respect to run time and rest time duration ($p<0.05$) [Table 3]. There was no significant difference in the endurance parameters recorded in the Normoxic Control group [Table 4].

There was deterioration in the mental performance of the HC group during hypoxia as seen in the increase in number of shocks initiated per unit distance traveled, whereas the HE group performed significantly better ($p<0.05$) than HC [Table 5].

Table 4: Physical performance of normoxic control (NC) rats of batch I

Variables	PE	E 1	E II
Speed cm/sec	12.56 ± 2.11	14.36 ± 1.92	14.02 ± 1.02
Distance cm	728.08 ± 124.08	834.02 ± 106.09	873.2 ± 81.49
Run time sec	52.31 ± 1.48	54.97 ± 1.13	54.93 ± 1.04
Rest time sec	6.16 ± 1.53	3.83 ± 0.48	5.02 ± 1.12
Stimuli No.	12.38 ± 1.11	10.45 ± 1.27	12.23 ± 1.18

Values are : Mean ± SEM, n = 7

Variables	OVER ALL	PE vs E I	PE vs E II	E I vs E II
Speed cm/sec	NS	---	---	---
Distance cm	NS	---	---	---
Run time sec	NS	---	---	---
Rest time sec	NS	---	---	---
Stimuli	NS	---	---	---

Table 5: Effect of hypoxia on mental performance in control and CHO-supplemented groups of batch I

Condition / Group	PE	E I	E II
HE	2.27 ± 0.458	1.902 ± 0.234	1.188 ± 0.269
HC	1.75 ± 0.296	2.525 ± 0.257	2.161 ± 0.349
NC	1.75 ± 0.201	1.30 ± 0.165	1.468 ± 0.225

Values are : Mean ± SEM, n = 7

	HE vs HC	HE vs NC	HC vs NC
PE	NS	NS	NS
E I	NS	NS	P < 0.05
E II	P < 0.05	P < 0.05	P < 0.05

Blood Glucose

The blood glucose levels of the hypoxic (Experimental and Control) groups during HA exposure were significantly lower ($p< 0.01$ and $p< 0.05$ respectively) in comparison to their pre-exposure values [Figure 3A]. The blood glucose levels of the Hypoxic Experimental (supplemented) group decreased by 18.64 % ($p<0.05$) from a pre-exposure value of 99.84 ± 4.28 mg/dl during the first week (E I). In the second week (E II), it had dropped by 32.27 % from the pre-exposure value ($p<0.01$). Similarly, the blood glucose levels of the Hypoxic Control group declined by 33.95 % during the second week (E II) from a pre-exposure value of 96.38 ± 2.48 mg/dl. The same trend was seen in the Normoxic Control group also, with a 23.22 % decrease from 95.53 ± 3.1 mg/dl ($p < 0.05$) [Figure 3A]. There was, however no significant difference in the blood glucose levels between the different groups at the three different time periods (PE, E I and E II).

Plasma Total Cholesterol

Plasma [TC] in both hypoxic groups decreased over time throughout the study [Figure 4A]. After 10 days (E II) of exposure to 6096 m, plasma [TC] of Hypoxic Experimental (supplemented) was 66.77 ± 5.48 mg/dl representing a 37 % decrease compared to basal (PE) values ($p < 0.01$). Plasma [TC] of the Hypoxic Control group after 10 days at HA was 75.02 ± 6.52 mg / dl representing a 28 % decrease which was not significant however. The plasma [TC] of the Normoxic Control group increased by 14 % from a pre-exposure value of 96.93 ± 2.67 mg/dl ($p < 0.05$) after 3 days (E I) and thereafter declined by 12 % ($p < 0.05$) to 84.76 ± 3.22 mg/dl after 10 days (E II) [Figure 4].

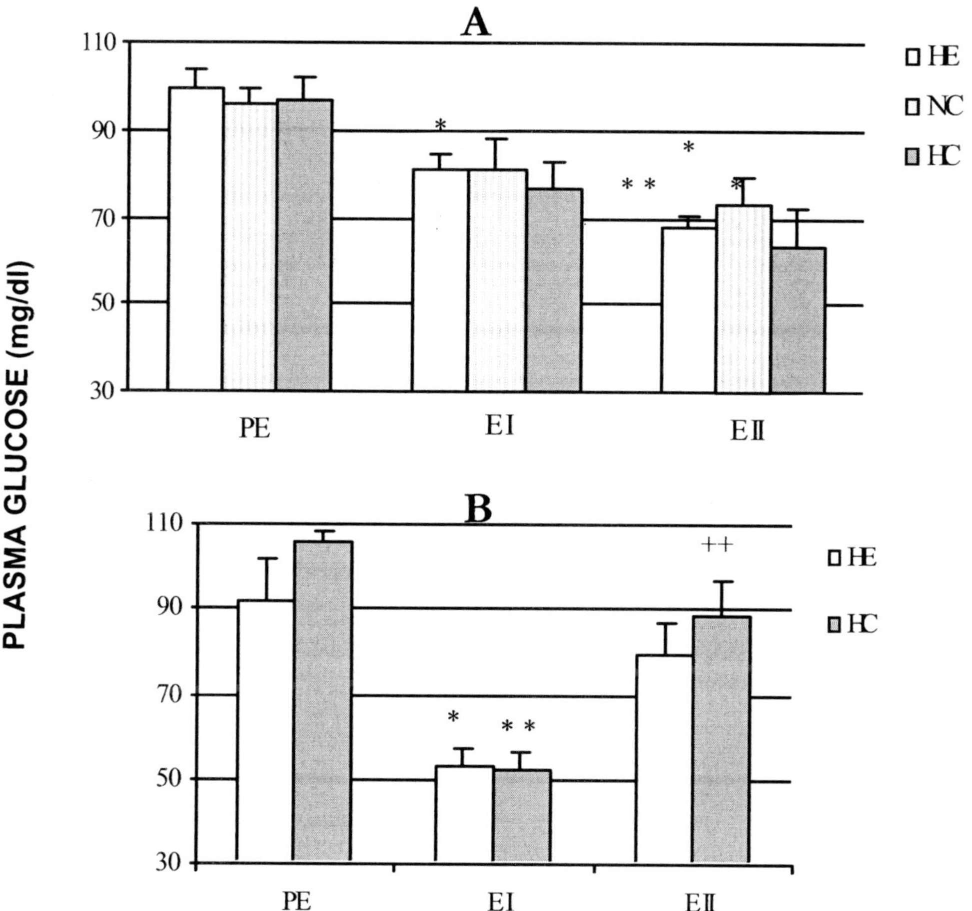

Figure 3: Effect of Hypobaric Hypoxia on Blood Glucose in Control and CHO-supplemented rats of Batches I [A] and II [B]. * P<0.05, significantly different compared to PE value; ** P<0.01, significantly different compared to PE value; ++ P< 0.01, significantly different compared to corresponding EI value.

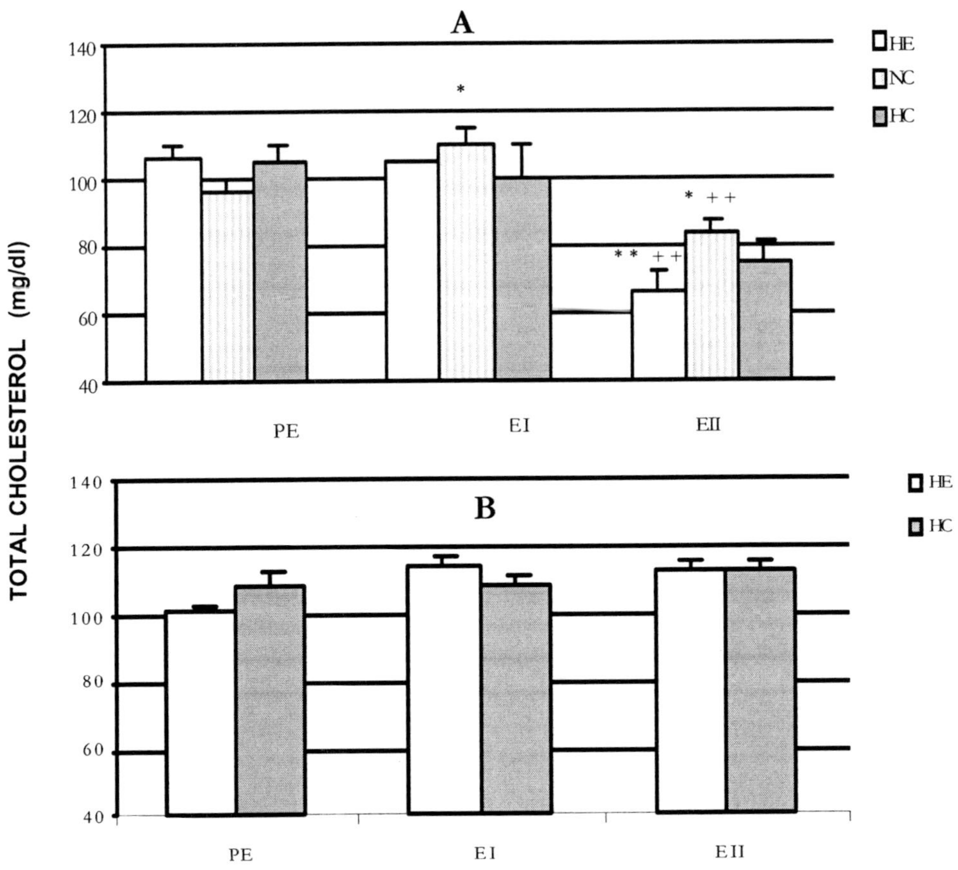

Figure 4: Effect of Hypobaric Hypoxia on plasma Total Cholesterol in Control and CHO-supplemented rats of Batches I [A] and II [B]. * $P<0.05$, significantly different compared to PE value; ** $P<0.01$, significantly different compared to PE value; ++ $P< 0.01$, significantly different compared to corresponding EI value;

Plasma [HDL-Cholesterol] and [VLDL + LDL-Cholesterol]

A similar decline was observed in the plasma [HDL-C] [Figure 5A] and plasma [VLDL + LDL-C] [Figure 6A] in Hypoxic Experimental (supplemented) group. The pre-exposure value of [HDL-C] and [VLDL + LDL-C] averaged 41.12 ± 4.24 mg/dl and 65.65 ± 4.04 mg/dl respectively. After 10 days at 6960 m, plasma [HDL-C] and [VLDL + LDL-C] were decreased by 19 and 18 % respectively to 33.39 ± 6.74 mg/dl and 33.82 ± 6.92 mg/dl respectively ($p< 0.01$). Plasma [HDL-C] of the HC group increased by 55 % from a basal value of 33.21 ± 2.93 mg/dl ($p< 0.05$) after 3 days at HA and by day 10, had declined to 35.80 ± 6.11 mg/dl. Plasma [VLDL + LDL-C] in the Hypoxic Control group showed a sharp decline during the first week, decreasing 33 % from a pre-exposure value of 71.76 ± 3.96 mg/dl ($p< 0.05$) and further decreasing during the second week by 45 % to 39.23 ± 6.13 mg/dl ($p< 0.05$). Plasma [HDL-C] in the Normoxic Control group increased from a pre-exposure value of 35.71 ± 2.09 mg/dl by 31 % to 51.56 ± 3.2 mg/dl ($p< 0.01$) after 3 days and were still elevated at 43.21 ± 1.92 mg/dl by the end of the experiment. In the Normoxic Control group, basal plasma [VLDL + LDL-C] (61.20 ± 2.49 mg/dl) declined to 58.81 ± 5.57

mg/dl in the first week, and further by 32 % to 41.89 ± 4.26 mg/dl ($p < 0.05$) by the second week.

Plasma Triglycerides

The plasma [TG] of all the groups declined over time [Figure 7A]. Plasma [TG] of both Hypoxic Experimental and Hypoxic Control declined by 30 % from pre-exposure values of 115.28 ± 9.54 mg / dl and 106.66 ± 5.14 mg / dl to 81.3 ± 15.74 mg /dl and 74.63 ± 5.89 mg / dl respectively, by the end of exposure. The plasma [TG] of the Normoxic Control group declined by 22 % from a pre-exposure value of 134.96 ± 11.88 mg / dl to 105.2 ± 14.53 mg / dl till the end of the experimental period. None of these decreases were significant, however.

Plasma Aspartate Aminotransferase

The plasma AST values of the Hypoxic Control group rose significantly by 69.28 % ($p < 0.05$) by the second week (E II) from a pre-exposure value of 12.6 ± 2.34 IU/L, while those of the Hypoxic Experimental and Normoxic Control groups did not register any significant change [Figure 8A].

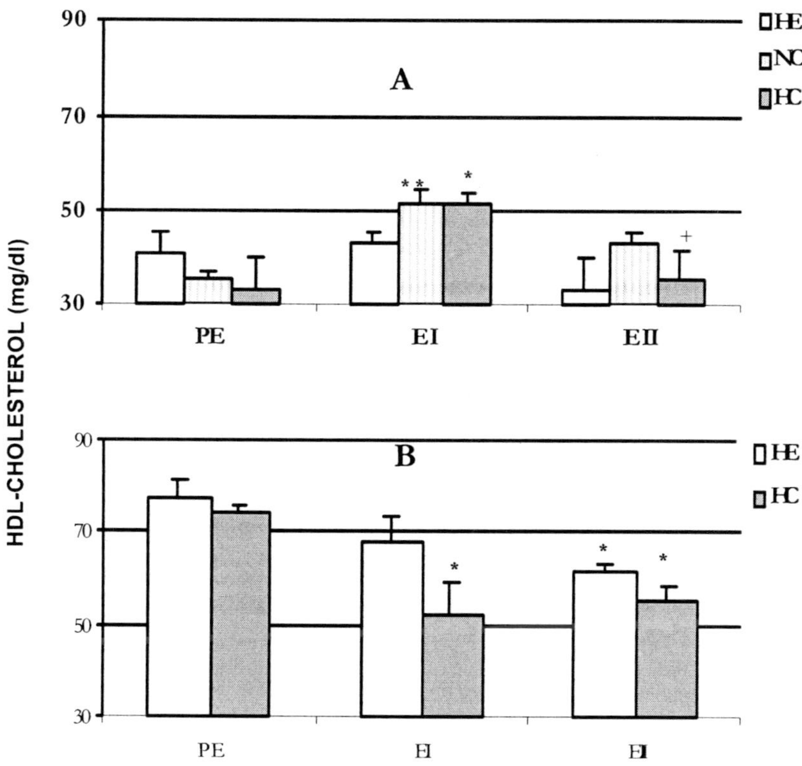

Figure 5: Effect of Hypobaric Hypoxia on Plasma HDL-Cholesterol in Control and CHO-supplemented rats of Batches I [A] and II [B]. * $P<0.05$, significantly different compared to PE value; ** $P<0.01$, significantly different compared to PE value; + $P< 0.05$, significantly different compared to corresponding EI value;

Plasma Alanine Aminotransferase

There was no significant change in the plasma ALT activity in any of the three groups throughout the study [Figure 9A].

Plasma Lactate Dehydrogenase

Plasma lactate dehydrogenase activity in both Hypoxic Control and Normoxic Control groups was raised significantly ($p < 0.01$) by the first week (E I) from a basal value of 80.95 ± 16.84 IU/L to 316.15 ± 56.26 IU/L, while it remained unchanged in case of the Hypoxic Experimental group [Figure 10A].

Muscle and Liver Glycogen

The muscle glycogen of the Hypoxic Experimental group was significantly higher ($p < 0.05$) compared to the Hypoxic Control group while there was no difference between the muscle glycogen values of the Hypoxic Experimental and Normoxic Control groups [Figure 11A]. The liver glycogen values of the Hypoxic Experimental and Normoxic Control groups were also higher than the Hypoxic Control values.

Batch II

This batch consisting of two groups viz. Hypoxic Experimental (supplemented), and Hypoxic Control, was subjected to hypobaric hypoxia ≅ 6096 m for 11 days continuously. These animals (n=20) were young rats, (age- 90 ± 5 days), weighing 150 ± 10 g.

Food Intake

The food intake of the both the groups was significantly reduced ($p < 0.001$) in comparison with their pre-exposure intakes and was apparent from day 2 of exposure itself [Figure 1B]. The Hypoxic Control group registered a 28.36 % drop in food intake by the end of the exposure period compared to the pre-exposure values whereas the Hypoxic Experimental group had a 38.42 % decrease in food intake compared to the pre-exposure values. The Hypoxic Experimental group consumed significantly more ($p < 0.001$) calories compared to the Hypoxic Control group on days 2 and 5 of the exposure period.

Body Weight

The body weights of both the groups showed considerable fluctuations throughout the exposure period, and did not show a significant decrease when compared to the last day of pre-exposure [Figure 2B]. In fact, they steadily increased throughout the exposure and were significantly higher on days 4, 9 and 11 of exposure compared to the second day. The Experimental and Control groups had a 4.6 and 6.1 % gain in body weight respectively from the last pre-exposure value throughout the 11-day exposure period.

Exercise Endurance Performance and Mental Performance

There was no significant difference in any of the parameters of endurance (running speed, distance traveled, running time, rest time and number of shock stimuli avoided) at the three different time periods in both the groups; i.e., the slight deterioration in performance of both the groups under hypoxic stress was not significantly different from the basal values [Tables 6, 7].

Table 6 : Effect of CHO supplementation in first and second weeks of exposure to hypobaric hypoxia on physical performance – batch II

Group	Endurance variables	PE	E I	E II
HE	Speed (cm/sec)	± 0.5	11.21 ± 1.15	± 1.41
	Distance (cm)	735.68 ± 43.35	659.71 ± 65.25	760.46 ± 84.85
	Run Time (sec)	53.2 ± 1.58	52.86 ± 4.08	51.43 ± 2.77
	Rest Time (sec)	6.43 ± 1.67	6.94 ± 4.09	± 2.71
	Stimuli (no.)	12.2 ± 1.26	10.38 ± 1.91	8.21 ± 1.69
HC	Speed (cm/sec)	± 0.63	± 1.07	± 1.82
	Distance (cm)	652.47 ± 39.46	± 72.15*	581.46 ± 110.01
	Run Time (sec)	51.57 ± 1.90	38.53 ± 5.39*	40.95 ± 3.99*
	Rest Time (sec)	8.20 ± 1.97	20.28 ± 4.93	18.92 ± 3.95*
	Stimuli (no.)	10.87 ± 1.46	8.74 ± 1.05	11.82 ± 1.63

Values are Means ± SEM, n= 10

* Significantly different from corresponding HE values ($p<0.05$)

Table 7. Effect of hypoxia on physical performance of CHO-supplemented (HE) rats of batch II

Variables	PE	E 1	E II
Speed cm/sec	11.75 ± 0.50	11.21 ± 1.15	12.72 ± 1.41
Distance cm	735.68 ± 43. 35	659.71 ± 65.25	760.46 ± 84.85
Run time sec	53.2 ± 1.58	52.86 ± 4.08	51.43 ± 2.77
Rest time sec	6.43 ± 1.67	6.94 ± 4.09	8.15 ± 2.71
Stimuli No.	12.20 ± 1.26	10.39 ± 1.91	8.21 ± 1.69

Values are : Mean ± SEM, n = 10

Variables	Over all	PE vs E I	PE vs E II	E I vs E II
Speed cm/sec	NS	---	---	---
Distance cm	NS	---	---	---
Run time sec	NS	---	---	---
Rest time sec	NS	---	---	---
Stimuli No.	NS	---	---	---

However, in comparison to Hypoxic Control, the Hypoxic Experimental group logged a significantly greater ($p< 0.05$) distance covered, longer run times in the first week; and significantly longer ($p< 0.05$) run times and lower rest times during the second week [Table 8].

Mental performance as seen by number of shocks initiated per unit distance traveled deteriorated during the hypoxic exposure period when compared to the corresponding pre-exposure values. The supplemented group avoided significantly more shocks ($p<0.05$) compared to the Control group during exposure [Table 9].

Table 8: Effect of hypoxia on physical performance of hypoxic-control (HC) rats of batch II

Variables	PE	E 1	E II
Speed cm/sec	11.01 ± 0.63	8.09 ± 1.08	9.81 ± 1.82
Distance cm	652.47 ± 39.46	453.31 ± 72.15	581.46 ± 110.01
Run time sec	51.47 ± 1.90	38.53 ± 5.39	40.95 ± 3.99
Rest time sec	8.20 ± 1.97	20.28 ± 4.93	18.92 ± 3.95
Stimuli No.	10.87 ± 1.46	8.74 ± 1.05	11.82 ± 1.63

Values are : Mean ± SEM, n = 10

Variables	Over all	PE vs E I	PE vs E II	E I vs E II
Speed cm/sec	NS	---	---	---
Distance cm	NS	---	---	---
Run time sec	NS	---	---	---
Rest time sec	NS	---	---	---
Stimuli No.	NS	---	---	---

Table 9 : Effect of hypoxia on mental performance in control and CHO-supplemented groups of batch II

Condition / Group	PE	E I	E II
HE	1.76 ± 0.246	1.73 ± 0.386	1.256 ± 0.361*
HC	1.68 ± 0.23	2.174 ± 0.264	2.387 ± 0.291

Values are : MEAN ± SEM, n = 10

* Significantly different from corresponding hc value (P < 0.05)

Blood Glucose

The blood glucose levels of the Hypoxic (Experimental and Control) groups during hypoxic exposure were significantly reduced ($p < 0.05$ and $p < 0.001$ respectively) in comparison with their pre-exposure values [Figure 3B]. The blood glucose levels of the Hypoxic Experimental group decreased by 42.4 % from a pre-exposure value of 91.98 ± 10.15 mg/dl to 53.12 ± 4.35 mg/dl in the first week, and was still depressed by 14 % by the second week (79.22 ± 8.01 mg/dl). Similarly, the blood glucose levels of the Hypoxic Control group decreased by 50.4 % from a pre-exposure value of 105.53 ± 3.23 mg/dl to 52.26 ± 4.38 mg/dl in the first week and recovered to 88.22 ± 8.19 mg/dl by the second week.

Plasma Cholesterol

Plasma [TC] of both the groups did not register any significant change during the exposure period with the plasma [TC] levels of both groups rising marginally during the exposure period [Figure 4B]. There was no significant difference between the [TC] levels of the two groups during the exposure period.

Plasma [HDL-C]

Plasma [HDL-C] of both groups declined significantly (p< 0.05) over the exposure period, with the Hypoxic Experimental group registering a lower decline [Figure 5B]. Basal plasma [HDL-C] of the Hypoxic Experimental group (77.49 ± 3.62 mg/dl) declined to 67.68 ± 5.64 mg/dl by the first week (E I) and further declined by 21 % to 61.08 ± 2.25 mg/dl (p< 0.05) by the end of the exposure period. The Hypoxic Control group on the other hand showed a decline of 26 % (p< 0.05) from pre-exposure concentrations of 73.94 ± 1.73 mg/dl to 54.99 ± 3.88 mg/dl by the end of the exposure.

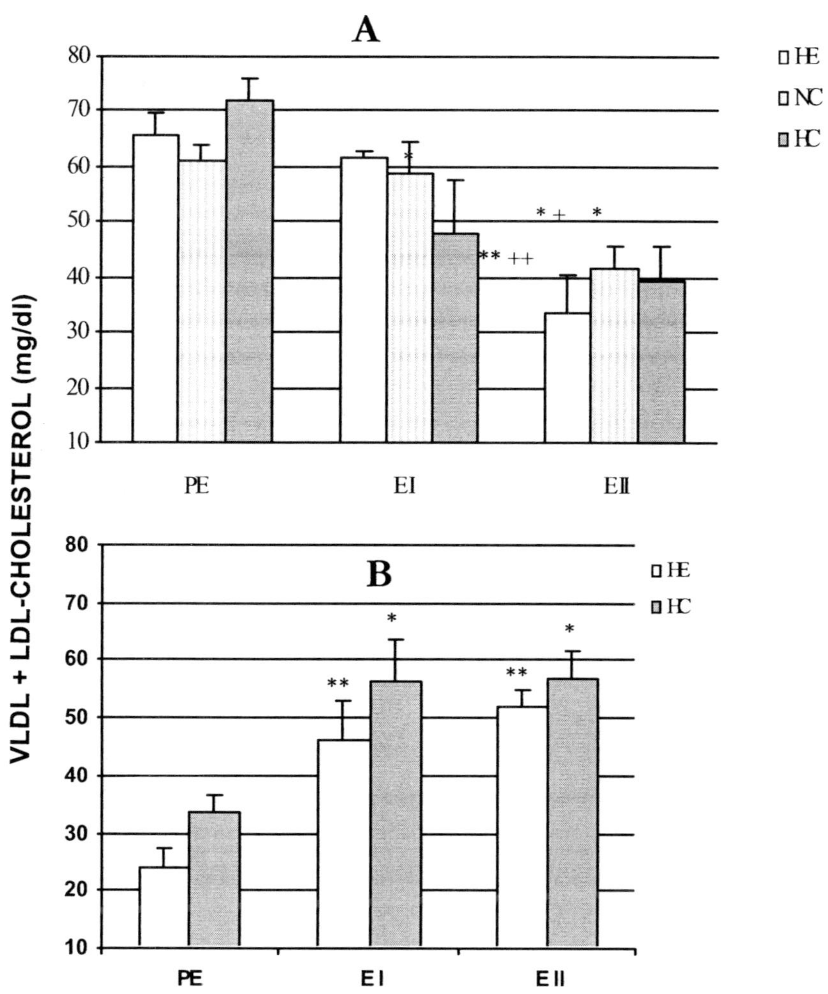

Figure 6: Effect of Hypobaric Hypoxia on Plasma [VLDL+LDL]-Cholesterol in Control and CHO-supplemented rats of Batches I [A] and II [B]. * P<0.05, significantly different compared to PE value; ** P<0.01, significantly different compared to PE value; + P< 0.05, significantly different compared to corresponding EI value; ++ P< 0.01, significantly different compared to corresponding EI value;

Plasma [VLDL + LDL-Cholesterol]

The plasma [VLDL + LDL-C] of the supplemented group increased significantly (p< 0.01) by 47.28 % from a PE value of 24.24 ± 3.13 mg/dl to 45.98 ± 6.89 mg/dl by the first week and further increased to 52.17 ± 2.95 mg/dl ($p < 0.01$) by the end of the exposure period [Figure 6 B]. Similarly, the plasma [VLDL + LDL-C] of the HC group also registered a significant ($p < 0.05$) 40.27 % increase from a pre-exposure value of 33.53 ± 3.24 mg/dl to 56.14 ± 7.29 mg/dl by the first week and did not change significantly in the second week. There was no significant difference between the VLDL + LDL-C concentrations of the two groups throughout the exposure period.

Plasma Triglycerides

The plasma [TG] in Hypoxic Experimental group was higher during the first week of exposure (93.16 ± 6.62 mg/dl) by 16 % compared to the pre-exposure value of 80.45 ± 6.42 mg/dl but then decreased by 18 % to 66.04 ± 13.59 mg/dl) by the second week of exposure [Figure 7 B]. The plasma [TG] of the Hypoxic Control group decreased by 8 % from a pre-exposure value of 74.4 ± 7.22 mg/dl to 68.75 ± 11.62 mg/dl by the first week and increased thereafter to pre-exposure values by the end of the exposure period. None of these changes were statistically significant however.

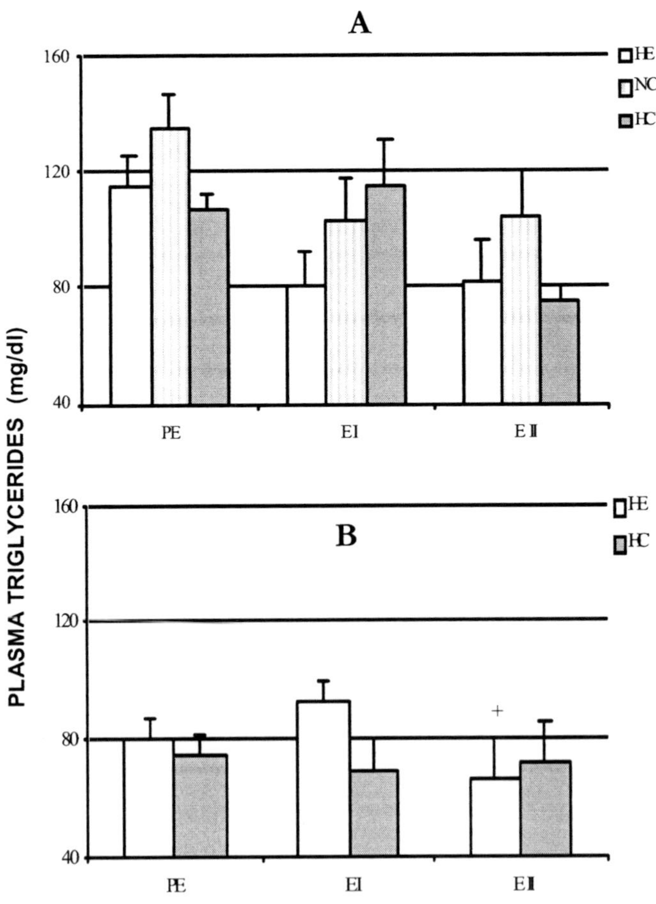

Figure 7: Effect of Hypobaric Hypoxia on Plasma Triglycerides in Control and CHO-supplemented rats of Batches I [A] and II [B]. + $P < 0.05$, significantly different compared to corresponding EI value;

Plasma Aspartate Aminotransferase

The plasma AST values in the Hypoxic Experimental group declined marginally from 13.96 ± 3.95 IU/L to 8.14 ± 1.43 IU/L by the second week (E II), but the decline was not statistically significant. The plasma AST values of the Hypoxic Control group rose marginally from a pre-exposure value of 9.3 ± 1.43 IU/L to 11.63 ± 2.6 IU/L by the end of the second week (E II). Overall, there was no significant change in the AST activity during the time period studied [Figure 8 B].

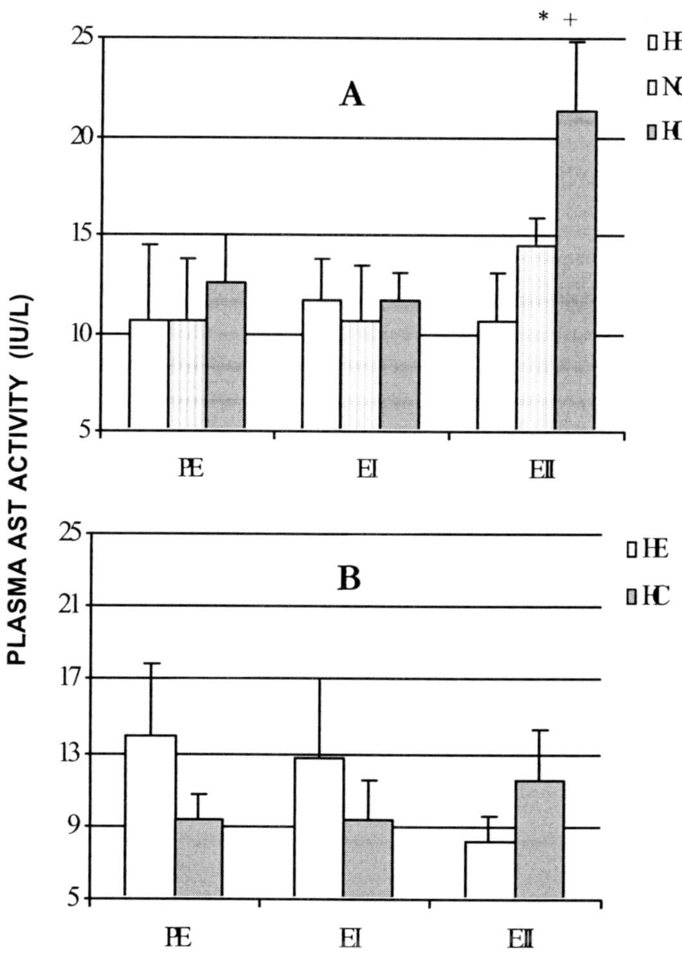

Figure 8: Effect of Hypobaric Hypoxia on Plasma Aspartate Aminotransferase (AST) in Control and CHO-supplemented rats of Batches I [A] and II [B]. * P<0.05, significantly different compared to PE value; + P< 0.05, significantly different compared to corresponding EI value;

Plasma Alanine Aminotransferase

The plasma ALT levels in the Hypoxic Experimental group rose during the exposure period from 27.92 ± 6.48 to 46.53 ± 5.52 IU/L but the increase was not significant. There was a similar trend observed in plasma ALT of Hypoxic Control group with the pre-exposure value (37.22 ± 5.07 IU/L) rising to 41.88 ± 5.00 IU/L by the end of the exposure period [Figure 9 B].

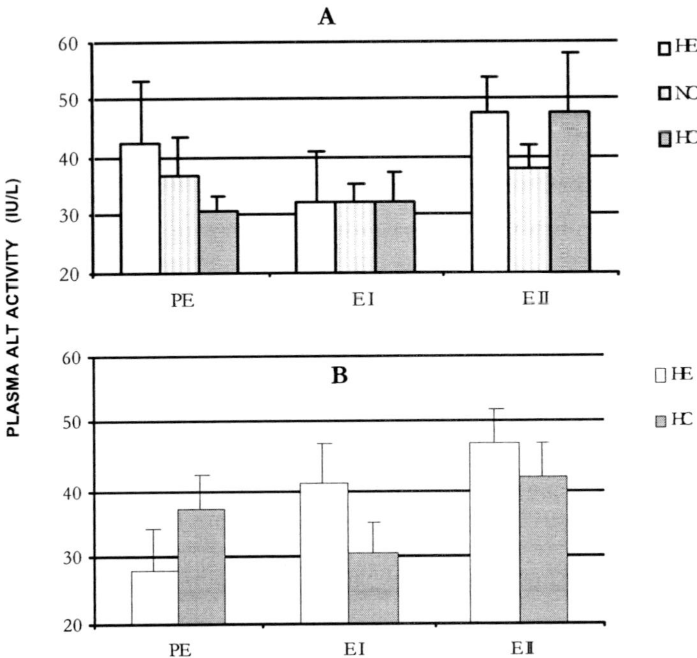

Figure 9: Effect of Hypobaric Hypoxia on Plasma Alanine Aminotransferase (ALT) in Control and CHO-supplemented rats of Batches I [A] and II [B].

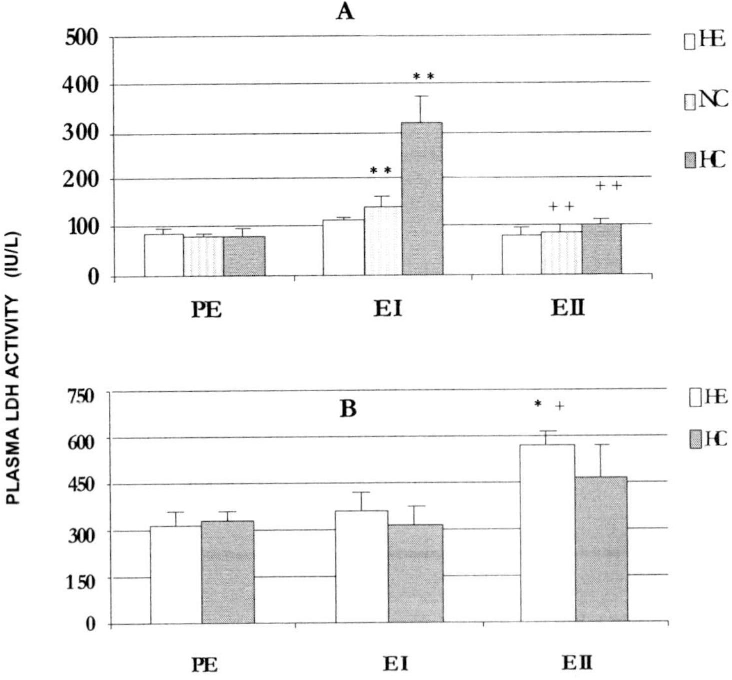

Figure 10: Effect of Hypobaric Hypoxia on Plasma Lactate Dehydrogenase (LDH) in Control and CHO-supplemented rats of Batches I [A] and II [B]. * P<0.05, significantly different compared to PE value; ** P<0.01, significantly different compared to PE value; + P< 0.05, significantly different compared to corresponding EI value; ++ P< 0.01, significantly different compared to corresponding EI value;

Plasma Lactate Dehydrogenase

The plasma LDH levels in the Hypoxic Experimental group were significantly increased ($p<0.05$) by 79.3 % to 567.19 ± 49.57 IU/L by the second week of exposure (E II) from a basal value of 316.24 ± 40.44 IU/L. The Hypoxic Control group also showed an increase of 41.5 % from a basal value of 330.81 ± 31.66 IU/L to 468.43 ± 108.91 IU/L by the end of the exposure period, but this increase was not significant [Figure 10 B].

Muscle and Liver Glycogen

The muscle and liver glycogen contents of both the Hypoxic Experimental and Hypoxic Control groups did not differ significantly [Figure 11 B]

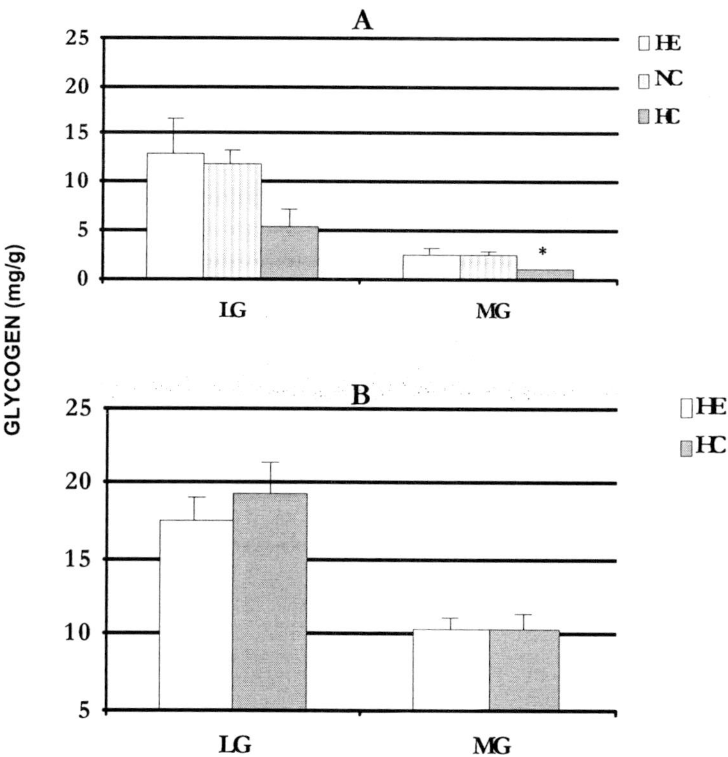

Figure 11: Effect of Hypobaric Hypoxia on Liver and Muscle Glycogen in Control and CHO-supplemented rats of Batches I [A] and II [B]. * $P<0.05$, significantly different compared to HE and NC values;

Discussion

Chronic exposure to simulated altitude in experimental animals of different age groups, with and without CHO supplementation, elicited complex physiological and biochemical responses. In the present study, chronic (continuous) exposure to simulated altitude resulted in significant anorexia as evidenced by their hypophagic response during the exposure period. The voluntary ingestion of diet was reduced which resulted in weight loss. This is in agreement with reports of anorexia in animals (Alippi *et al*, 1983; Singh *et al*, 1996; 1997a;

Vats *et al*, 1999) (Consolazio *et al*, 1969; Hannon *et al*, 1976), who attributed this decrease to loss of appetite. The anorexia was maximum during the first week and not much of an improvement was seen toward the end of the exposure protocol, with food consumption being only 70% compared to Pre-exposure intakes.

The HC group of Batch I lost ~35% body mass while the HE group had a loss of ~29% by the end of the exposure period, a feature noted in our earlier studies (Singh *et al*, 1996; 1997a). The HE group lost marginally lesser weight compared to the HC group, and this could be attributed to the increased intake of CHO in the diet. In batch II, both groups did not lose BW and continued to gain weight, albeit sluggishly and with a lot of fluctuations. In young rats, weight gain is much more rapid, and this failure to support normal weight gain during hypoxia clearly demonstrates the severe effects of hypoxia on growth rate.

The exact causes for this weight loss, whether discomfort, decreased availability of palatable food, or changes in nutrient preferences and eating habits, are difficult to explain. Several investigators have used an animal model to study the direct effects of hypoxia on body and muscle growth. Many studies have reported a decrease in the growth rate of rats at least during the first days of exposure to HA (Bigard *et al*, 1991; 1996; Klain and Hannon, 1970; Pugh, 1962; Purshottam *et al*, 1977; Schnakenberg *et al*, 1971; Singh *et al*, 1996; 1997a). The depression of growth rate has been attributed to anorexia, loss of body water, a direct effect of hypoxia on protein metabolism, or impaired absorption of nutrients (Schnakenberg *et al*, 1971). In the present study, the absorption of nutrients was not done and faecal matter not reported, and protein levels in the diet were maintained constant. Thus, the gain in body weight was used as an indirect indicator of the severe effect of hypoxia on depression in food intake.

Schnakenberg and Burlington (1970) studied the effects of high CHO, protein and fat diets and HA on growth and caloric intake of rats. However, the high protein content of the diet had a further anorectic effect. Bigard *et al* (1996) studied the effect of different dietary protein levels on growth rate and body composition during long-term (26 days) exposure to severe hypoxia (6,000 m) in rats. They observed marked anorexia in response to HA exposure for all protein diets. They concluded that hypobaric hypoxia per se (i.e., independently of anorexia) decreased the growth rate and that increased protein intake had no beneficial effect on the preservation of lean body weight.

Blood Glucose

The blood glucose levels of all the hypoxic groups were significantly decreased during the hypoxic exposure. The hypoxic groups as well as the NC group were significantly hypoglycemic when compared to their PE blood glucose levels. In batch II, both the hypoxic groups were significantly hypoglycemic compared to PE by E I and subsequently had an increase in blood glucose so that they approached PE values by the end of the exposure period.

The fall in blood glucose levels of the batch I hypoxic groups ranged from 32-34 % with the HC group having a greater decrease. The fall in blood glucose levels in the Batch II hypoxic groups was greater, ranging from 42-50 %, again with the HC group showing a greater decrease.

Many investigators have reported changes in blood glucose levels and glucose tolerance at high altitude. A depressed utilization of glucose at high altitude has been reported (Picon-Reategui, 1966; Blume and Pace, 1967). A depressed oxidation of glucose and its conversion to fatty acids were also observed in high altitude exposed rats (Picon-Reategui, 1966). Dogs exposed to 18,000 ft and 24,000 ft simulated altitudes, show increased glucose tolerance (Kelly and Mc Donald, 1948; Keyes and Kelley, 1949) while rats, under similar conditions, show decreased glucose tolerance and glycosuria (Van Middlesworth, 1946). Our earlier studies showed a decrease in blood glucose levels in rats subjected to continuous simulated hypobaric hypoxia (6960 m) for 21 days (Singh *et al*, 1996).

In man, decreased glucose tolerance at an altitude of 5340 m was observed (Forbes, 1936), while a study at 3500 m reported increased tolerance (Schaffler and Flury, 1948). A study by Williams (1975) reported a rise in fasting blood glucose levels on acute exposure to hypoxia, followed by a fall towards control values by the end of the week. In acclimatized low landers, fasting blood glucose levels were found to be consistently lower than at sea level by some workers (Stock *et al*, 1978), but unchanged by others (Sawhney *et al*, 1986). Even after 10 months stay at altitude, persistently raised glucose levels were found by Singh *et al* (1974), whereas Srivastava *et al* (1975) found increased fasting blood glucose levels up to the tenth month of stay and thereafter a progressive decrease even below the normal sea level values by the end of a two year stay. Fasting blood glucose has repeatedly been reported to be lower in highlanders than in low landers (Calderon and Llenara, 1965; Hurtado, 1964; Picon-Reategui, 1962; Picon-Reategui, 1970) as well as in rats exposed for various periods of time to simulated altitude (Davidson and Aoki, 1970; Ou, 1974). Consolazio *et al* (1972) found no difference in glucose tolerance of lowlanders at an altitude of 4300 m. During acute exposure to altitude, the increase in hematocrit and semi-starvation imposed by hypoxia-induced anorexia (Hannon, 1966) may serve to lower the whole blood glucose concentration. Studies in experimental animals have shown a reduction in blood glucose during acclimatization to high altitude (Blume and Pace, 1967).

Though there is a lot of variation and controversy reported in literature on the effects of hypoxia on blood glucose, all our studies consistently demonstrated a hypoglycaemic effect of chronic short-term hypoxia.

Plasma Lipids

With the exception of the HE group in Batch I in which there was a significant decrease by the end of exposure, none of the other hypoxic groups registered any significant change in plasma [TC] during the hypoxic exposure. With reference to plasma [HDL-C], the batch I HE group did not show any significant decrease, and the HC group had a significant increase at E I followed by a significant decrease by E II. Both the hypoxic groups of batch II registered a significant decrease in plasma [HDL-C] during the hypoxic exposure. The hypoxic groups of batch I had a significant decrease in plasma [VLDL + LDL-C] while those of batch II had a significant increase in plasma [VLDL + LDL-C] during hypoxic exposure.

The NC group of batch I followed a pattern similar to the HC group. The plasma [TC] initially had a significant increase followed by a significant decrease. The plasma [TC] levels by the end of the exposure period were significantly lower when compared to the pre-exposure levels. The plasma [HDL-C] also increased significantly at E I whereas the plasma [VLDL + LDL-C] had decreased significantly by the end of the study period.

With the exception of the batch II HE group that had an initial increase followed by a significant fall in plasma [TG], all the other hypoxic groups had a tendency to decrease, but did not register any significant changes in plasma [TG] throughout the exposure protocol.

The reduction in plasma [TC], [TG] and [VLDL + LDL-C] noticed in the batch I hypoxic groups as also the NC group are well supported by the numerous studies documenting the effects of exercise on plasma lipids (Superko, 1991; Stray-Gunderson *et al*, 1991; Ratliff *et al*, 1990; Brown, 1993; Hartung, 1993).

The transient increase of plasma [TG] in the batch II HE group at E I could have been due to the fact that the HE group was consuming a higher relative percentage of CHO compared to HC by means of the supplement. Thus, the consumption of CHO could have contributed to the increased accumulation of plasma [TG] (Grundy, 1986; 1988; 1990). The decrease in plasma [TG] noticed in all the other groups could have been due to the effects of exercise.

Lipid metabolism is reportedly altered with exposure to high altitude (Bason *et al*, 1969; Consolazio *et al*, 1968; De Mendoza *et al*, 1979; Krzywicki *et al*, 1969; Whitten and Janoski, 1969). Weight loss attributable to loss of body fat (Krzywicki *et al*, 1969) or lean body mass (Consolazio *et al*, 1968) has been reported with long-term exposure to high altitude. Also, workers have reported increased circulating TG levels (Whitten and Janoski, 1969); and reduced (De Mendoza *et al*, 1979) or unchanged (Whitten and Janoski, 1969) plasma cholesterol concentrations on exposure to HA. Previous studies have reported diverse effects on plasma lipid profiles (Bason *et al*, 1969; De Mendoza *et al*, 1979; Nestel *et al*, 1979; Whitten and Janoski, 1969; Srivastava *et al*, 1977; Klain and Hannon, 1968; Ferezou *et al*, 1988). Thus, the effect of exposure to HA on lipid metabolism appears to be a complex processes involving multiple responses by the body.

The reduction in plasma [TC], [TG] and [VLDL + LDL-C] noticed in the batch I hypoxic groups as also the Normoxic group are well supported by the numerous studies documenting the effects of exercise on plasma lipids (Superko, 1991; Hartung, 1993). Bailey *et al*, (2000) have reported the effect of exercise training in hypoxia in healthy men. They found decreased resting plasma concentrations of FFA, total cholesterol, HDL-C and LDL-C.

Loss of body weight has been reported to decrease fasting blood [TG] (Olefsky *et al*, 1974). Loss of ~ 11 Kg in normal and hypertriglyceridemic individuals resulted in a decrease in plasma [TG] and TC (Olefsky *et al*, 1974). Thus, weight loss alone can be effective in lowering plasma [TG]. In the present study, the HE and HC groups in batch I had a BW loss of 23 and 25 % respectively. Thus the decrease in plasma [TG] seen in the present study could be due to this weight loss. The lower decrease of plasma [TG] seen in batch II could have been due to the fact that they did not lose weight. Also, the effects of exercise cannot be ruled out.

Decreased plasma [TC], [LDL-C], [TG] and essentially unchanged [HDL-C] and [VLDL-C] has been reported by Ferezou *et al*, (1988) and Quatrini *et al*, (1983). The findings of increased LDL-C and VLDL-C along with decreased cholesterol FFA, LDL-C and VLDL-C in young rats exposed to hypobaric hypoxia are in agreement with the reports of Tomasova *et al*, (1987). Bason *et al*, 1969, reported increase in plasma [TC] levels after a 3-week stay at 3800 m altitude. Long term residence has also been reported to alter cholesterol concentrations in socio-economically matched high (3500 m) and low (1000 m) altitude natives of Peru showed the low altitude residents had higher total cholesterol concentrations, predominantly [LDL-C] (De Mendoza 1979). Srivastava *et al*, 1977 observed a hypocholesterolemic effect of moderate altitude in low landers on prolonged stay of two years. In a later study (Srivastava *et al*, 1992) conducted at both moderate (3050 m) and extreme altitude (4800-6000 m), they observed a general increase over SL values in circulating [TG] at 3050 m and a relative decrease in extreme HA. They also observed an increased [LDL] and [VLDL-C] and decreased [HDL-C] after 3 months at extreme HA indicating an increased risk factor for atherogenesis. However, a further 3-month stay resulted in normalization of values. Increase in fasting plasma [TG] accumulation with a concurrent decrease in plasma [TC] and [HDL-C] during a 40-day sojourn to HA was reported by Young *et al* (1989). These varied responses of high altitude effects on blood lipid profile may be due to various different altitudes studied, duration of exposure, diet and exercise employed in the different studies.

Muscle and Liver Glycogen Content

Chronic exposure to HA resulted in a decrease in muscle and liver glycogen (batch I) in the Hypoxic Control compared to Normoxic Controls. Muscle glycogen contents of CHO supplemented group in Batch I were at par with the Normoxic groups. The hepatic glycogen stores of the Hypoxic Experimental group were at par with the Normoxic Control group and higher than the Hypoxic Control group. In batch II, both the supplemented and Control groups had adequate muscle and liver glycogen stores. The varied responses could be indicative of glycogen recovery, especially in the batch II comprising of younger animals.

Evans (1934) observed an increase in glycogen, mostly in the liver, in fasted rats exposed for twenty-four hours to a half atmospheric pressure. These findings were confirmed by Lewis *et al* (1942) not only in rats, but also in rabbits and in monkeys. But Van Middlesworth (1946) reported different results. Timiras *et al* (1958) exposed well-fed rats to an altitude of 3800 m for seven and half hours and observed markedly decreased glycogen content in liver, heart and skeletal muscle. However, fasting rats exposed to altitude retained higher concentration of glycogen as compared to that at sea level. Prolonged exposure of two to six months brought the glycogen levels to the same concentration as at sea level, but after ten months glycogen concentration decreased again. Reduced liver glycogen has also been found in adult rats exposed to simulated altitude of 4800 m for 6 weeks (Davidson and Aoki, 1970) and 5400 m for 3 months (Ou, 1971; Ou, 1974) as well as in new born rats after 2 weeks at 4,700 m (Burgos *et al*, 1970). This has been attributed to a reduction in the activities of the rate limiting gluconeogenetic enzymes (Ou, 1974) and in gluconeogenesis by the liver (Freminet, 1976)

The cardiac glycogen content, however, remained high throughout two months of exposure period (Srivastava and Prakash, 1966). Mc Nulty *et al* (1996) reported a decrease in myocardial glycogen concentration under hypoxia, which recovered on subsequent re-oxygenation. The rats born at high altitude had lower body weight, smaller size and decreased hepatic and skeletal muscle glycogen content (Timiras *et al*, 1958). Exercise results in depletion of muscle glycogen reserves and a reduction in maximum sustainable exercise intensity (Hultman, 1967; Phinney *et al*, 1980). In contrast, exercise after altitude acclimatization is associated with greater endurance exercise capacity, less muscle glycogen utilization (Young *et al*, 1982) and less muscle lactate accumulation (Green *et al.*, 1989) than exercise of the same relative intensity at sea level.

The altitude-induced decrease in both liver and muscle glycogen is also consistent with results of previous studies (Blume and Pace, 1967; Taguchi *et al*, 1985; Bigard *et al*, 1996). Bigard *et al*, (1996), demonstrated that glycogen stores in the muscle, particularly Soleus, were altered by both decreased energy intake and hypoxia per se. Enhancement of protein in the diet had further deleterious effects on glycogen stores (Bigard *et al*, 1996). Van Liere and Stickney (1963) have reported marked elevation in liver glycogen of fasted rats, raising the possibility of increased interconversion of either protein or fat to carbohydrate in excess of oxidative requirements.

Exercise Performance

Hypobaric hypoxia resulted in a deterioration in endurance performance compared to the basal values. Supplementation with CHO however ameliorated this deterioration and the Hypoxic Experimental (supplemented) groups performed better compared to their respective Hypoxic Control groups.

The reduction in work capacity and physical performance under hypoxia has been studied by many workers (Cymerman *et al*, 1985; Pugh *et al*, 1964, Srivastava *et al*, 1992). A reduction in treadmill exercise performance of rats was reported by Altland *et al* (1969) at sea level after acclimatization to a simulated altitude of 7,600 m, 5 hr daily for 6 weeks. Cymerman *et al*, 1989, have also reported a reduction in work capacity and physical performance in human volunteers under hypoxia. As glycogen stores within muscles are depleted, there is an increase in demand for blood glucose by the muscles, reducing the availability of glucose to the brain. Prolonged exercise has been shown to lower blood glucose below 3mmol/L when volitional fatigue occurs (Casey *et al* 2000). Glucose is the preferred substrate of the brain, and it is possible that a reduction in blood glucose availability may impair cognitive function and contribute to central fatigue during exercise. Studies have shown that performance on tests of cognitive function is significantly impaired at low blood glucose levels (Martin and Benton, 1999) and there is a deterioration of selective or sustained attention, memory, and both auditory and visual information processing systems.

In the present study, the Runimex was used to evaluate mental performance. The number of shocks initiated per 100 cms traveled is an indication of learning ability and memory. This was recorded in both batches. When the number of shocks initiated was compared between groups, it was found that the HE groups avoided more shocks during the exposure period compared to either their own pre-exposure values or the HC, which performed poorly as the exposure progressed.

Exposure to hypobaric hypoxia is known to cause reductions in mental performance, and rapidly produces decrements in learning and memory and cognitive performance both in rats (Shukitt-Hale *et al*, 1994; Drago *et al*, 1990; Ando *et al*, 1987; Kadar *et al*, 1998; Boismare *et al* 1980) and men (Stivalet *et al*, 2000; Leifflen *et al*, 1997; Takagi and Watanabe, 1999).

Leiberman *et al* (1991) reported deficits in reaction times, vigilance, memory, and reasoning ability. Subjects of a simulated ascent to Mt. Everest as well as climbers experienced word aphasia (difficulty in speaking), and apraxia (difficulty in manual dexterity), neurological impairments in tasks such as memory recall and rapid finger tapping (Hornbein *et al*, 1989, Regard *et al*, 1989), and impairment of memory (Cavaletti, 1987; Regard *et al*, 1989). Complex task performance also deteriorates, and they are performed more slowly and with greater number of errors (Leiberman *et al*, 1991). The degree of hypoxia and duration of exposure (Leiberman *et al*, 1991) influence these adverse changes.

The underlying mechanisms in the brain responsible for mood and performance deficits at high altitudes are not known. Some workers speculate that alterations in those neurotransmitters whose synthesis requires oxygen like catecholamines and serotonin might be involved (Gibson and Duffy, 1981). More recent behavioural studies in rats point towards changes in acetylcholine formation and release (Shukitt-Hale *et al*, 1991; 1993a; 1993b). In addition, the reduced food intake and body weight loos associated with hypoxia at high altitudes may aggravate the direct chemical effects of HA on brain chemistry and function.

Studies on tyrosine administration, a catecholamine precursor, to stimulate transmitter production have demonstrated improved performances in rats under stressful conditions (Ahlers et al, 1994; Luo et al, 1992; Rauch and Leiberman, 1990) and improved cognitive performance in soldiers exposed to stressful situations (Ahlers et al, 1994; Leiberman et al, 1990).

Raising the level of blood glucose has been found to improve memory in healthy young adults (Benton *et al*, 1996); improved vigilance (Benton *et al*, 1994) and performance of an intelligence test (Benton *et al*, 1996). A higher baseline blood glucose has been associated with a better recall of word lists (Benton *et al*, 1994; Martin and Benton, 1999) and increased vigilance (Benton *et al*, 1994). When an association between baseline blood glucose levels and subsequent performance has been reported, in every instance a higher level of blood glucose has been associated with better performance. As equilibrium develops between plasma and brain glucose, high levels of blood glucose might result in higher brain glucose levels.

An association between acetylcholine-mediated neurotransmission and memory is well accepted (Kopelman, 1986). Glucose is the main source for the acetyl groups used in the formation of acetyl CoA, which is a precursor of acetylcholine. Brain acetylcholine levels have been reported to be lowered after a24-hr fats, and these can be restored by either feeding or the administration of glucose (Kuntscherova, 1972; Messier *et al*, 1990). The administration of glucose in the present study resulted in an improved performance under hypoxia compared to the non-supplemented animals.

HEPATIC FUNCTION

The HE and NC groups of Bath I did not register and significant change in AST and ALT activity, while in the HC group plasma AST levels increased significantly towards the end of the hypoxic exposure. The plasma LDH levels of all three groups were increased (significantly for HC and NC) by the first week, and were comparable to pre-exposure values by end of exposure period.

In batch II, there were no significant changes in either plasma AST or ALT levels during the entire study period. The plasma LDH levels were significantly increased only in the HE group toward the end of the exposure.

Essentially normal hepatic function has been reported in highlanders living at an altitude of 4540 m in Peru (Berendsohn, 1962) and 4000 m in Bolivia (Capderou *et al*, 1977); and in newcomers during the first week at 3500 m (Ramsoe *et al*, 1970). Srivastava et al (1973), did not find any change in the activities of SGOT and SGPT in lowlanders stationed for 2 years at 3500-4000 m. On the other hand, serum malic dehydrogenase (MDH), SGPT, SGOT and aldolase were measured in rats exposed to simulated HA of 25,000 ft by Nelson *et al* (1967) and found that they were significantly increased by day 2 of exposure. Similar effects of hypoxia were demonstrated by other workers (Nelson, 1966; Highman and Altland, 1960, 1966). The effect of exercise on plasma enzyme levels has been studied extensively and many investigators have demonstrated the existence of a relationship between the magnitude of plasma enzyme elevation and intensity and duration of the exercise. Loegering and Critz (1971) studied the effects of hypoxia and muscular activity on plasma enzyme levels (Plasma GOT, Plasma LDH, Plasma CPK) in dogs and observed an elevation in all after exposure to hypoxia. However, Sridharan *et al* (1994) found a depression in plasma AST activity in rabbits exposed to 7,000 m for 6 hrs. The increased AST activity in Hypoxic Control group of batch I in our chronic study is in agreement with the results obtained by Nelson, 1966; Nelson *et al*, 1967; Highman and Altland 1960, 1966; Loegering and Critz, 1971. As there was no alteration in the protein levels in the diet, the effects observed could be due to alterations in membrane permeability itself.

Hypobaric hypoxia of 7,000 m for 6 hours was found to increase plasma LDH activity in adult rabbits (Sridharan *et al*, 1994). Other workers have reported decreased lactate dehydrogenase/ citrate synthase activity ratios in the skeletal muscle in hypoxic groups compared to control groups (Tanaka *et al*, 1997). Bigard *et al* (1992) reported increased LDH activity in skeletal muscles of rats after endurance training. When there is an increased anaerobic metabolism, there will be accumulation of lactate, thereby provoking an increase in LDH activity.

In summary, chronic exposure to simulated altitude equivalent to 6096 m for 11 days, with and without CHO supplementation, in rats of different age groups resulted in a significant reduction in food intake, loss of body weight, depressed growth rate and lowered blood glucose levels in all the hypoxic groups. The responses of plasma lipids under hypoxia were quite complex. With the exception of one supplemented group that showed a significant decrease, there was no significant change in the TC during the hypoxic exposure. HDL-C concentrations were significantly decreased by the end of the exposure period in all the hypoxic groups. The VLDL-C+ LDL-C concentrations were significantly decreased in the older batch while it was significantly increased in the younger batch of animals. The plasma TG showed a tendency to decrease in all the groups. The increased VLDL-C + LDL-C and decreased HDL-C concentrations constitute an increased risk factor for atherogenesis. The Normoxic control displayed a response typical of the effects of exercise on plasma lipids. The plasma ALT activity did not register any significant changes in any of the groups during hypoxic exposure while AST levels were increased significantly in older hypoxic control group. The LDH levels were increased in all the hypoxic groups but were significant only in the case of the control group in the older batch, and the supplemented group in the younger batch. Supplementation with CHO significantly ameliorated the reduced exercise endurance caused by hypoxic exposure in both younger and older rats.

References

Ahlers ST, JR Thomas, J Schrot, and D Shurtleff. Tyrosine and glucose modulation of cognitive deficits resulting from cold stress. 1994. Pp 301-320 in *Food Components to Enhance Performance, An Evaluation of Potential Performance-Enhancing Food Components for Operational Rations*, BM Marriot, ed. A report of the Committee on Military Nutrition Research, Food and Nutrition Board. Washington DC: National Academy Press.

Alippi RM, Barcelo AC, Rio ME, Bozzini CE. Growth retardation in the early developing rat exposed to continuous hypobaric hypoxia. *Acta Physiol Lat Am*; 33(1); 1983.

Altland PD, B Highman, and MP Dieter. Reduced exercise performance of rats at sea level after altitude acclimatization: changes in serum enzymes, glucose, corticosterone and tissue structure. *Inter J Biometeorol*; 13: 173-181, 1969.

Ando S, Kametani H, Osada H, Iwamoto M and Kimura N. Delayed memory dysfunction by transient hypoxia, and its prevention with forskolin. *Brain Res*; 405 (2): 371-374, 1987.

Askew EW. Nutrition and performance under adverse environmental conditions, in *Nutrition in Exercise and Sport*, Hickson JF Jr. and Wolinsky, I., eds., CRC Press, Boca Raton FL., 1989, 367.

Bailey DM, Davies B, Milledge JS, Richards M, Williams R, Jordinson M, Calam J. Elevated plasma cholecystokinin at high altitude: metabolic implications for the anorexia of acute mountain sickness. *High Alt Med Biol* 2000 Spring; 1(1): 9-23.

Bason R and CE Billings. Effects of high altitude on lipid components of human serum. *Arch Environ Health* 19: 183-185, 1969.

Benton D, Owens DS, Parker PY. Blood glucose influences memory and attention in young adults. *Neuropsychologia*; 32: 595-607, 1994.

Benton D, Parker PY, Donohoe RT. The supply of glucose to the brain and cognitive functioning. *J Biosoc Sci*; 28: 463-479, 1996.

Berendsohn S. Hepatic function at high altitudes. *Arch Internal Med* 109: 56-64, 1962.

Bigard AX, A Brunet, CY Guezennec and HM Monod. Skeletal muscle changes after endurance training at high altitude *J Appl Physiol* 71: 2114-2121, 1991.

Bigard AX, Brunet A, Serrurier B, Guezzennec CY, Monod H. Effects of endurance training at high altitude on diaphragm muscle properties. *Pflugers Arch Dec*; 422(3)239-44, 1992.

Bigard AX, P Douce, D Merino, F Leinhard, and CY Guezzennec. Changes in dietary protein intake fail to prevent decrease in muscle growth induced by severe hypoxia in rats. *J Appl Physiol* 80 (1): 208-215, 1996.

Blume FD and Pace N. Effect of translocation to 3,800 m altitude on glycolysis in mice. *J Appl Physiol* 23: 75-79,1967.

Boismare F, Le Poncin-Lafitte M, Rapin JR. Blockade of the different enzymatic steps in the synthesis of brain amines and memory (CAR) in hypobaric hypoxic rats treated and untreated with L. Dopa. *Aviat Space Environ Med* 51(2): 126-128, 1980.

Boyer SJ, and D Blume. Weight loss and changes in body composition at high altitude. *J Appl. Physiol* 57 : 1580-1585, 1984.

Brooks GA, GE Butterfield, RR Wolfe, BM Groves, RS Mazzeo, JR Sutton, EE Wolfel, and JT Reeves. Increased dependence on blood glucose after acclimatization to 4,300 m. *J Appl Physiol* 70: 919-927, 1991.

Brown WV. Lipoproteins: what, when and how often to measure? *Heart Dis Stroke* 1: 21, 1992.

Burgos MH, EO Zangheri and IM Parish. The rat hepatocyte after exposure to high altitude: structural and chemical changes. *Quart J Exptl Physiol*; 55: 54-58, 1970.

Burstein M et al *J Lipid Res* 11: 583, 1953.

Butterfield GE, J Gates, S Fleming, GA Brooks, JR Sutton and JT Reeves. Increased energy intake minimizes weight loss in men at high altitude. *J Appl Physiol* 72:1741-1748, 1992.

Butterfield GE. Maintenance of body weight at altitude: In search of 500 Kcal/day, In: *Nutritional Needs in Cold and in High Altitude Environments*, 1996, pp 357-378 Washington DC. National Academy Press (BM Marriott and SJ Carlson, eds.)

Caldiron R and LS Llenara. Carbohydrate metabolism in people living in chronic hypoxia. *Diabetes*; 14: 100-105, 1965.

Capderou A, Polianski J, Mensch Dechem J, Drout L, Antezana G, Zetter M and Lockhart A. Splanchnic blood flow, O2 consumption, removal of lactate and out put of glucose in highlanders. *J Appl Physiol: Respiratory Environmental and Exercise Physiology*; 43: 204-2110, 1977.

Casey A, Mann R, Banister K, Fox J, Morris PG, McDonalds IA, and Greenhaff PL. Effect of carbohydrate ingestion on glycogen resynthesis in human liver and skeletal muscle, measured by 13C MRS *Am J Physiol*; 278 (1): E 65-75, 2000

Castonguay TW, Hirsch E, and Collier G. Palatability of sugar solutions and dietary selection? *Physiol Behav* 27: 7-12, 1981.

Cavaletti G, R Morooney, P Garavaglia, and G Tredici. Brain damage after high altitude climbs without oxygen. *Lancet* 1: 101, 1987,

Consolazio CF, CO Matoush, HL Johnson, and TA Daws. Protein and water balances of young adults during prolonged exposure to HA (4200 m). *Am J Clin Nutr* 21 : 154-161, 1968.

Consolazio CF, Matoush LO, Johnson HL, Krzywicki HJ, Daws TA and Isaac GJ. Effects of high-carbohydrate diets on performance and clinical symptomatology after rapid ascent to high altitude. *Fed. Proc.* 28, 937, 1969.

Consolazio CF, HL Johnson, HJ Krzywicki and TA Daws. Metabolic aspects of acute altitude exposure (4300 m) in adequately nourished humans. *Ann J Clin Nutr* 25:23-29, 1972.

Cymerman A, JT Reeves, JR Sutton, PB Rock, BM Groves, MK Malconian, PM Young, PD Wagner and CS Houston. Operation Everest II: Maximal Oxygen uptake at extreme altitude. *J Appl Physiol* 66 : 2446-2453, 1989

Davidson MB and Aoki. Fasting glucose homeostasis in rats after chronic exposure to hypoxia. *Am J Physiol*; 219: 378-383, 1970.

De Mendoza S, H Nucete, E Incichen, E Salazar, A Zerpa, CJ Glueck. Lipids and lipoproteins in subjects at 1000 and 3500 m altitude. *Arch Envir Health* 34: 308-310, 1979.

Drago F, Grassi M, Valerio C, Spadaro F, D' Agata V, Lauria N. Effects of vinburnine on experimental models of learning and memory impairments. *Pharmacol Biochem Behav*; 37 (I) : 53-57, 1990.

Dramise JG, Inouye CM, Christensen BM, Fults RD, Canham JE and Consolazio CF. Effects of a glucose meal on human pulmonary function at 1600 m and 4300 m altitudes. *Aviat. Space. Environ. Med.* 46:365, 1975

Evans G. The effect of low atmospheric pressure on the glycogen content in the rat. *Am J Physiol*; 110: 273-277, 1934.

Ferezou J JP Richalet, T Coste and C Rathat. Changes in plasma lipids and lipoprotein cholesterol during a high altitude mountaineering expedition. *Eur J Appl Physiol* 57: 740-745, 1988.

Forbes WH. Blood sugar and glucose tolerance at high altitude. *Am J Physiol*; 116: 309-316, 1936.

Freminet A. *Etude Dynamique du Metabolisme du lactate Chez le Rat* (These de doctorat is Sciences) Orsay, France: Universite Paris-sud, 1976. No. 1326.

Gibson GE and DE Duffy. Impaired synthesis of acetylcholine by mild hypoxic hypoxia or nitrous oxide. *J Neurochem.* 36:28-33, 1981.

Gill MB and LGCE Pugh. Basal Metabolism and Respiration in men living at 5800 m (19000 ft). *J Appl Physiol* 19: 949-954, 1964.

Green HJ, Sutton J, Young PM, Cymerman A, Houston CS. Operation Everest II: muscle energetics during maximal exhaustive exercise. *J Appl Physiol* 66: 142-150, 1989.

Grundy SM. Comparison of monounsaturated fatty acids and carbohydrates for lowering plasma cholesterol *N Eng J Med* 314: 745, 1986.

Grundy SM, Florentin L, Nix D, and Whelan MF. Comparison of monounsaturated fatty acids and carbohydrates for reducing raised levels of plasma cholesterol in man *Am J Clin Nutr* 47: 965, 1988.

Grundy SM. Cholesterol and coronary disease: future directions *JAMA* 264: 3053,1990.

Guilland JC and J Klepping. Nutritional alterations at high altitude in man. *Eur J Appl Physiol Ocupp Physiol* 54:517-523. 1985.

Hannon JP. A comparative review of certain responses of men and women to high altitude. In: *Proceedings, Symposia on Arctic Biology and Medicine.* VI. The physiology of work in cold and altitude, eds. Helfferick, Arctic Aeromedical Laboratory, Alaska, pp 113-245. 1966.

Hannon JP, GJ Klain, DM Sudman and FJ Sullivan. Nutritional aspects of high altitude exposure in women. *Ann J Clin Nutr* 29 : 604-613, 1976.

Hansen JE, Hartley LH and Hogan RP. Arterial oxygen increase by high-carbohydrate diet at altitude, *J Appl Physiol*, 33 : 441, 1972

Hartung GH. High density lipoprotein cholesterol and physical activity: an update: 1983-1991, *Sports Med* 1993.

Highman B and PD Altland. Serum enzyme rise after hypoxia and effect of autonomic blockade. *Am J Physiol* 199: 981-986, 1960.

Highman B and PD Altland. Effect of dimethyl sulfoxide in rats exposed to high altitude. *Life Sci* 5: 1839-1847, 1966.

Hornbein TF, BD Towns, RB Schoene, JR Sutton and CS Houston. The cost on the central nervous system of climbing to extremely high altitudes. *N. Engl. J Med* 321:1714-1719, 1989.

Hultman E. Physiological role of muscle in man, with special reference to exercise. *Circ Res*; 20-21 (Suppl-1); 99-114, 1967.

Hurtado A. Animals in high altitudes: resident man. *Handbook of Physiology. Adaptation to the environment.* Washington DC: Am Physiol Soc 1964, sect 4, chpt 54, p 843-860

Kadar T, Dachir S, Shukitt-Hale B, Levy A. Sub-regional hippocampal vulnerability in various animal models leadind to cognitive dysfunction. *J Neural Transm* 105 (8-9): 987-1004, 1998.

Kayser B. Nutrition and energetics of exercise at altitude. Theory and possible practical applications. *Sports Med* 17: 309-323, 1994.

Kelly VC, Mc Donald RK. Effects of acute exposure to simulated altitude on dextrose tolerance and insulin tolerance. *Am J Physiol*; 152: 250-256, 1948.

Keyes GH, Kelly VC. Glucose tolerance of dogs as altered by atmoshpheric decompression. *Am J Physiol*; 158: 358-366, 1949.

Klain GJ and JP Hannon. Effects of high altitude on lipid components of human serum. *Proc Soc Exptl Biol Med* 129: 646-649, 1968.

Klain GJ, and Hannon JP. High altitude and protein metabolism in the rat. *Proc Soc Exp Biol Med* 134: 1000-1004, 1970.

Kopelman MD. The cholinergic neurotransmitter system in human memory and dementia : A review. *Q J Exp Psychol*; 38A: 535-573; 1986.

Kuntscherova J. Effect of short term starvation and choline on the acetylcholine content of organs of albino rats. *Physiol Bohemoslov*; 21: 655-660, 1972.

Krzywicki HJ, CF Consolazio, LL Matoush, HL Johnson, and RA Barnhart. Body composition changes during exxposure to altitude. *Federation Proc.* 28: 1190-1194, 1969.

Leiberman HR, LE Banderet B Shukitt-Hale. Tyrosine protects humans from the adverse effects of acute exposure to hypoxia and cold.*Abstr Soc Neuro* 16: 272, 1990.

Leiberman HR, B Shukitt-Hale, LE Banderet, and JF Glenn. Exposure to hypobaric hypoxia: A method for the comparison of neuropsychologic tests in humans. *Abstr Soc Neuro* 17: 1233, 1991.

Leifflen D, Poquin D, Savourey G, Barraud PA, Raphel C, Bittel J. Cognitive performance during short acclimation to severe hypoxia. *Aviat Space Environ Med* 68 (11): 993-997, 1997.

Lewis RA, Tharne GW, Koepf GF, and Dorrance SS. The role of the adrenal cortex in acute anoxia. *J Clin Invest*; 21:33-46, 1942.

Loegering DJ, and Critz JB. Effect of hypoxia and muscular activity on plasma enzyme levels in dogs. *Am J Physiol.* 220 (1): 100-104, 1971.

Luo S, L Villamil, CJ Watkins and HR Leiberman. Further evidence tyrosine reverses behavioura deficits caused by cold exposure. *Abstr Soc Neuro* 18(1): 716, 1992.

Martin PY and D Benton. The influence of a glucose drink on a demanding working memory task. *Physiol Behav* 67(1) 69-74, 1999.

McNulty PH, Chin NG, Liu WX, Jagasia D, Letsou GV, Baldwin JC, Soufer R. Autoregulation of myocardial glycogen concentration during intermittent hypoxia. *Am J Physiol.*; 271: R 311-319, 1996.

Messier C, Durkin T, Mrabet O, Destrade C. Memory improving action of glucose: Indirect evidence for a facilitation of hippocampal acetylcholine synthesis. *Behav Brain Res* 39: 135-143; 1990.

Montgomery H. determination of glycogen. *Arch Biochem Biophys;* 67: 378-386; 1957.

Nelson BD. Hepatic lysosomes and serum enzymes in rats exposed to high altitude. *Am J Physiol* 211: 651-655, 1966.

Nelson BD, Highman B, and PD Altland. Oxidative phosphorylation during altitude acclimatisation in rats. *Am J Physiol* 213 (6): 1414-1418, 1967.

Nestel PJ, M Podkolinski, and NH Fidge. Marked increase in high density lipoproteins in mountaineers. *Atherosclerosis* 34: 193-196, 1979.

Olefsky JM, GM Reaven, JW Farquhar. Effect of weight reduction on obesity: studies of carbohydrate metabolism. *J Clin Invest* 53: 64-76, 1974.

Ou LC. *Tissue Metabolic Function and Adaptive Change in Acclimatization to Chronic Hypoxia* (Ph.D. Thesis) Hanover NH: Dartmouth College, 1971.

Ou LC. Hepatic and renal gluconeogenesis in rats acclimatized to high altitude. *J Appl Physiol*; 36: 303-307, 1974.

Phinney SD, Hortom Es, Sims EAH, Hanson JK, Danforth Jr E, LaGrange BM. Capacity for moderate exercise in obese subjects after adaptation to a hypocaloric ketogenic diet. *J Clin Invest;* 66: 1152-1161, 1980.

Picon-Reategui E. Studies on the metabolism of carbohydrates at sea level and at high altitudes. *Metabolism*; 11 1148-1154, 1962.

Picon-Reategui E. Effect of chronic hypoxia on the action of insulin in carbohydrate metabolism *J Appl Physiol* 29: 560-563, 1966.

Picon-Reategui E, ER Buskirk and PT Baker. Blood glucose in high altitude natives and during acclimatization to altitude. *J Appl Physiol*; 29: 560-563, 1970.

Pugh LGCE. Physiological and medical aspect of the Himalayan Scientific and Mountaineering Expedition 1960-61. *Br Med J* 2: 621-627, 1962

Pugh LG, MB Gill, S Lahiri, J S Milledge, MP Ward and JB West. Muscular exercise at great altitude. *J Appl Physiol* 19 : 431-440, 1964.

Purshottam T, U Kaveeshwar, and HD Brahmachari. Altitude tolerance in rats in relation to carbohydrates and fats in their diet. *Aviat Space Environ Med* 48: 438-442, 1977.

Quatrini U, Licciardi A. [Initial observations on lipid metabolism in the albino rat raised under normobaric hypoxic hypoxia] [Italian]. *Boll Soc Ital Biol Sper Apr* 30; 59(4): 549-52, 1983

Rauch TM and HR Leiberman. Pre-treatment with tyrosine reverses hypothermia induced behavioural depression. *Brain Res Bull* 24: 147-150, 1990.

Ramsoe K, S Jarnum, R Dreisig, J Tauber, N Tygstrup, and H Westergaard. Liver function and blood flow at high altitudes. *J Appl Physiol*; 28: 725-727, 1970.

Ratliff R, Knehans A, and Mc Carthy M: Effects of frequency of exercise training on plasma lipids and lipoproteins *Med Sci Sports Exercise* 22: (Abstr) S48, 1990.

Regard M, O Oelz, P Brugger, D. Biol and T. Landis. Persistent cognitive impairment in climbers after repeated exposure to extreme altitude. *Neurology*. 39: 210-213, 1989.

Reynolds RD, Howard MP, Deuster P, Lickteig JA, Conway J, Rumpler W and Seale J. Energy intakes and expenditures at Mt. Everest. *FASEB J.* 6, A, A1084, 1992.

Richalet JP. *Paper presented at 3rd International Hypoxia Symposium*, Banff, Alberta, Canada, 1983.

Roberts AC, GE Butterfield, Cymerman A, JT Reeves, EE Wolfel, and GA Brooks. Acclimatization to 4300 m altitude decreases reliance on fat as a substrate. *J Appl Physiol* 81: 1762-1771, 1996.

Roberts AC, JT Reeves, GE Butterfield, RS Mazzeo, JR Sutton, EE Wolfel and GA Brooks. Altitude and β-blockade augment glucose utilization during submaximal exercise. *J Appl Physiol* 80: 605-615, 1996.

Rose MS, CS Houston, CS Fulco, G Coates, JR Sutton and A Cymerman. Operation Everest II: Nutrition and body composition. *J Appl Physiol* 65 : 2545-2551, 1988.

Sawhney RC, Malhotra AS, Singh T, Rai RM, Sinha KC. Insulin secretion at high altitude in man. *Int J Biometeorol*; 30: 231-238, 1986.

Schaffler K, Flury M. Glucose tolerance in high mountains. *Helv Physiol Pharmacol Acta*; 6: 596-600, 1948.

Sclafani A. Carbohydrate taste, appetite and obesity: An overview. *Neurosci Biobehav Rev* 11:131-153, 1987.

Schnakenberg DD and RF Burlington. Effect of high carbohydrate, protein and fat diets and high altitude on growth and caloric intake of rats. *Proc Soc Exp Biol Med* 134:905-908, 1970.

Schnakenberg DD, Krabill LF and Weiser PC. The anorexic effect of high altitude on weight gain, nitrogen retention and body composition of rats. *J Nutr* 101: 787-796, 1971.

Shukitt-Hale B, LE Banderet, and HR Leiberman. Relationship between symptoms, mood and performance, and acute mountain sickness at 4700 m. *Aviat Space Environ Med* 62: 865-869, 1991.

Shukitt-Hale B, MJ Stillman, A Levy, JA Dcvine and HR Leiberman. Nimodipine prevents the in vivo decrease in hippocampal extracellular acetylcholine produced by hypobaric hypoxia. *Brain Res* 621: 291-295, 1993a.

Shukitt-Hale B, MJ Stillman, BE Marlowe, DI Welch, RL Galli, JA Devine, A Levy, and HR Leiberman. Hypobaric hypoxia adversely affects spatial memory in an exposure-dependant fashion. *Abstr Soc Neuro* 19:363, 1993b.

Shukitt-Hale B, Stillman MJ, Welch DI, Levy A, Devine JA, Lieberman HR. Hypobaric Hypoxia impairs spatial memory in an elevation-dependant fashion. *Behav Neural Biol*; 62(3): 244-52, 1994.

Singh I, Malhotra M, Khanna PK, Nanda R, Purshottam T, Upadhyay T, Radhakrishna U, Brahmachari H. Changes in blood cortisol, blood antidiuretic hormone, and urinary catecholamines in high altitude pulmonary edema. *Int J Biometeorol*; 30: 33-41, 1974.

Singh SB, Sharma A, Sharma KN and Selvamurthy W. Effect of high altitude hypoxia on feeding responses and hedonic matrix in rats. *J Appl Physiol* 80 (4), 1133-1137, 1996.

Singh SB, Chatterjee A, U Panjwani, A Vij, D K Yadav, Khemchandra, K N Sharma and W Selvamurthy. Hypobaric hypoxia and hedonic matrix in rats. *Japanese J Physiol* 47(4), 327-333, 1997a.

Singh SB, Sharma A, Yadav DK, Tyagi AK, Verma SS, Srivastava DN, Sharma KN and Selvamurthy W. High altitude effects on human taste intensity and hedonics. *Aviat. Space Environ Med.* 68:1123-1128, 1997b.

Sridharan K, Patil SK, Upadyay TN, Mukherjee AK. Effects of pyridoxine supplementation on blood glucocorticoids level, aspartate aminotransferase activity and glucose tolerance pattern under acute hypoxic stress. *Biol Neonate;* 66(2-3): 106-11, 1994.

Srivastava KK, Prakash O. Animal metabolism and nutritional requirements under physiological stress- Effect of high altitude. *Df Sci J;* 16: 125-140, 1966.

Srivastava KK, Rao YB, Chander A, Malhotra MS. Serum Aspartate and Alanine aminotransferases in lowlanders during prolonged exposure to high altitudes and in natives of high altitude area. *Indian J Exp Biol* 1973 Mar; 11(2): 130-1, 1973.

Srivastava KK, Kumria MML, Grover SK, Sridharan K, Malhotra MS. Glucose tolerance of low landers during prolonged stay at high altitude and among high altitude natives. *Aviat Space Environ Med*; 46: 122-126, 1975.

Srivastava KK, SK Bharadwaj and MS Malhotra. Effect of prolonged stay at an an altitude of 4000 m on blood cholesterol of lowlanders. *Ind J Exptl Biol* 15: 557-558, 1977.

Srivastava KK. *Studies on High Terrestrial Altitudes, Adaptations to 15000-20000 ft. in Man.* Technical Report No. DIPAS/ 3/92, Min. of Def., New Delhi, 1992.

Stivalet P, Leifflen D, Poquin D, Savourey G, Launay JC, Barraud PA, Raphel C, Bittel J. positive expiratory pressure as a method for preventing the impairment of attentional processes by hypoxia. *Ergonomics*; 43 (4): 474-485, 2000.

Stock MJ, Chapman C, Stirling JL, Campbell IT. Effects of exercise, altotude and food on blood hormone and metabolite levels. *J Appl Physiol*; 45: 350-354, 1978.

Stray Gundersen J, Denkee MA, and Grundy SM. Influence of lifetime cross-country skiing on plasma lipids and lipoproteins *Med Sci Sports Exercise* 23: 695, 1991.

Superko HR. Exercise training, serum lipids, and lipoprotein particles: is there a change threshold? *Sci Sports Exercise* 23: 677, 1991.

Taguchi S, Hata Y, Itoh K. Enzymatic responses and adapatations to swimming, training and hypobaric hypoxia in post-natal rats. *Jpn J Physiol*; 35(6): 1023-32, 1985.

Takagi M, and S Watanabe. Two different components of contingent negative variation (CNV) and their relation to changes in reaction time under hypobaric hypoxic conditions. *Aviat Space Environ Med* 70 (1): 30-34, 1999.

Tanaka M, Mizuta K, Koba F, Ohira Y, Kobayashi T, Honda Y. Effects of exposure to hypobaric hypoxia on body weight, muscular and haematological characteristics, and work performance in rats. *Jpn J Physiol*; 47(1): 51-7, 1997.

Timiras PS, Hill R, Krum AA, Lis AW, Hwang CA, Lem GY. Carbohydrate metabolism in fed and fasted rats exposed to an altitude of 12470 feet. *Am J Physiol*; 193: 415-424,1958.

Tomasova H, Lisy V, Trojan S, Stastny F. Effect of short-term or intermittent hypobaric hypoxia on plasma lipids in young rats. *Physiol Bohemoslov*; 36(4): 361-4, 1987.

Trinder P. *Ann Clin Biochem*, 6: 24, 1969.

Van Liere EJ, Stickney JC. Chemical changes in the blood during hypoxia. In: *Hypoxia*. The University of Chicago Press, Chicago. Pp 61-75, 1963.

Van Middlesworth L. Glucose ingestion during severe anoxia. *Am J Physiol*; 146: 491-495, 1946.

Vats P, AK Mukherjee, MML Kumria, SN Singh, SKB Patil, S Ranganathan, K Sridharan. Changes in the activity levels of glutamine synthetase, glutaminase, and glycogen synthetase in rats subjected to hypoxic stress. *Int J Biometeorol*; 42: 205-209, 1999.

Whitten BK and AH Janoski. Effects of high altitude and diet in lipid components of human serum. *Federation. Proc.* 28: 983-986. 1969.

Williams ES. Mountaineering and the endocrine system. In: Clarks C, Ward M, Williams E, eds. Mountain Medicine and Physiology. *Proceedings of a Symposium for Mountaineers, Expedition Doctors and Physiologists*, Alpine Club, London. pp 38-44, 1975.

Young AJ, WJ Evans, A Cymerman, KB Pandolf, JJ Knapik, and JT Maher. Sparing effect of chronic high-altitude exposure on muscle glycogen utilization. *J Appl Physiol* 52: 857-862, 1982.

Young PM, MS Rose, JR Sutton, HJ Green, A Cymerman, CS Houston. Operation Everest II: Plasma lipid and hormonal responses during a simulated ascent of Mt. Everest. *J Appl Physiol* 66(3): 1430-1435, 1989.

In: Trends in Dietary Carbohydrates Research
Editor: M. V. Landlow, pp. 179-219
ISBN 1-59454-798-X

Chapter 8

EFFECTS OF PREBIOTICS IN DOG AND CAT NUTRITION: A REVIEW

M. Hesta, J. Debraekeleer, G. P. J. Janssens and R. De Wilde
Laboratory of Animal Nutrition, Ghent University, Faculty of Veterinary Medicine, Merelbeke, Belgium

ABSTRACT

Prebiotics are substrates for bacteria already present in the large intestine. An overview is given on the effects of prebiotics on the gastrointestinal (GI) tract (faecal characteristics, flora, digestibility, gastrointestinal dimensions and potential side effects), metabolism (lipid, carbohydrate and nitrogen metabolism), immune system and palatability in dogs and cats. Potential clinical benefits and topics for future research are discussed.

GENERAL ASPECTS

Introduction

Traditionally, nutrition of pet animals has focused on nutrient requirements and the prevention of nutritional deficiencies. Later on, more emphasis is put on the link between metabolic and skeletal disorders and excessive intake of nutrients such as energy and calcium. Only recently, research is directed towards functional feeding, i.e. the beneficial effects of higher intake of specific nutrients on health and live expectancy. Hence the interest in research with feed additives such as prebiotics and antioxidants has increased.

The terms probiotics, prebiotics and synbiotics are briefly defined hereafter and will be discussed in some detail later on. The main emphasis of this review will be on prebiotics in dogs and cats. The effect of prebiotics on other species will not be reviewed due to the large differences in gastrointestinal tract. When data on dogs and cats are not available or limited, effects found in man or rodents will be discussed briefly.

- *Probiotics* are live microbial feed supplements that beneficially affects the host by improving the intestinal microbial balance [1].
- *Prebiotics* are growth substrates for potentially beneficial bacteria already present in the colon [2].
- *Synbiotics* are a combination of both pro- and prebiotics. The prebiotic aids in the establishment of the probiotic organism in the complex colonic environment [1].

With this in mind, more and more pet food manufacturers supplement their feeds with prebiotics. Especially diets intended to be fed in case of diseases such as gastrointestinal disorders, renal insufficiency and recovery may be supplemented with prebiotics including fructo-oligosaccharides (FOS) and mannanoligosaccharides (MOS).

There is high interest in improving the intestinal flora and its beneficial effects. However, probiotics may encounter difficulties in surviving gastric acid and bile acids, need to be capable of adhering to the intestinal epithelium and of competing with other bacteria for nutrients and ecological sites. Their effect may be transient, i.e. when the treatment is stopped; the added bacteria are rapidly washed out of the large intestine. It is believed that these difficulties can be partly overcome by the use of prebiotics [2].

The fermentative capacity of the dogs' and cats' gastro-intestinal (GI) tract is generally believed to be limited due to its anatomical structure and the carnivorous nature of the diet.

Definitions and Structure

The concept of *prebiotics* was highlighted by Gibson and Roberfroid [2] as: "a non digestible food ingredient that beneficially affects the host by selectively stimulating the growth and/or activity of one or a limited number of bacteria in the colon and thus improves host health". *Non-digestible oligosaccharides* (NDO) in general and FOS in particular are classified as prebiotics [2]. Oligosaccharides are natural components of plants and vegetable products. Some products of animal origin, such as milk, may also contain one or more types of oligosaccharides or their glycoconjugates [3].

Criteria for the classification of a food ingredient as prebiotic [4].
A prebiotic should: – Neither be hydrolysed, nor be absorbed in the proximal gastrointestinal tract. – Be a selective substrate for potentially beneficial commensal bacteria in the large intestine; it should stimulate bacteria to proliferate, become metabolically active, or both. – Change the colonic microenvironment into a healthier one. – Induce gastro-intestinal or systemic effects that are beneficial to the host.

Oligosaccharides can be classified according to the characteristics of [3]:

- Their monomeric sugar unit
- The type of bond between the monomeric sugars
- The chain structure (linear, branched, substitutes)
- The linkage to non-carbohydrates (conjugates)

The polysaccharide inulin and the following oligosaccharides: fructo-oligosaccharide (FOS), isomalto-oligosaccharides (IMO), galacto-oligosaccharides (GOS), xylo-oligosaccharides (XOS), manno-oligosaccharides (MOS), lactulose, lactosucrose (LS) will be discussed in detail (Table 1, Figure 1).

Table 1: Chemical structure of non-digestible oligosaccharides.[5]

Name	Formula	n
Fructo-oligosaccharides (obtained by transfructosylation)	α-D- glu-(1-2)- [β-D- fru- (1-2)-]n	2-4
Fructo-oligosaccharides (obtained by inulin hydrolysis)	β-D- fru-(1-2)- [β-D- fru- (1-2)-]n and α-D- glu-(1-2)- [β-D- fru- (1-2)-]n	1-9 2-9
Isomalto-oligosaccharides	[α- -D- glu- (1-6)-]n	2-5
Galacto-oligosaccharides	α-D-glu (1-4)-[β-D- gal- (1-6)-]n	2-5
Xylo-oligosaccharides	[β-D- xyl- (1-4)-]n	2-9
Lactulose	β-D- gal-(1-4)- α-D-fru	
Lactosucrose	β-D- gal-(1-4)-α-D- glu-(1-2)- β-D-fru	
Soybean-oligosaccharides	[α-D- gal-(1-6)-]n -α-D-glu (1-2)- β-D-fru	1-2

glu: glucose, fru: fructose, gal: galactose, xyl: xylose, n: number of monomers.

Fructans: Fructo-oligosaccharides (FOS) and Inulin

Most plants use starch or sucrose as storage carbohydrates but approximately 15% of the flowering plants store fructans [6]. Fructans are carbohydrates with fructosyl-fructose bonds instead of glucose. They can be linear *β-2,1-linked inulins* or branched *β-2,6-levans* forming fructose oligomers or polymers. Inulin consists mainly or exclusively of β-2,1-fructosyl-fructose linkages and is mainly of plant origin. Levans are mainly produced by many bacteria and some fungi. Both inulin and levans usually have a terminal glucose molecule because they are synthesised from sucrose [7]. Fructans are produced by several mono- and dicotyledonous plant families like *Liliaceae, Amaryllidaceae, Gramineae and Compositae*, including vegetables such as asparagus, garlic, leek, onion, artichoke, Jerusalem artichoke, scorzonera, and chicory roots [7,8]. In plants, fructans are used as carbon storage but they are also involved in plant protection against water deficit caused by drought or low temperature.[6] Indeed, fructan-accumulating plants are abundant in climate zones with seasonal drought or frost but are nearly absent in tropical areas. Starch synthesis decreases dramatically when temperature drops below 10°C but photosynthesis and fructan production are less sensitive to low temperature [6].

Chicory is used as the main inulin source for food industry but agave and Jerusalem artichoke are also used [7]. Fructans are classified according to their degree of polymerisation (DP), which is based on the number of fructosyl units (osyl units). Inulin has a high DP (<60, average of 12) and is strictly speaking no longer an oligosaccharide. By partial enzymatic hydrolysis of inulin under controlled conditions, oligofructose is formed. Oligofructose has a DP of < 9 (average: 4.8) [2]. Chicory-derived inulin (DP>10) is fermented (*in vitro*) at least twice as slowly as oligofructose and will reach more distal parts of the large intestine [9]. FOS can also be produced from sucrose by transfructosylation using the enzyme β-fructofuranosidase and contains between 2 and 4 β-1-2 fructosyl units linked to a terminal α-

D-glucose residue. They are 1-kestose (GF2), 1-nystose (GF3) and 1^F-fructosylnystose (GF4) [5].

Hussein et al [10]. analysed 25 pet food ingredients for short chain fructans. FOS were not detected in corn, corn distiller's solubles, hominy, milo, brown and white rice and brewer's rice, rice hulls, seaweed and soybean meal. But wheat by-products contained the highest concentrations (4-5.07mg/g dry matter) of total FOS followed by peanut hulls, alfalfa meal, barley and wheat (Table 2). Data on longer chain FOS and inulin concentration of typical pet food ingredients are not available.

Table 2: Concentration of FOS in 25 pet-food ingredients.[10]

Ingredients	Total FOS[1] concentration	Ingredients	Total FOS[1] concentration
Alfalfa meal	2.24	Peanut hulls	2.4
Barley	1.95	Rice bran	0.14
Beet pulp	0.05	Soybean hulls	0.12
Canola meal	0.04	Wheat	1.36
Corn gluten feed	0.09	Wheat bran	4.00
Corn gluten meal	0.34	Wheat germ	4.68
Oats	0.36	Wheat middlings	5.07
Oats groats	0.12		

[1] mg/g dry matter; as a mixture of GF2 (1-kestose), GF3 (1-nystose) and GF4 (1^F-fructosylnystose)

Iso-malto-oligosaccharides (IMO)

IMO consist of α-D-glucose residues linked by α(1-6) glycosidic bonds. The mixtures may also contain oligosaccharides with both α(1-6) and α(1-4) glycosidic bonds [11]. IMO is not completely indigestible but is partially digested by intestinal enzymes; however, the bulk of IMO passes into the large intestine.

Galacto-oligosaccharides (GOS)

GOS consist of β1-6 linked galactopyranosyl units linked to a terminal glucopyranosyl residue trough a α 1-4 glycosidic bound. They are used in infant formulas and are naturally present in very low quantities in human milk. They can be produced from lactose via glycosyltransferase by β-galactosidase [5].

In Japan, a different class of GOS, isolated from soybean whey, is used. These alpha-GOS consist of α 1-6 linked galactose units bound to a terminal sucrose molecule [1]. Raffinose (fructose-galactose-glucose) and stachyose (fructose-galactose-galactose-glucose) are non-digestible (50%) oligosaccharides extracted from soybean whey, a by-product of soy protein production [12]. Raffinose and stachyose are also found in pulses (*Phaeseolus vulgaris, Pisum sativum, Lens esculenta*). Alpha-galactosides can be found in leguminous seeds [13].

Xylo-oligosaccharides (XOS)

Xylo-oligosaccharides consist of 2 to 7 units of β1-4 -D linked xylans (5 carbon sugar). Commercially XOS is prepared by enzymatic hydrolysis of xylan polymers rich products such as corncob, bagasse, cottonseeds, brewery and distillers grains. The structure depends on the rate of substitution by arabino- and glucurone side chains [3]. XOS are much more acid resistant compared to other prebiotics [1].

Manno-oligosaccharides (MOS)

A linear chain of D-mannopyranose units linked by β 1-4 bonds is found in the endosperm of tagua palm while a slightly branched mannan is found in the commercial seaweed: red algae (*Porphyra umbilicalis*). These plant mannans differ particularly from yeast mannans, which are highly branched and contain 1-2; 1-3 and 1-6 linkages [14]. MOS play a role in pathogen resistance. Lectins bind to epithelial cells of the gut by attaching to the oligosaccharide component of glycoconjugate receptors. Lectins are carbohydrate-binding (Figure 1).

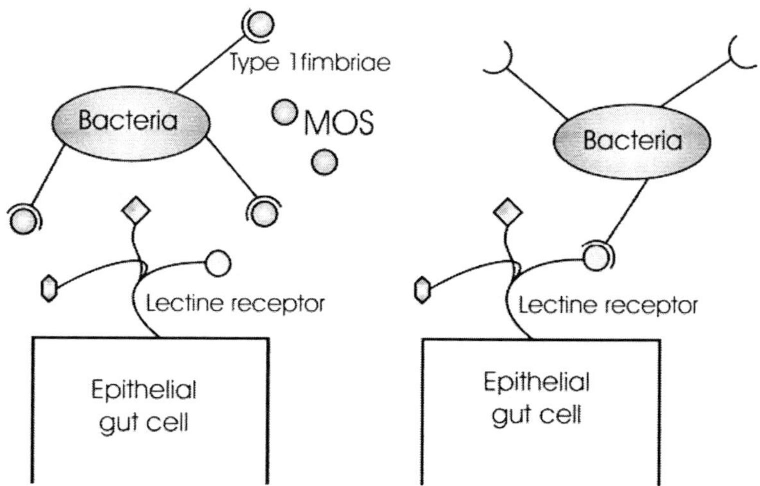

Figure 1: Influence of MOS in pathogen resistance.

Digestibility

In mammals, the activity of small intestinal carbohydrase enzymes is largely restricted to the cleavage of the α(1-4) glucosidic bond, which is the predominant type of linkage between glucose molecules in starch [3]. The β-2,1 osidic bond, including the first glucose-fructose bond of FOS, cannot be hydrolysed by mammalian digestive enzymes (α-glucosidase, maltase, isomaltase, sucrase), which are specific for α-osidic linkages. Substances such as FOS, IMO, soybean oligosaccharides and XOS, will therefore not by digested by pancreatic and small intestine (SI) enzymes and arrive almost intact in the large intestine [15]. FOS largely resist acidic and enzymatic hydrolysis by the digestive system of mammals but can be degraded by specific microbes. FOS and XOS can be fermented by *Bifidobacteria* at the highest rate; by *Lactobacilli*, most *Bacteroides* and *Pepto-streptococcus* at a lower rate but not by *Eubacteriaceae*, most *Clostridia*, *E. coli* and *Staphylococcus* [3]. The resistance to intestinal hydrolytic digestion depends on the extent of polymerisation. IMO with a DP of more than 3 have a good resistance. The β2-1 links of fructans are completely resistant but β2-6 links may be partially hydrolysed at low pH [16].

The fact that prebiotics are not enzymatically digested in the SI is generally accepted but difficult and time consuming to prove experimentally [15] and has therefore been proven *in vivo* only for a few prebiotics [17]. In ileostomy patients, an average of 88% of inulin and oligofructose was recovered at the terminal ileum after dietary supplementation.[17] Additional indications for the poor enzymatic digestibility and small intestinal absorption in people are the lack of increase in serum glucose/insulin concentration after ingestion and the fact that short-chain fructans are not detected in the urine after supplementation with different doses [18 in 15, 19].

In one study, ileal digestibility of the soybean oligosaccharides stachyose and raffinose in dogs was very variable: ileal digestibility of stachyose ranged from 20.9 to 60.8% after addition of conventional soybean meal at 18.55 or 37.1% and total tract digestibility was 100% [20].

The addition of 6% α-gluco-oligosaccharide or maltodextrine-like glucose-based oligosaccharide (MD) to a basal diet reduced the ileal digestibility of carbohydrate by 5.5 and 4.3% points respectively but the effect was not significant ($p=0.08$) [21]. The decrease in ileal digestibility of glucose on the contrary (4.6 and 4.8% points for α-gluco-oligosaccharide and MD respectively) was significant ($p<0.05$). These data indicate that α-gluco-oligosaccharide and MD resist hydrolytic digestion and intact molecules may enter the large intestine.

Prebiotics as Dietary Fibre

Dietary fibre can be classified according to its chemical structure, rate of fermentation, its digestible and indigestible fractions, solubility or ability to disperse in water, as well as its water-holding capacity and viscosity. The degree of fermentation of fibre depends on its physical and chemical structure. In most cases, soluble fibre is rapidly fermentable (e.g. pectins and gums), whereas insoluble fibre such as cellulose and most hemicellulose is slowly fermentable. Fermentation leads to production of lactic acid, short chain fatty acids (SCFA) and gases. All fibre types hold water to some degree but soluble fibre has a greater water-holding capacity and may form gels and viscous solutions [22]. Insoluble, non-fermentable fibre types have a bulking effect and decrease transit time. Inulin and oligofructose can be regarded as soluble and fermentable dietary fibre, behaving in the same way and having similar effects [23,24].

Over the years several definitions of dietary fibre have been used based on different concepts. There are 3 main views [13]:

- The first is a botanical view where dietary fibre is regarded mainly as plant cell wall constituents.
- The second is based on a chemical view and methods for measurements of dietary fibre in the food.
- The third is based on physiological and nutritional consequences. The definition includes all polysaccharides and lignin that resists digestion in the upper GI tract.

Recently the definition has been expanded to oligosaccharides not digested in the small intestine.

Non-starch polysaccharides from plant cell walls, lignin, gums, microbial polysaccharides, inulin, resistant starch and oligosaccharides are all components that vary in chemical structure and properties but are included in the last definition.

Classical analysis methods like AOAC [25] or Englyst methods do not detect oligosaccharides because of their ethanol/water solubility but specific enzymatic or HPLC methods have been developed to determine oligosaccharides in food. Pure inulin is detected by AOAC or Englyst method but the results are unreliable and the recovered fraction is too low. The methods revealed to be even less reliable when results of analysing a known inulin concentration in food (10%) were compared with the analytical results of pure inulin [24,13]. An official method (997.08) for quantification of inulin type fructans in plants and food products has been accepted by the Association of Official Analytical Chemists [25,23].

Physical and chemical properties such as viscosity (soluble fibre), water-binding capacity, particle size and effects of fermentation on GI health may be important for local and systemic responses of fibre [13].

Due to their capacity to form viscous solutions, some water-soluble polysaccharides may increase the volume and viscosity of the intestinal chyme, delay gastric emptying and promote satiety [13]. They can reduce emulsification and assimilation of lipids, decrease the digestion of protein, fat and carbohydrate by hindering the diffusion of digestive enzymes towards the substrates, and slow the release of hydrolysis products, resulting in lower postprandial nutrient levels in the general circulation.

Certain fibre types can adsorb or entrap bile acids and phospholipids leading to increased bile acids excretion and higher cholesterol turn over.

Adsorption and retention of water contributes to the bulking effect of fibre in the colon and the dilution of cytotoxic substances.

Particle size plays a role in transit time, fermentation and faecal excretion. The rate of fermentation is proportional to the external surface area in contact with the bacteria.

Rapidly fermentable fibres are involved in physiological effects on the colon mucosa and function but also in post–absorptive actions on liver and other tissues through metabolism products [13].

Effects in the Gastro-Intestinal Tract

Introduction

Mammalian digestive carbohydrase enzymes cleave the $\alpha(1\text{-}4)$ glucosidic bond, the predominant linkage between glucose molecules in starch. NDO cannot be degraded by these enzymes, but there is evidence that NDO can be degraded in the distal part of the ileum by microbial enzymes [3]. Although the effect of inulin and oligofructose is likely to be minimal in the SI, by adding non-digestible material the dry weight and volume of the ileal chyme is likely to be increased. In contrast to some other soluble fibre types, such as pectin, which are used for their jelly forming properties, oligofructose and inulin do not appear to increase viscosity, nor do they bind bile acids [26, 27]. These properties depend on the length of the chains and the degree of methylation.

Carbohydrate fermentation produces SCFA, lactate, hydrogen, carbon dioxide and methane. The SCFA are absorbed in the colon and can be used for energy; this also reduces the osmotic load in the colon, which decreases risk of osmotic diarrhoea [27]. The possible effects of prebiotic supplementation are presented in table 3 and figure 2.

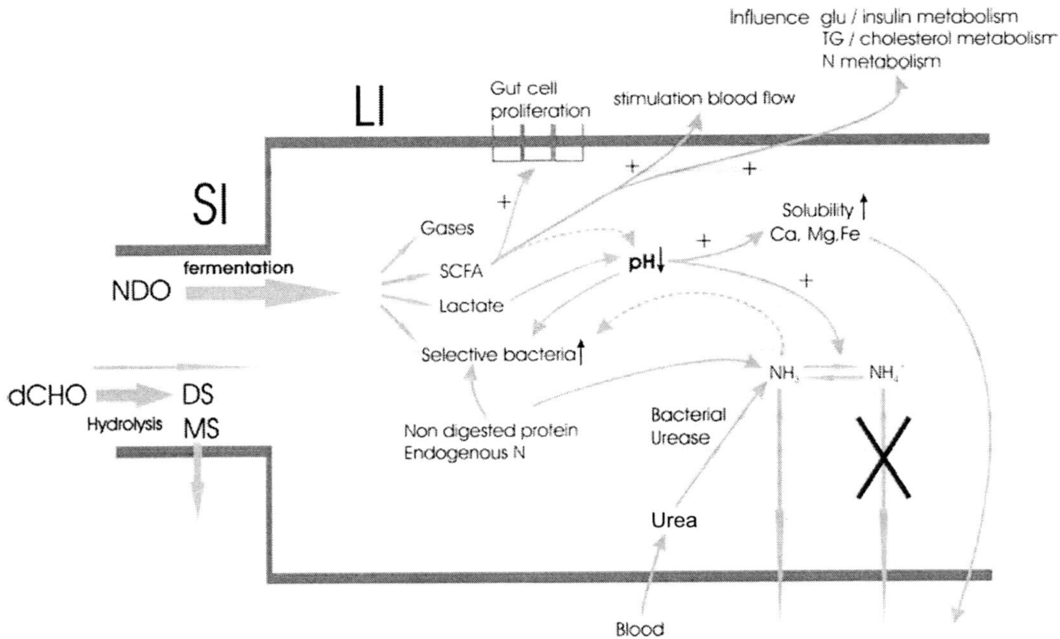

Figure 2: Possible influences of NDO SI: small intestine, LI: large intestine; dCHO: digestible carbohydrates, DS disacchairdes, MS: monosaccharides, Glu: glucose, TG: triglycerides

Dry Matter Intake and Palatability

When fed *ad libitum*, the dry matter (DM) intake as % of body weight was significantly lower in dogs receiving a food supplemented with 1.5% scFOS than in those receiving a food to which 6% of cellulose was added [29]. Increased satiety was suggested to be the consequence of a slower gastric emptying and transit time.

A linear decrease in DM intake was also noted with increasing pectin (P) content in exchange for cellulose (C) (10% supplement consisting of 100% C, 66% C + 33% P, 33% C + 66%P and 100% P respectively) in dogs fed at maintenance energy requirements [30].

Supplementation with α-gluco-oligosaccharides (a branched-chain [α 1-2, α1-4 and α1-6] glucose polymer, average DP of 5) or maltodextrine-like glucose-based oligosaccharide (MD) (α and β: 1-4, 1-6, 1-2, 1-3 linkages) at 6% did not decrease DM intake in dogs [21]. At lower addition rates, (0.5% FOS, MOS or XOS) (0.7% scFOS) oligosaccharides did not reduce DM intake when the food was given at maintenance energy requirements [31,32,33].

When cats were fed *ad libitum*, supplementation with FOS (2%) did not significantly influence feed intake [34]. Likewise, oligofructose supplemented cats fed at maintenance energy intake did not have a reduced feed intake [35].

Table 3: Claimed gastrointestinal effects of prebiotics in humans.[17]

Fermentation in the large bowel
– Production Of SCFA And Lactate
– Gas, Mainly CO2 And H2
– Increased Biomass
– Increased Faecal Energy And Nitrogen
– Mild Laxative properties
Microflora
– Selective increase in Bifidobacteria and Lactobacilli
– Reduction of clostridia
– Increased colonisation resistance to pathogens
– Potential benefit in preventing pathogen invasion
Small intestine
– Osmotic effect of low molecular weight prebiotics (DP 3, 4) which may cause diarrhoea
– Improved Ca, Mg and Fe absorption
– Interaction with mucus to change binding sites for bacteria, lectines etc.
Mouth
– Protection against caries
Others
– Bile acid metabolism: no consistent changes reported
– Variable effect on microbial enzymes with potential to affect carcinogenesis
– Stimulation of apoptosis

In dogs, fed at maintenance energy requirements, NDO do not seem to decrease palatability or DM intake at inclusion rates normally found in commercial feeds. For most cats, sweeteners do not improve the palatability of the diet [36]. But since NDO, like FOS, have a limited sweetening effect [37] palatability problems are not likely to be seen in cats if introduced gradually. For dogs, sugar taste does not reduce palatability [36].

Characteristics of Chymus and Faeces

Water and Dry Matter Content

2.3.1.1 Faecal Consistency Scores

In dogs, low inclusion rates of oligosaccharides (0.5% FOS, MOS or XOS) (0.7% scFOS) did not change faecal consistency scores [31,32,33]. Higher inclusion rates (1g/KG BW or 5.88% diet) of MOS, TGOS and lactose did not have a negative effect on stool quality but lactulose, at the same inclusion rate, tended to decrease faecal consistency compared to the control diet [38]. Supplementation of 3% FOS, MOS or RS did not reduce faecal consistency scores [39]. In addition, consistency problems were not noted after a 10% supplementation of an IMO containing product (65% of IMO) during only 3 days [40].

On a 10% pectin diet, looser stools were seen more frequently compared to the cellulose diet [30]. Soft, unformed stools were seen when an enteral solution was supplemented with

6% α-gluco-oligosaccharide or MD. The loose stools were partially caused by the consumption of an enteral solution but stool quality further decreased by the addition of α-gluco-oligosaccharide and especially by the addition of MD [21]. In a preliminary study, 10% (DM) FOS supplementation was associated with runny faeces in dogs. Therefore FOS was mixed with beet fibre at a 4 to 1 ratio and incorporated at 5 or 10% DM [41].

In cats, a 2% FOS supplementation to a commercial canned diet did not change faecal consistency [34]. Yet, inclusion rates of 6 and 9% of oligofructose decreased faecal consistency as compared to the control and 3% supplementation [35].

2.3.1.2 Dry Matter Content and Production

In general, dietary fibre can increase faecal bulk by increasing bacterial cell mass, undegraded fibre residue, faecal water or a combination of these factors [42]. Faecal water content can be increased by the physical water-holding properties of fibre and possibly by the osmotic effect of SCFA produced during fermentation [43,42]. During rapid fermentation, the reabsorption capacity for SCFA's will be exceeded, resulting in an acid faecal pH and increased water and electrolyte loss [27]. In rats, the increased faecal dry weight excretion of 24 hours indicated that 41-47% of the carbon atoms from oligofructose were incorporated into newly synthesised bacteria [37]. In rats and humans, bulking index (increase in fresh faecal weight in g / g of indigestible carbohydrate eaten) for oligofructose and inulin was around one, which is similar to easily fermentable fibres such as pectin [44]. Van Loo et al. [12] mentioned a slightly higher bulking effect (1.5-2g/g NDO ingested).

In dogs, faecal wet weight was significantly increased at the highest incorporation rate of FOS + beet fibre (8.2%FOS+2% beet fibre) and tended to increase at the lower incorporation rate (4% FOS + 1% beet fibre) compared to the basal diet. Faecal moisture content was significantly increased at both incorporation rates (linearly) but DM production was not altered [41]. (Table 4)

Ileal flow (g DM/day) did not change but faecal moisture content (%) increased and DM output (gDM/day) decreased linearly as pectin content increased (10% cellulose, 3.33% pectin + 6.67% cellulose; 6.67% pectin+ 3.33% cellulose; 10% pectin) [30]. This was suggested to be related to the higher water-holding capacity and fermentability of pectin.

Indeed, MOS supplementation (5.88%) increased faecal moisture content (%) compared to the basal diet but unbound water content (measured by centrifugation) was lowest. This increased water-binding might have influenced the solubility of nutrients (see paragraph on digestibility) [38].

Stool bulk increased by 28.5% during LS supplementation in dogs. Faecal water content increased significantly after LS supplementation (1.5g/day) and was normalised 7 days after the treatment was stopped [45].

Inulin supplementation (7% DM) significantly increased stool volume (g/day). This was the consequence of increased moisture content of the faeces, not of increased DM excretion. At the same time the daily water consumption was increased by 39% [46].

A linear increase of wet faecal production ($p=0.042$) was noted with two doses of lactulose (2.3 and 6.5% DM) [47]. Once again, faecal DM production was not changed but there was a trend ($p=0.088$) for a lower DM content.

Inclusion rates of more than 2% chicory (a natural source of inulin) increased faecal volume.[48] Faecal weight (g/day) was significantly increased by the addition of 6% α-gluco-oligosaccharide or MD to a highly digestible dog diet. Faecal DM excretion (g/day) was only increased by MD addition probably because of incomplete fermentation (see carbohydrate digestibility) [21].

Table 4: Effect of NDO on faecal production and moisture content in dogs.

Reference	Supplement	Suppl. rate	Faecal prod.* g/day	DM%	Faecal prod. gDM/ day
[47]	Lactulose	1g/MJ 3g/MJ	79→80.7 79→93.3	33.6→32 NS 33.6→29 NS	
[51]	FOS	1%	144.7→137 NS	32.2→33 NS	
[41]	FOS + sugar beet fibre	4+1%DM 8.2+2%DM	139→180 NS 139→222	29→25.3 29→22	40.3→45 NS 40.3→48 NS
[46]	Inulin	7%DM	65.6→96.0	34.4→27	22.6→25.9 NS
[21]	α-gluco OS MD	6% DM	35→64.8 35→79.4		16→20 NS 16→26.7
[50]	FOS	1g/day 3g/day	NS NS		44→48 44→34
[31]	FOS MOS XOS	0.5%DM	350→340 NS 350→330 NS 350→350 NS		33.4→34.9 NS 33.4→35.5 NS 33.4→36.7 NS
[32]	FOS†	0.7%DM	248→241 NS 288→232	39.4→40.7 NS 39.1→40.1 NS	98→98 NS 113→93
[33]	FOS MOS	0.5%	167→166 NS 167→165 NS	38→39 NS 38→38.2 NS	
[30]	pectin	10%DM		49.5→35	40→23.7
[45]	lactosucrose	0.25%	435→576	25.7→23.1	
[38]	MOS, TGOS, Lactose, Lactulose	5.88%		35,7→31.6 →36.1 NS →36.3 NS →32.1 NS	

*(g/day) OS: oligosaccharide; †results of two identical experiments. Absolute figures cannot be compared between the studies because not all references included body weights or food intakes; NS: non-significant

The addition of FOS or IMO to a protein supplemented diet significantly increased or tended to increase faecal production but faecal moisture content was not significantly changed. On the other hand, faecal dry matter production was significantly increased in two of the three protein and NDO supplemented groups [49].

Surprisingly, in one study, faecal output, on "as is" and "dry matter" basis was decreased after 0.7% (DM) scFOS supplementation compared to the control diet (p respectively: 0.06 and 0.05) [32]. Dry matter and organic matter digestibility of the control diet were 76.8 and 87% respectively and were not significantly influenced by the addition of FOS. The moisture content was not changed [32]. The effect may also depend on the dose used. Supplementation of 1g oligofructose per day increased dry faecal output but 3g/day decreased dry faecal output [50].

Lactulose (5.88%) tended to decrease faecal consistency scores but moisture content (%) was not changed [38]. Faecal production and moisture content were unchanged after 1%

oligofructose supplementation or 0.5% FOS, MOS or both in dogs [33,51]. Small amounts of oligosaccharides (0.5% FOS, MOS or XOS) did not change faecal DM output and ileal DM flow compared to the control diet [31]. Faecal moisture output tended to be slightly decreased in the oligosaccharide supplemented groups.

In cats, information is scarce. In one study, faecal DM production was 23% higher after FOS supplementation (2%) compared to the control diet [34], which was not seen in dogs except for MD supplementation at 6% [21] and FOS or IMO supplementation to a protein supplemented diet. [49]. Lactosucrose supplementation in cats slightly increased faecal water content and stool weights were increased by 10.4 and 6.6% seven and fourteen days after supplementation respectively, although statistical significance was not reached [52]. A higher moisture content induced an increased fresh faecal production after oligofructose (6 and 9%) supplementation compared to the control diet and 3% supplementation. Daily faecal dry matter production was not increased after 3 or 6% inulin or 3% oligofructose supplementation compared to the control diet [35].

The bulking indexes calculated from literature are given in table 5. The results are slightly inconsistent even within one animal species. In cats, the bulking index for oligofructose (3%) in one experiment [35] was 1.7 compared to 4.76 in another experiment [66]. However, the diets used in both experiments were quite different (maintenance versus renal diet). When the same diets were used, the differences were moderate (0.6-1.7 for oligofructose). On the other hand, a clear dose effect can be noted as the bulking index increases with increasing prebiotic dose. In dogs, bulking indexes of about 1 were noted for oligofructose. For dogs, similar bulking indexes as in humans (1-2g/g NDO) can be used for oligofructose and inulin although the practical use is probably limited.

Table 5: Calculated bulking indexes.

Reference	Species	Supplement	Doses	Bulking index*
[46]	Dogs	inulin	7%	1.89
[47]	Dogs	Lactulose	1g/MJ	0.44
[47]	Dogs	Lactulose	3g/MJ	1.23
[35]	Cats	Oligofructose	3%	-0.6
[35]	Cats	Oligofructose	3%	1.74
[66]	Cats	Oligofructose	3.1%	4.76
[35]	Cats	Oligofructose	6%	2.3
[35]	Cats	Oligofructose	9%	2.5
[35]	Cats	Inulin	3%	1.05
	Cats	Inulin	6%	2.36
[49]†	Dogs	Oligofructose	3%	1.02
	Dogs	IMO	3%	3.03
[39]	Dogs	Oligofructose	3%	0.89
	Dogs	IMO	3%	-0.08
	Dogs	RS	3%	1.67

* Calculated as the increase in daily faecal wet weight in g per daily NDO intake in g.

† Differences per protein supplement: MBM (meat and bone meal): 1.05 (or FOS:-0.46 IMO: 2.56); GM (greaves meal): 3.13 (or FOS 2.43 IMO: 3.83); PM (poultry meal): 1.89 (or FOS: 1.08 IMO: 2.7). IMO: isomalto-oligosaccharide, RS: resistant starch.

The effect of NDO on faecal consistency is dose dependent. Low doses do not seem to decrease faecal consistency but high doses may induce runny faeces. The duration of the adaptation period may also play a role since lower doses may cause consistency problems in unadapted animals. In addition, the composition of the basal diet is important as well. Depending on the source of NDO and the dose, NDO supplementation seems to increase faecal volume because of an increased moisture content of the faeces in dogs. This increased moisture is probably the consequence of an increased water-holding capacity of the supplement. This may be accompanied by higher water consumption. In most studies, DM production was not changed. With lower supplementation doses, the effect on faecal volume and moisture content was not significantly changed.

pH

Due to fermentation and consequently production of lactic acid and SCFA, intestinal pH can be decreased.

In dogs, mean ileal pH of 7.1 was not changed by supplementation of 0.5% FOS, MOS or XOS in the dog [31].

The already low faecal pH (6.3) did not further decrease after LS supplementation [45]. The same was true for the supplementation of 1% of oligofructose (faecal pH: 6.1) [51], 3% of chicory or 1% of FOS (faecal pH: 5.7-5.9) [48] and 0.7% scFOS (faecal pH6.5-6.3) [32] in dogs. Probiotic and synbiotic supplementation had no effect either [32]. A high faecal pH (6.8-7.1) on a protein supplemented diet was not decreased by 3% FOS or IMO [49].

The faecal pH decreased from 6.9-7.1 after feeding the basal diets, a diet supplemented with TGOS or lactose to 6.6 after adding 5.88% MOS to the diet [38]. Faecal pH also decreased from 7.14 to 6.61 after the addition of lactulose both at 0.1 or 3.0 g/MJ ME [47]. FOS supplementation (0.5%) did not reduce faecal pH but unexpectedly MOS supplementation tended ($p=0.088$) to increase faecal pH from 6.76 to 7.27 [33].

In cats, faecal pH was decreased from 6.3 to 6.1-6.0 after LS supplementation although statistical significance was not reached [52]. Faecal pH was decreased from 6.37 and 6.21 in the control and 3% oligofructose group to 5.99 and 5.73 after 6 and 9% supplementation respectively [35]. Nevertheless, inulin (3 and 6%) and oligofructose (3%) did not reduce the faecal pH compared to the control diet (6.86) in another experiment [35].

The change in faecal pH generated by the supplementation of NDO seems to depend on the initial pH. The faecal pH can be decreased if rather high before supplementation, but if the initial pH is low no further decrease should be expected. If with an initially high faecal pH no decrease is seen after the addition of NDO, it may be possible that the decrease in pH is restricted to the more proximal large intestine, especially if rapidly fermentable NDO are used.

Short Chain Fatty Acids

During the fermentation of carbohydrates, short chain fatty acids (SCFA) (mainly acetate, propionate and butyrate) and lactate are produced along with gases. This allows the host to recuperate part of the energy of the NDO but these fermentation products may also play a role in regulating cell metabolism as well as cell division and differentiation [7]. As up to 95% of produced acids are rapidly absorbed in the colon, faecal concentrations are not representative of the situation in the large intestine.

In vitro tests with faecal/cecal inoculum from humans or rats, indicated that inulin increased the production of acetate and butyrate, whereas GOS increased acetate and propionate production and XOS increased acetate production only [12].

An *in vitro* test with canine faecal inoculum showed a high total SCFA production after FOS supplementation. However, compared to human *in vitro* tests, the production of individual SCFA (acetate, propionate, butyrate) was slightly lower in dogs [53]. In cats the SCFA production after supplementation of FOS was high compared to other substrates, but total SCFA production seemed slightly lower compared to the dog experiment [54]. Vickers et al. [55] compared fermentation of four inulin products, FOS, MOS, soy fibre, beet pulp and cellulose in an *in vitro* test with dog faeces. Total SCFA, butyrate and acetate production were highest for the 4 inulin products and FOS. FOS and two of the four inulin products produced significantly higher amounts of propionate. Lactate production was higher after inoculation with FOS and 1 of the inulin products compared with the other substrates. In ruminants, faster fermentation results in the formation of relatively more propionate and less acetate [56]. Indeed, the acetate/propionate ratio decreased 6 hours after onset of fermentation for inulin, FOS and soy fibre but increased when using beet pulp, MOS and cellulose in dogs. The author suggested that the substrates with a lower acetate/propionate ratio might be degraded more rapidly [55].

The produced butyrate is used as an oxidative fuel for the colonocytes but also influences cell maturation, cell differentiation and apoptosis [57]. Butyrate acts as a metabolic fuel for the large intestinal mucosa in rats but this has not yet been proven in dogs [55]. However, results of Drackly et al [58] suggest that butyrate is oxidised at a relatively high rate by jejunal canine enterocytes and showed that oxidation of glucose and propionate was decreased when a combination of substrates (glucose, propionate, butyrate and glutamine) was available for enterocytes. The oxidation of glutamine and propionate in the colonocytes was also decreased after using the combined substrate. In contrast to other species, butyrate was a major fuel for canine colonocytes but glucose appeared to be an obligatory fuel. Acetate and ketone bodies were not tested [58].

Ileal Concentrations / Productions

Silvio et al. [30] measured ileal SCFA concentrations in dogs fed diets where cellulose was substituted by the rapidly fermentable fibre pectin. Total SCFA (μmol/g) concentrations were higher with the cellulose diets but because data on ileal DM content and water-holding capacity were not available this might be misleading. Ileal acetate and propionate proportion increased with increasing pectin content whereas isobutyrate and isovalerate decreased. With low inclusion rates of oligosaccharides (0.5% FOS, MOS or XOS) significant changes in ileal SCFA proportions were not noted [31]. However, ileal butyrate proportion tended to decrease after oligosaccharide supplementation compared to the control ($p=0.07$) but tended to increase in FOS and XOS compared to MOS ($p=0.07$). The proportion of propionate tended to be higher in MOS compared to FOS or XOS ($p= 0.09$) Total ileal VFA concentrations (on DM as well as wet weight) were not affected by treatment [31].

Faecal Concentrations/Productions

In dogs, faecal butyric acid concentration was significantly decreased after 14 days of LS supplementation but other VFA concentrations were not changed [45]. (Table 6)

Swanson et al. [32] showed some significant changes in faecal SCFA concentration after scFOS supplementation (0.7%DM) but the results were inconsistent between two consecutive experiments: in a first experiment propionate and lactate concentration were significantly increased and butyrate tended to be increased (p=0.06); in a second experiment only butyrate was significantly increased and lactate tended to be increased (p=0.06). Neither experiment demonstrated an effect on faecal acetate or total SCFA concentration. In the second experiment isobutyrate and isovalerate concentration as well as total BCFA concentration (μmol/g DM) were significantly decreased but this was not noted in the first experiment.

Faecal VFA concentrations were not different after MOS, TGOS, lactose or lactulose supplementation (5.88%) in dogs but tended to increase after a 24h incubation period after MOS and lactulose supplementation [38]. With lower supplementation rates of FOS, MOS or FOS+MOS (0.5%), faecal SCFA and BCFA were not altered in dogs [33].

In cats, faecal acetic acid content decreased after 6% inulin supplementation compared to the control diet and 3% inulin or oligofructose supplementation. Faecal valeric acid content and total VFA excretion increased after 6% inulin supplementation compared to the control diet. The ratio acetic to propionic acid decreased after inulin supplementation (3 and 6%) [35].

In vitro tests with dog or cat faecal inoculum seem to affect total or individual production of SCFA after FOS or inulin supplementation. *In vivo* pectin supplementation influenced the proportion of ileal acetate and propionate but significant effects on ileal SCFA proportion were not seen for NDO. Though there were some tendencies and the effect of NDO on ileal proportions of SCFA was only tested in one experiment. Data on faecal SCFA concentrations and productions are inconsistent. Faecal production or concentrations of SCFA do not necessarily reflect changes in SCFA production in the large intestine as up to 95% of the SCFA are rapidly absorbed. Consequently, without *in situ* (proximal and distal large intestine) or portal blood measurements it is impossible to know the exact pattern of acid production after NDO supplementation in dogs or cats.

Ammonia/ammonium Concentration/production

Increased colonic luminal ammonia concentrations can promote tumorigenesis by stimulating cell proliferation [59]. Dietary fibre may be protective by dilution of ammonia, by increasing the passage of ammonia through the colon, by inducing a lower colonic pH and consequently less absorption of ammonia (absorption mainly by non–ionic diffusion; more acidic pH: more ammonium (NH_4^+): less absorption) or by the 'nitrogen sink': bacteria may scavenge ammonia nitrogen for protein synthesis if a suitable energy source is available (fermentable dietary fibre) [59]. Bacterial protein synthesis depends on an energy (fermentable fibre) and a nitrogen source. Nitrogen can be provided by undigested protein, mucins, bile, cell debris, enzymes, passive diffusion of blood urea [60]. Ammonia in the colon can be generated from urea by bacterial urease but also from bacterial deamination of amino acids, peptides and proteins. The protein content of the diet as well as the protein digestibility will play an important role. Martineau and Laflamme [61] compared the effect of a dry and a canned dog diet on faecal putrefactive compounds. Faecal ammonia concentrations were significantly higher in the high protein canned diet (41.4 versus 24.8%DM) although the soluble fibre content of the canned diet was higher (5.3 versus <0.6%DM). Dietary protein quantity or composition might be responsible for the higher ammonia concentration but diets differed also in nutrients other than protein and ingredients.

Table 6: Faecal concentrations of SCFA

Ref.	NDO	Suppl. rate	BA	AA	PA	VA	Total SCFA	IV	IB	BCFA	LA
32	scFOS	0.7% DM	↑ (p=0.06)	NS	↑	NS	NS[1]	NS	NS	NS[2]	↑
	scFOS	0.7% DM	↑	NS	NS		NS[1]	↓	↓	↓[2]	↑ (p=0.06)
33	FOS, MOS, FOS+MOS	0.5%AF 0.5+0.5%					NS[1]			NS[2]	
45	Lactosucrose	1.5g/day (0.25% AF)	↓	NS	NS	NS	NS	NS	NS		
38	MOS TGOS Lactose Lactulose	5.88%					↑[3*] NS[3] NS[3] ↑[3*]				

BA Butyric acid, AA Acetic acid, PA: propionic acid, VA: valeric acid, IB: iso-butyric acid, IV iso-valeric acid, BCFA: branched chain fatty acid; LA: Lactic acid.

[1] AA+PA+BA.

[2] VA+IV+IB.

[3] after a 24hour incubation period.

[*] significantly different from the basal diet in period II but not in period I.

Another important factor is the collection of the faecal samples. They should be as fresh as possible as ammonia is volatile and concentrations will decrease over time.

In dogs, ileal ammonia concentrations linearly decreased with increasing pectin supplementation (substituted for cellulose) [30]. This may indicate an enhanced rate of ammonia use by bacteria because of the higher pectin fermentability or a higher ammonia production in the less fermentable cellulose diet. Ileal protein digestibility (dietary protein content 21%DM) was not affected by fibre source. Strickling et al. [31]. both measured ileal and faecal ammonia concentration and noted no differences after low inclusion rates of oligosaccharide (0.5% FOS, MOS or XOS) in a high protein diet (30%DM).

Faecal ammonia concentration decreased significantly after 14 days of LS supplementation to a moderate protein diet (25.7% as fed) [45]. Faecal ammonia concentrations decreased after MOS supplementation (5.88%) compared to the basal diet and lactulose supplementation but TGOS and lactose concentration did not induce changes [38]. Surprisingly, the basal diet had a rather high protein content (36.6% as fed). In the same experiment faecal ammonia concentrations were different between the basal diets given at two different periods. Ammonia production after a *24-h in vitro* faecal incubation period was not different between the different supplements (TGOS, MOS, lactose and lactulose) but when compared to the basal diet, ammonia production increased after lactulose supplementation and a similar trend was noted for the other supplements [38].

Faecal ammonia concentrations may be decreased but if faecal volume is increased, ammonia production is not necessarily lower. Faecal ammonium (NH4+) production was not decreased after 1% of oligofructose supplementation to a rather high protein diet (28.8%DM) in dogs [51]. Faecal pH (6.1) was not influenced by oligofructose, implying that there was no conversion from ammonia to ammonium (NH4+). In an earlier study of the same author [47], faecal pH (7.14) was higher and ammonium excretion (9.1mmol/day compared to 16.6mmol/day in the previously mentioned experiment, control diets) lower, pointing to the importance of a negative correlation between pH and ammonium excretion. In this study, ammonia excretion was not influenced by adding the lactulose supplement to an even higher protein diet (35.3%DM) either.

Faecal ammonia concentration did not change after supplementation of FOS, MOS (0.5%) or both to a protein rich diet [62].

Swanson et al. [32] noted a significant increase in faecal ammonia concentration in one experiment but no effect in another experiment after scFOS supplementation (0.7%DM) to a moderate protein diet (23.8%) in dogs. Faecal ammonia excretion was not changed by adding FOS or IMO (3%) to a protein supplemented diet except for the greaves meal supplemented diet where ammonia excretion was increased by oligosaccharide supplementation [49].

In cats, Terada et al. [52] noted a significantly decreased faecal and urinary ammonia concentration after LS supplementation. Moreover the ammonia concentration in the surrounding air was decreased significantly.

The inconsistent results on the influence on ammonia concentration after prebiotic supplementation can be caused by the fact that faecal ammonia concentrations are not a clear reflection of ammonia production since the absorption of ammonia depends on the local pH - ammonia (NH_3) can only be absorbed as ammonia and not as ammonium (NH_4^+) and NH_4^+ is formed at lower pH conditions - and the rate of incorporation into bacterial proteins depends on the availability of fermentable energy. A study in rats [59] showed decreased ammonia concentrations in the caecum but three times greater concentrations in the colon after supplementing a low (8%) as well as a high protein (24%) diet with pectin (8%). This was partly explained by a decreased protein absorption in the SI and by an increased number of colonic microorganisms and consequently increased hydrolysis of urea to ammonia/ammonium by bacterial urease. Consequently, faecal concentrations are not necessarily a good indication of ammonia production as even within the different parts of the large intestine differences can be generated.

Ammonia concentration can be influenced by protein digestibility, protein amount (amount of protein that enters the large intestine) and fibre content (dilution, transit time) which might explain the differences between the experiments.

Other Faecal Metabolic/ putrefactive Products

Fewer aberrant crypt foci (early colonic preneoplastic lesions) induced by azoxymethane were seen in rats after 10% oligofructose or inulin supplementation compared to the placebo group [63]. It was suggested that this was the result of *Bifidobacteria* who contain relatively less enzymes such as β-glucuronidase, azoreductase, nitro and nitrate reductase. These enzymes can convert precancerous substances into cancerogens. However the bulking effect could also contribute to the antineoplastic effect due to a decreased exposure to cancerogens [64,4].

Mull and Perry [3] suggested the use of FOS in elderly dogs to reduce the production of putrefactive substances and bad smelling flatus. Bad faecal odour may be inconvenient for dog and cat owners and might be a potential indicator for a decreased GI health of the animal.

The main faecal odourous substances generated by bacterial degradation of endogenous and undigested protein are presented in table 7.

Table 7: Main faecal odour components. [65]

Ammonia	
Aliphatic amines	agmantine, cadaverine, phenylethylamine, putrescine, tyramine
Branched chain fatty acids	isobutyrate, isovalerate
Indoles	indole, 3-methylindole (skatol), 2-methylindole, 2,3-methylindole, 2,5-methylindole
Phenols	phenol, p-cresol, 4-ethylphenol
Volatile sulphur-containing compounds	dimethyl disulfide, diethyl disulfide, di-n-propyl disulfide, di-n-butyl disulfide

Pathogenic and less desirable bacteria are responsible for the production of faecal odour components [65]. On the other hand, the growth or activity of one or a limited number of desirable bacteria in the colon can be selectively stimulated by prebiotics [2].

A few studies in dogs or cats have investigated the effect of NDO on the excretion of these putrefactive substances.

In dogs, faecal phenol, ethylphenol, indole and skatol concentration significantly decreased after 14 days of LS supplementation (1.5g/day) [45].

Swanson et al. [33] measured four indoles (indole, 2-methyl indole, 3-methyl indole, 2.3-dimethyl indole) in freshly collected faecal samples but only indole was quantifiable in all faecal samples. A tendency for a 50% decrease in indole concentration was noted for FOS

(0.5%) (p=0.075) and FOS (0.5%) + MOS (0.5%) (p=0.082). In a second experiment [32] scFOS supplementation (0.7%) also tended to decrease indol concentration (p= 0.07).

Due to high variability, potential differences in faecal total phenol concentrations could not be shown. Individual phenols (phenol, p-creasol, 4-ethylphenol) were not present in all faecal samples although most samples contained at least one of them. The combined concentration of indoles and phenols was significantly decreased (approximately 50%) in FOS (0.5%) and FOS+MOS compared to the control diet [33].

FOS supplementation (0.7%DM) did not affect concentrations of phenol and 4-ethylphenol in freshly collected faecal samples in dogs [32]. However, in a first experiment, total phenols and total indoles and phenols decreased or tended to decrease (p=0.07) respectively but this was not repeatable in a second experiment. There were no significant effects (p>0.1) on faecal concentrations of biogenic amines (agmantine, cadaverine, histamine, phenylethylamine, putrescine, spermidine, spermine, tryptamine, tyramine, total biogenic amines, total monogenic amines and decylamine) by the addition of FOS and/or MOS [32,33]. Faecal samples were also incubated for determination of volatile sulphur containing components. Dimethyl disulphide (DMDS) and dimethyl trisulphide (DMTS) were only detected in trace amounts. A treatment effect was noted for hydrogen sulphide in a first but not in a second experiment. After 24h of fermentation, FOS supplementation showed the lowest hydrogen sulphide concentrations followed by the control and synbiotic (FOS + *Lactobacillus acidophilus*) treatment. The highest concentrations were noted after the probiotic treatment (*Lactobacillus acidophilus*) [32]. Faecal emission of H_2S was not changed after supplementation with FOS, IMO or resistant starch [39].

In cats, Terada et al. [52] noted a significantly decreased ethylphenol and indole concentration in the faeces of cats supplemented with LS. Phenol, p-cresol and skatol concentrations were not changed. Emission of H_2S and dimethyldisulphide were not changed after FOS supplementation [66].

Although similar trends were noted for some substances (decreased indol, total indols and phenols concentrations), data on other substances are inconsistent especially in the experiment of Swanson et al. [32] where 40 dogs were divided over 2 experiments and different results were seen for the 2 experiments.

One should also hold in mind that faecal concentrations give an idea of the odorous potential but not on the odour production since the odour components are volatile and their emission depends on several environmental components e.g. temperature, pH, moisture of the faeces and atmospheric humidity [67].

Flora

Although fibre fermentation is not highly contributing to energy supply in dogs and cats, fibre fermentation may contribute to intestinal health [68]. The microflora of the gastrointestinal tract are diverse and complex. Some bacteria are pathogenic whereas others may be health promoting (Table 8). Health promoting groups may inhibit harmful bacteria, stimulate immune function, aid in digestion and absorption of food and synthesise vitamins. Harmful groups may produce toxins, carcinogens or putrefactive substances.

Table 8: Predominant human faecal bacteria, classified due to their generally beneficial, harmful or pathogenic effects.[2]

Potentially harmful pathogenic bacteria	Potentially health promoting bacteria
Ps. aeruginosa	*Lactobacilli*
Proteus	*Eubacteria*
Staphylococci	*Bifidobacteria*
Clostridia	
Veillonellae	
Enterococci	
E. coli	
Streptococci	
Bacteriodes	

Fructans may increase *Bifidobacteria* and *Lactobacilli* populations, suppress putrefactive bacteria and reduce toxic fermentation products [69 in 50]. Toxic metabolites can be formed during fermentation by *E. coli, Clostridia* (ammonia, amines, nitrosamines, phenols, indole, aglycones and secondary bile acids), *Bacteroides spp*., *Streprococcus faecalis* (nitrosamines, aglycones, sec. bile acids) and *Proteus* (ammonia, amines, indole) [69 in 50]. Secondary bile acids are produced by bacteria from primary bile acids by dehydroxylation [70].

Total anaerobes and aerobes indicate general fermentative activity. *Bifidobacteria* and *Lactobacilli* indicate a more remedial, beneficial bacterial population and have been associated with decreased faecal concentrations of potentially pathogenic bacteria and decreased levels of putrefactive and carcinogenic compounds. *Bifidobacteria* are believed to stimulate immune system [71]. Most *Bacteroides*, a predominant colonic bacterial genus, are considered neither beneficial, neither detrimental. *Bacteroides* are polysaccharide utilisers [2].

The selective growth of beneficial bacteria can be at the expense of other bacteria such as *Bacteroides*, *Clostridia* or other coliformes. This could be in part by the lower pH of the local environment but according to Teitelbaum and Walker [4] supplemental mechanisms are likely.

The bacterial diversity in the dog intestine was similar to human intestine [72] and was confirmed by Benno et al. [73] Compared to humans and dogs, healthy cats have higher numbers of bacteria in the proximal part of the SI [74,75]. Total bacterial count was approaching 10^6 CFU/ml, regardless of the diet (commercial dry or canned diet) [74,75,79]. Aerobes were more numerous than anaerobes [74].

The older pet population tended to have a less desirable large intestinal microbial flora compared to younger animals. Beagle dogs of more than 11 years, harboured significantly less *Bifidobacteria, Lactobacilli*, *Bacteroides*, *Eubacteria*, *Peptostreptococci*, total anaerobes and total bacteria in the large intestine (colon and/or caecum and/or rectum) compared to younger dogs (<12 months). On the other hand, lecithinase negative *Clostridia* (alpha toxin is a lecithinase) and *Streptococci* were significantly increased in the rectum of older dogs. The microflora of the stomach, duodenum, jejunum and ileum showed no differences between the age groups [73]. Dietary composition also plays a role as *C. perfringens* numbers were increased by protein enriched diets and *Bifidobacteria* and *Lactobacilli* by fermentable carbohydrates [80].

Small Intestinal Flora

In healthy dogs, total aerobic and anaerobic bacterial concentrations were not changed in duodenum and ileum after 1.5% of scFOS supplementation nor did total coliformes and *lactobacillus spp* [29]. However, *Clostridium spp.* were significantly increased in the ileum but not in the duodenum of dogs supplemented with FOS. A fibre blend consisting of 6% beet pulp, 2% of gum talha and 1.5% FOS, did not change the Clostridial concentrations [29].

Strickling et al. [31] also measured ileal bacterial colony forming units (*C. perfringens*, *Bifidobacteria*, *Lactobacilli*, aerotolerant anaerobes, *E. coli* and Coliformes) and did not note significant differences after rather low inclusion rates (0.5%) of FOS, MOS or XOS after 21 days of supplementation.

Duodenal, proximal jejunal fluid and tissue were sampled by laparotomy in dogs with small intestinal bacterial overgrowth (SIBO) due to Ig A deficiency: FOS supplementation (1%) decreased aerobic and facultative anaerobic counts compared to the control group. Counts of anaerobic bacteria in fluid samples were not different between the 2 groups but in tissue samples the counts were lower in the FOS supplemented group [81]. Consequently, FOS supplementation might be applied in clinical nutrition in dogs with SIBO.

In cats, FOS supplementation (0.75%DM) did not induce changes in the flora (aerobic, anaerobic and total bacterial counts) of duodenal juice collected trough oral endoscopy [74]. Bacterial counts of individuals varied considerably over time though consuming the same diet. Comparison of the prevalence of common bacterial species/groups (*E. faecalis*, *C. perfringens*, *Bacteroides*, *Pasteurella*, *Streptococcus spp.*, unidentified gram-negative rods, *E. coli*, *Neisseria spp.* and *Staphylococci*) showed no influence of FOS supplementation [74].

Large Intestinal and Faecal Flora

Dogs

Microbial N, estimated by measuring purine content of faeces and bacterial isolates from faeces, were increased by 1.5% of scFOS supplementation compared to 6% of cellulose, when expressed as a percentage of N intake or total N output. [29]. Total faecal count of dead and live bacteria was not increased by 1% of oligofructose supplementation in dogs [51].

In dogs, several experiments *in vivo* with different fermentable fibre supplementation investigated the effects on the large intestinal and/or faecal flora. The results will be discussed by bacterial group (Table 9).

Beynen et al. [51] showed significant increases in total counts of aerobic and anaerobic bacteria after 1% of oligofructose supplementation in dogs.

Howard et al. [29] compared several fermentable fibres (6% beet pulp, 1.5% scFOS) and a fibre blend (6% beet pulp + 2% gum talha and 1.5% FOS) with 6% cellulose in dogs and noted no differences for total anaerobes, total coliformes in proximal and distal colon; however total aerobic bacteria tended to increase in the distal colon after FOS supplementation (p=0.1). In two experiments with 0.7% sc FOS supplementation, faecal concentrations of total anaerobes did not change but in one of the two experiments, total aerobes significantly increased [32]. Swanson et al. [33] noted a trend for a lower total aerobe population after MOS supplementation (0.5%) (p=0.054) and lower anaerobe population after MOS+FOS supplementation (both 0.5%) (p=0.088) compared to the control diet.

Table 9: Effect of prebiotica on large intestinal/ fecal flora in dogs

Reference	prebiotic	Total aerobes	Total anaerobes	*Bifidob.*	*Lactob.*	*Clostridia*	*Bacteroides*	Coliformes	others
[51]	1% oligofructose	↑	↑	↑	↑NS	↑	=		*Streptococci*↑
[21]	6%GlucoOS, MD	=	=	=	=		=		
[29][†]	1.5% FOS Fibre blend[a]	↑ (NS) =	= =	Not present	= =	= =		= =	
[48]	0; 1.5; 3; 5% chicory or 1% FOS or 3% chicory			↑		= ↓			
[31]	0.5% FOS, MOS, XOS		=[*]		=	=, ↓ (MOS↔ FOS;XOS)		=	
[32]	0.7% sc FOS	↑ or =	=	↑ or =	↑NS or =	↓NS or =		=	
[33]	0.5%MOS, FOS	↓NS (MOS)	↓NS (MOS+FOS)	=	↑NS (MOS)	=		=	
[45]	0.27% lactosucrose			↑	=	↓[b]	=		
[82]	1% FOS			Present in 4/18 samples		=	=	=	

NS: statistical non-significant changes.

[*] aerotolerant anaerobes.

[†] in distal colon.

[a] 6% beet pulp, 2% gum talha and 1.5% FOS.

[b] Lecithinase positive.

In other studies faecal counts of total aerobes, anaerobes or aerotolerant anaerobes, were not changed after NDO supplementation [21,21,45].

Terada et al. [45] noted a 5-fold increase of faecal *Bifidobacteria* after 7 and 14 days of LS supplementation (0.27% DM) compared to non-supplementation. Beynen et al. [51] showed significant increases in bifidobacterial counts after 1% of oligofructose supplementation in dogs. Faecal concentrations of *Bifidobacteria* increased significantly ($p<0.05$) after 3% of chicory or 1% of FOS addition to a dry dog diet [48]. In another experiment, chicory was added at 3 levels (0; 1.5; 3 and 5%) and all inclusion rates significantly increased *Bifidobacteria* concentrations [48]. In one of two experiments, *Bifidobacteria* counts were significantly increased after 0.7% scFOS supplementation [32]. Viable *Bifidobacteria* were not found at any of the four parts of the intestinal tract (duodenum, ileum, proximal and distal colon) using a fructose-6-phosphate-phosphoketolase assay in dogs fed beet pulp, FOS, cellulose or a fibre blend [29]. Furthermore, *Bifidobacteria* were not isolated in faecal samples in labrador dogs [76]. In an earlier study, *Bifidobacteria* were also not detected in conventionally housed dogs but were a predominant species in dogs housed in a locked environment or dogs in a conventional environment after being in the locked environment for one month [72]. Moreover, Benno et al. [73] found *Bifidobacteria* in caecum, colon and rectum of all young animals (<12 months) and in rectum of all older animals (>11years). *Bifidobacteria* were found in 7 of the 8 older animals in colon and caecum but in lower concentrations compared to the younger animals.

The inconsistent effect on *Bifidobacteria* may be due to absence or very low number of *Bifidobacteria*, being excluded by competition with other taxa such as *Lactobacilli*. The authors also indicated that the agar used (Beerens agar) may be the appropriate choice for human samples but may not be suitable for canine studies [76]. *Bifidobacterium spp.* were isolated in only 4 of 18 faecal samples from 6 dogs during 3 periods whereas *Lactobacillus* spp. were isolated in 12 of 18 faecal samples. However only 2 dogs had faecal *Lactobacilli* consistently [82]. Because of the inconsistent isolation, the effect of FOS (1%) on *Bifidobacteria* and *Lactobacilli* could not be determined in this experiment. Most likely, *Bifidobacteria* should already be present to show an effect of prebiotics on the Bifidobacterial count. If one starts with *Bifidobacteria* negative dogs, a synbiotic, containing *Bifidobacteria* as a probiotic, could be used instead of a prebiotic. On the other hand, in *Bifidobacteria* bearing dogs, extra proliferation is possible after supplementation with prebiotics.

Although *Bifidobacteria* were present, an increase was not seen after the addition of alpha-gluco-oligosaccharide or maltodextrin–like oligosaccharide supplementation (6%) to a highly digestible enteral diet [21]. *Bifidobacteria* populations were not changed after low inclusion rates of FOS, MOS or both (0.5%) [33].

When different strains of *Bifidobacteria* were tested for growth on oligofructose, all species grew well but growth rates of *B. pseudolongum*, *B. infantis* and B. *catenulatum* were highest. Two of these species with a high growth rate were not found in the dog and B. *pseudolongum* comprises only a small part of total *Bifidobacteria* species (2/41 *Bifidobacteria* strains isolated). *B. adolescentis* compromises the greatest part of all *Bifidobacteria* in the canine (29/41 *Bifidobacteria* strains isolated) [77] but this strain had the lowest growth rate on oligofructose. An increase in *Bifidobacteria* in the canine is expected but not in the same amounts as in other experimental animals. In humans, although numbers of *Bifidobacteria* are increased in response to oligosaccharide supplementation, they rarely exceed $10^{9.5}$ bacteria per g faeces [7].

In the faeces of dogs, *Lactobacilli* outnumbered *Bifidobacteria* [77]. Indeed, in the study of Greetham et al. [76] *Lactobacilli* and no *Bifidobacteria* were isolated in faecal samples of labrador dogs. *Lactobacillus murinus* appeared to be predominant in 2 of 4 faecal samples but was also isolated in the other 2 samples. When *L. murinus* was present, a lower variety of other *Lactobacilli* were observed suggesting a form of competitive exclusion.

Beynen et al [51] showed a trend for an increased *Lactobacilli* count (p=0.08) after 1% of oligofructose supplementation in dogs. In one of the two experiments with 0.7% sc FOS supplementation *Lactobacilli* counts tended to increase (p=0.08) [32]. MOS supplementation tended to increase faecal *Lactobacillus* counts (p=0.126) but FOS supplementation did not induce changes [33].

In several other experiments with NDO there were no changes in faecal *Lactobacilli* counts [21,29,31,45].

Beynen et al. [51] showed a significantly increased *Clostridia* count after 1% of oligofructose supplementation in dogs, whereas faecal *Clostridia (Lecithinase positive: C. perfringens group A*) concentration decreased significantly after 7 and 14 days of LS supplementation. Moreover, the occurrence of *Clostridia* (*lecithinase positive*) decreased from 100% before and after 7 days of supplementation to 88% after 14 days of supplementation [45].

Other results are more inconsistent. Three % of chicory or 1% of FOS addition to a dry dog diet decreased faecal *Clostridia* concentrations. However, in another experiment by the same author, chicory was added at 3 levels (0; 1.5; 3 and 5%) and none of the inclusion rates reduced *Clostridia* concentrations [48]. In one of the 2 experiments with 0.7% scFOS supplementation, *C. perfringens* tended to decrease (p= 0.08) [32]. *C. perfringens* tended (p=0.09) to be lower when MOS was supplemented compared to FOS or XOS (0.5%) but when all oligosaccharide supplementations (0.5% FOS, MOS or XOS) were compared to the control, differences regarding *C. perfringens* were not noted.[31] FOS, MOS or supplementation of both, did not change *Clostridia perfringens* populations [33].

Beynen et al. [51] showed significant increases in *Streptococci* counts after 1% of oligofructose supplementation in dogs. Faecal bacterial counts of *Bacteroidaceae*, *Eubacteria*, *Peptococcaceae*, *Enterobacteriaceae*, *Streptococci*, *Staphylococci*, *Bacilli* and yeasts did not change significantly after LS supplementation [45]. Alpha-gluco-oligosaccharide or maltodextrin–like oligosaccharide supplementation (6%) did not change faecal *Bacteroides* counts [21]. The concentrations of total *Enterobacteriaceae*, *Staphylococci*, *Bacteroidaceae*, yeasts and moulds were not influenced by 1% of oligofructose supplementation [51]. Howard et al. [29] compared several fermentable fibres (6% beet pulp, 1.5% scFOS) and a fibre blend (6% beet pulp + 2% gum talha and 1.5% FOS) with 6% cellulose in dogs and noted no differences for total coliformes. Oligosaccharide supplementation (0.5% FOS, MOS or XOS) did not changes faecal bacterial counts of *E. coli* and coliforms compared to the control diet [31]. *E. coli* populations were not changed by FOS, MOS or both [33]. There was also no diet effect on *Bacteriodes* and *E. coli* concentrations; however, there was an effect of diet sequence on *Bacteroides* counts [82].

Probiotic or synbiotic supplementation (10^9 L. acidophilus, human strain and FOS) did not induce any significant change in faecal bacterial counts of *Bifidobacteria*, *Lactobacilli*, *C. perfringens*, *E. coli*, total aerobes and anaerobes [32].

Cats

Experiments with NDO are scarce in cats. Sparkes et al. [74,95] investigated the effect of dietary FOS supplementation (0.75%) on faecal flora in cats. Mean counts of faecal bacteria did not differ significantly due to FOS supplementation although a trend for a higher number of total anaerobes (p=0.1) and total bacteria (p=0.16) could be noted. There was an increased prevalence of *Lactobacilli* on the FOS diet (p=0.037). Mean counts of *Lactobacilli* and *Bacteroides* were significantly increased (p= 0.017 and 0.045 respectively) and *E. coli* and *C. perfringens* counts decreased after FOS supplementation (p=0.034 and 0.085 respectively). The percentage-prevalence of *E. coli* and *C. perfringens* was decreased after FOS supplementation [95].

In cats, *Bifidobacteria* were isolated in only one of the 12 cats [95]. Mitsuoka and Kaneuchi [77] also noted no detectable numbers of *Bifidobacteria* in faecal samples of cats. Terada et al. [52] noted a significantly increased frequence of occurrence of *Bifidobacteria* from before (0%) to 7 or 14 days (100%) after LS supplementation in cats. Seven days after termination of the supplementation, the occurrence was again decreased to 13%. Itoh et al. [78] also showed high numbers of *Bifidobacteria* in cat faeces and the strains were identified as *B. adolescentis*.

On day 14 of LS supplementation, the frequency of occurrence of *Clostridia* (lecithinase negative) and *Spirochaetaceae* were significantly decreased. Lactosucrose supplementation (50mg/kg BW) significantly increased *Lactobacilli* counts while *Clostridia* (lecithinase positive) and *Enterobactericeae* were significantly decreased in cats. *Bacteroides* counts were slightly but significantly increased on day 14 and *Staphylococci* and *Fusobacteria* were decreased on day 7 but not on day 14 of administration. Counts of total bacteria, *Eubacteria*, *Peptococcaceae*, *Spirochaetaceae*, *Streptococci*, *Bacilli*, *Corynebacteria*, yeasts and moulds were not changed [52].

Dogs and Cats

In the small intestine, NDO supplementation had no effect on bacterial flora in healthy dogs and cats but in dogs with small intestinal bacterial overgrowth, FOS supplementation might have a positive influence. In the large intestine the effect of NDO supplementation on total aerobes and anaerobes, Bifidobacteria, Lactobacilli and Clostridia was not consistent. This may be attribute to several factors:

Diet composition is probably a very important factor for microbial activity in non-ruminant animals. For example, in the experiment of Strickling et al. [31], soybean meal was used as an ingredient of the basal diet but soybean contains α-galacto-oligosaccharides and added oligosaccharides may have an additive or a masking effect.

On the other hand, Russell [48] compared different chicory supplementation rates (0; 0.5; 2 and 4%) with three different soy supplementation rates (0; 6 and 12%). It was concluded that there was no interaction between chicory and soy for the bacterial concentrations. The increased Bifidobacteria concentrations were independent of the soy inclusion level.

Another dietary factor is the purity of the used NDO supplement and this is not only important for the absolute amount of NDO that is supplemented. An in vitro test showed that several Salmonella species oxidised and grew on FOS-50 (28% FOS, 16% glucose and fructose and 5% sucrose) as good as glucose and this in contrast to pure FOS (>90% FOS).

[83,84] However, in in vivo studies, the glucose and fructose residues will be absorbed in the upper part of the intestinal tract.

Not only the NDO content of the basal diet may be important but protein content may also play an important role. High levels of dietary protein will stimulate production of putrefactive compounds (ammonia, amines, phenols and indoles). High protein / low fermentable fibre diets will stimulate protein fermentation and will often result in an alkaline pH in the colon and is often associated with more pathogenic bacteria. Since fructans may increase beneficial bacteria and reduce faecal odour components, these effects may be more pronounced in case of high protein / low fibre diets [50].

Faecal concentrations do not accurately reflect fermentations in the proximal colon, especially if low doses of highly fermentable supplements are used like scFOS. These may be rapidly fermented in the proximal colon, beneficially affecting microbial populations in the proximal colon without changing populations in lower regions [33].

Age of the animals may also play a role as shown by Benno et al. [73] This may be an explanation for the different results in the two experiments of Swanson et al. [32] In general, the dogs used in the first experiment were older (6.3years; 0.9-10.8 years) compared to the second experiment (2.2years; 0.9-5.9years) although the difference in age was non-significant.

Pathogen challenge tests are also needed before conclussions on pathogen resistence can be made.

Apparent Digestibility

Apparent Dry Matter Digestibility

The amount and type of fibre in a pet food is an important factor in regard to digestibility of nutrients. In general, slowly fermentable fibre will decrease DM digestibility compared to feeds without added fibre or rapidly fermentable fibre sources. An increased level of fibre will also decrease DM digestibility [22].

In dogs, 1.5% scFOS (DM basis) significantly increased DM digestibility compared to 6% cellulose (87.3% versus 83.55%). A fibre blend consisting of 6% beet pulp, 2% gum talha (kind of gum arabic) and 1.5% FOS, showed a DM digestibility intermediate between cellulose and FOS [29]. The authors suggested a slower gastric emptying and intestinal transit to be responsible for the higher DM digestibility. The slower gastric emptying and intestinal transit was suggested by the stimulation of a hormone: peptide YY, through an increased SCFA production.

Ileal DM digestibility was unaffected by exchanging cellulose for pectin [30]. Ileal and total tract digestibility were not changed by 6% DM supplementation of α-gluco-oligosaccharide or MD to a highly digestible dog diet [21]. However, *large intestinal and total tract* DM digestibility were increased as pectin content of the diet (max. 10%DM) increased (from 81.3 to 88.3% for total tract digestibility). Cellulose will increase faecal weight whereas pectin contributes less to faecal output [30]. A 7 % supplementation rate of inulin tended to decrease apparent DM digestibility in dogs (from 88.8 to 87.5%).[46] FOS and IMO also tended to decrease or significantly decreased apparent DM digestibility in different protein supplemented diets [49].

Other experiments with FOS and beet fibre supplementation (4 or 8.2%DM FOS + respectively 1 or 2% beet fibre), oligosaccharide supplementation (0.5% FOS, MOS or XOS, 1% FOS), chicory supplementation (3 or 5%) did not reduce apparent ileal, large intestinal or total DM digestibility [31,41,48]. FOS supplementation (0.5%) did not influence ileal and total tract DM digestibility but there was a trend for a lower ileal DM digestibility after MOS supplementation although statistical significance was not reached (p=0.149!) [33].

MOS significantly reduced apparent digestibility coefficients (ADC) of DM (81.9%) compared to the basal diet (89.5%), TGOS (87.2%), lactose (87.3%) and lactulose (86.5%) supplementation (5.88% diet). In the MOS supplemented dogs the faecal water-binding capacity was increased, suggesting a changed nutrient solubility with as a consequence lower digestibility coefficients [38].

Most experiments show no effect on DM digestibility. If measured, apparent ileal digestibility was not reduced. With increased supplementation rates, a decreased DM digestibility might be due to an increased water-binding capacity.

Apparent Organic Matter Digestibility

Ileal and /or total tract OM digestibility was not changed by the addition of 6% of α-gluco-oligosaccharide or MD to a highly digestible enteral diet or FOS and/or MOS supplementation (0.5%) ($p>0.05$) [21,33]. Apparent organic matter digestibility was significantly decreased by a 7% inulin supplementation to a dog diet [46]. FOS and beet fibre supplementation (4 or 8.2%DM FOS + respectively 1 or 2% beet fibre) did not change apparent organic matter digestibility in dogs [41].

Apparent Protein Digestibility

Fibrous foods may decrease apparent protein digestibility because of increased faecal nitrogen from increased faecal biomass. When calculating apparent digestibility (total tract), one assumes that all faecal N is of dietary origin however significant amounts of bacterial N are formed due to fermentation in the large intestine. Bacterial protein is then confounded with dietary protein resulting in a lower apparent protein digestibility [22].

Apparent total tract digestibility of protein was decreased linearly with increased pectin content (substituted for cellulose) in dogs (Table 10). However ileal protein digestibility was unchanged but large intestinal protein 'digestibility' was decreased. Total tract protein digestibilities do not take the 'nitrogen sink' (increased microbial populations) after fibre fermentation in the large intestine into account and should be interpreted carefully [30]. Similarly, apparent ileal protein digestibility was not decreased by the addition of 6% α-gluco-oligosaccharide or MD to highly digestible enteral dog diet but total tract digestibility was significantly decreased after α-gluco-oligosaccharide and MD supplementation respectively [21]. Interestingly, an increased ileal protein digestibility was noted after oligofructose supplementation to dogs (3g/day) without changes in total tract digestibility [50].

Table 10: Apparent protein digestibility in dogs.

Reference	Supplement	Dosis	Total tract digestibility	Ileal digestibility
[41]	FOS + sugar beet fibre	4+1%DM 8.2+2%DM	87.8→86.3% (NS) 87.8→83.8%	
[46]	inulin	7%DM	90.9→88.3%	
[21]	α-gluco OS maltodextrine	6%DM	92.3→90.1% 92.3→87.9%	80.8→82%(NS) 80.8→87%(NS)
[50]	oligofructose	3g/day		61→72.4%
[30]	Pectine	10%DM	83 → 73.6%	68.5→67.5%(NS)
[33]	FOS MOS FOS+MOS	0.5% 0.5% 0.5+0.5%	75.9→75.2%(NS) 75.9→75.7%(NS) 75.9→77.7% (NS)	66.2→64.7% (NS) 66.2→53.7% (NS) 66.2→60.8% (NS)
[38]	MOS TGOS lactose lactulose	5.88%	91.3*→79.8% 91.3→85.9% (NS) 91.3→86.2% (NS) 91.3→84.4%	

* basal diet I (82.5%) significantly different from basal diet II (91.3%); NS: statistically non-significant difference.

In other experiments ileal digestibility coefficients were not measured but similar decreases in total tract digestibility coefficients were seen. A 7% inulin supplementation significantly decreased apparent protein digestibility. This was assumed to be the consequence of bacterial proliferation although microbial measurements were not made [46]. FOS supplementation (8.2%DM) together with beet fibre (2%) significantly decreased apparent protein digestibility compared to the control diet in dogs. A lower inclusion rate (4% FOS + 1% beet fibre) showed results intermediate between control and high inclusion rates [41]. FOS and IMO supplementation decreased apparent protein digestibility in protein supplemetented dogs. At the same time estimated bacterial N content was significantly increased. When apparent N digestibility was corrected for the increased bacterial N content, significant effects disappeared except for the greaves meal supplemented group [49]. MOS significantly reduced apparent digestibilities of crude protein compared to the basal diet, TGOS, lactose and lactulose supplementation (5.88% dict). However, when compared to basal diet I, none of the supplementations showed reduced protein digestibilities. Protein digestibility of basal diet I and II were significantly different from each other [38]. A lower ileal protein digestibility was seen after MOS supplementation (0.5%) although statistically significant difference was not reached (p= 0.173) [33]. The authors suggested a binding and agglutination of proteins by mannans as a possible cause of the lower digestibility.

Nitrogen digestibility and N balance were unaffected by the addition of 1.5% of scFOS in dogs [29]. Nitrogen excretion in faeces or urine was not influenced by 1% of oligofructose addition in dogs [51]. With lower inclusion rates (0.5% FOS, MOS or XOS) ileal, large intestinal and total-tract protein digestibility coefficients were also unchanged [31,33]. Apparent digestibility coefficients of nitrogen were not different when 3% of chicory or 1% of FOS was compared to a basal diet. Similarly, higher inclusion rates of chicory (5%) did not reduce these digestibility coefficients [48]. Low oligosaccharide (stachyose and raffinose) soybean meal (18.55 and 37.1% incorporation rate) did not change protein and amino acid digestibilities at the ileum or total tract compared to conventional soybean meal in dogs [20].

In cats, total-tract protein digestibility coefficients decreased after inulin or oligofructose supplementation and concurrently estimated bacterial N increased. When the N digestibility was corrected for the larger bacterial N content, differences were no longer seen [35].

With high inclusion rates of NDO, a decreased total tract digestibility coefficient of protein was seen in several experiments but ileal digestibility of protein was not decreased when measured. The decreased apparent protein digestibility is most certainly due to the higher biomass of the faeces due to the addition of fermentable fibres. Consequently, total tract digestibility coefficients should be evaluated very carefully when fermentable fibre is added to the diet.

Apparent Fat Digestibility

Ileal and total tract fat digestibility were not changed by the addition of 6% α-gluco-oligosaccharide or MD to a highly digestible enteral diet [21]. Similarly, FOS and beet fibre supplementation (4 or 8.2%DM FOS + respectively 1 or 2% beet fibre) did not change apparent fat digestibility in dogs [41]. Crude fat digestibility was not reduced by supplementations of MOS, TGOS, lactose and lactulose (5.88% diet) [38].

However, Diez et al. [46]. noted a decreased fat digestibility after a 7% inulin supplementation (from 95.9 to 94.1%) to dogs but the reduction was more pronounced when guar gum (91.0) was added. A decreased apparent fat digestibility was also noted in meat and bone meal and FOS or IMO supplemented dogs [49]. In cats, a decreased fat digestibility was noted after 3 and 6 % inulin and 3% oligofructose [35].

Surprisingly, an increased ileal fat digestibility (94.6–92.4%) was noted after oligofructose supplementation to dogs (3g/day) without an effect on total tract digestibility [50].

A reduction of total tract digestibility of fat is not common and is not of clinical importance since the reduction is very small and probably not of ileal origin. The decrease might be the consequence of fat in the bacterial cell membranes.

Apparent Starch Digestibility

Ileal starch digestibility was decreased when cellulose was substituted for pectin in dogs (max.10% of pectin)(ileal starch digestibility: 98.6% versus 96.24%). At the same time ileal flow was significantly increased by pectin. Pectin not only increased the amount of fermentable fibre presented to the large intestine but also increased starch fermentation. Because of increased large intestinal starch fermentation, total tract digestibility was not changed by pectin addition. A decreased intestinal transit time with, as a consequence, a decreased time for digestion and/or increased digesta viscosity with as a result a lesser enzyme access were suggested as possible causes of the decreased small intestinal starch digestibility [30].

Ileal glucose ($p<0.05$) and carbohydrate ($p=0.08$) digestibility were decreased by the addition of 6% α-gluco-oligosaccharide or MD to a highly digestible dog feed from 97 to 92% and from 94 to 89% respectively. The diet contained 26.1 to 29.1% glucose on DM basis [21]. Total tract digestibility of glucose and carbohydrate were significantly reduced by the addition of MD (98 and 96.8% respectively) compared to the control diet (99.9 and 99.2%

respectively) or α-gluco-oligosaccharide supplementation. Probably MD was not completely fermented in the large intestine as was suggested by an *in vitro* study with human faecal samples. α-Gluco-oligosaccharide seemed to be fermented extensively [21]. MOS significantly reduced apparent digestibilities of N-free extract compared to the basal diet, TGOS, lactose and lactulose supplementation (5.88% diet) (mean of 92.5 to 83.1% after MOS supplementation). In the MOS supplemented dogs the faecal water-binding capacity was increased, suggesting a changed nutrient solubility with, as a consequence, lower digestibilities [38].

Inulin supplementation (7%) did not reduce apparent N free extract digestibility in dogs [46].

Prebiotics might affect ileal carbohydrate digestibility, which can be corrected by an increased large intestinal fermentability in some cases. Consequently, a lack of effect on apparent digestibility does not contradict an effect on ileal digestibility. In most experiments, the differences in digestibilities were rather small and the digestibilities were still very high except for MOS supplementation in the experiment of Zentek et al. [38].

Apparent Fibre Digestibility

Apparent ileal, large intestinal and total-tract ADF digestibilities all increased with increasing pectin content (substituted for cellulose) from 12.4; 41.6 and 48.8% to 66; 84.5 and 94.1% respectively. ADF measures primarily the insoluble component of fibre. TDF digestibilities are more suitable to evaluate both pectin and cellulose effects on fibre (both soluble and insoluble) digestibility. Apparent ileal digestibility was unchanged but apparent large intestinal and total-tract TDF digestibility were increased with increased pectin concentrations from –10.4 and 37.7 for cellulose to 38.7 and 69% for pectin respectively [30]. In dogs, ADF digestibility tended to increase from 23.3 in the control diet to 37.9% after inulin supplementation (7%DM) [46].

Apparent Mineral Absorption

Fibres may affect mineral availability: some fibres reduce; others enhance mineral absorption and use. Several properties of fibres have been evaluated for their effect on mineral availability: water-holding capacity, viscosity, cation exchange capacity, particle size, tannin and oxalate content, presence of phytates, uronic acid and phenolic groups. A direct relation between the *in vitro* properties of fibres and *in vivo* effect on mineral availability does not exist [22].

In rats, absorption of the minerals Ca, Mg and Fe was stimulated by inulin type fructans and TGOS. In humans, calcium absorption was increased by inulin type fructans [12].

Apparent mineral absorption of Ca and Mg were significantly increased from 8.6 and 14.0% to 16 and 23.4% respectively after 1% of oligofructose supplementation in adult dogs. Phosphorus absorption remained unchanged [51]. A dose dependent increase of apparent Ca and Mg absorption was noted in adult dogs after lactulose supplementation (0.1 or 3g /MJ ME) (from 11.5 to 21.1% of intake for Ca; 23.3 to 35.5% intake for Mg) [47]. Once again apparent P absorption was not changed. In rats, the increased calcium and magnesium absorption was explained by a lower ileal pH (7.5 versus 7.0) after lactulose feeding [85]. This decreased pH increased *in vitro* solubility of these minerals. The solubility of phosphorus is less sensitive to a decrease of ileal pH within the physiological ranges, explaining the lack of effect on P absorption. Beynen et al. [51] suggested a lowering of the ileal pH as a cause of increased apparent Ca and Mg absorption. However, calcium and magnesium absorption may also be increased due to an increased colonic absorption as was shown in rats by oligofructose supplementation [86]. This may be due to an increased SCFA production or again by a decreased luminal pH. In one experiment of Beynen et al. [47] faecal pH was significantly decreased but the other experiment [51] showed no effect on faecal pH. This does not exclude an effect in the more proximal part of the large intestine. Productions of SCFA were not measured in these experiments.

On the other hand, apparent absorption rates of calcium, phosphorus, magnesium, sodium and potassium were not changed with higher inclusion rates (1g/kg BW or 5.88% diet) of TGOS, MOS, lactose or lactulose in adult dogs [38]. Mineral absorption depends on the physiological needs of the animal (breed, age, reproduction).

Gastrointestinal Dimensions and Transport of Nutrients

During the fermentation of carbohydrates, SCFA (mainly acetate, propionate and butyrate) and lactate are produced. The produced butyrate is used as an oxidative fuel for the colonocytes but also has an influence on cell maturation, cell differentiation and apoptosis [57]. (See short chain fatty acids).

Small Intestine

The small intestine of dogs fed a diet supplemented with fermentable fibre (4.2% beet pulp and 1% oligofructose) had more surface, more mucosal mass and were heavier compared to a non-fermentable fibre (cellulose 3.6%) group. The capacity for carrier mediated glucose uptake was also greater in the fermentable fibre group compared to the non-fermentable fibre group [87].

Dogs fed a diet supplemented with 6% of beet pulp, had a heavier ileal gut wall compared to FOS (1.5%), Solka floc®[1] (6%) or a fibre blend (6% beet pulp, 2% gum talha, 1.5% FOS). However, the differences were related to heavier body weights [88]. Duodenal villi height tended (p=0.1) to be higher in dogs consuming a high fermentable fibre diet (beet pulp 6%, gum arabica 2% and FOS 1.5%) compared to a cellulose diet (7%).

Jejunal villi were significantly higher in the high fermentable fibre (beet pulp, gum arabica and FOS) group compared to the low fermentable fibre (cellulose). Duodenal, jejunal and ileal crypt depth and ileal villi height were not different between two supplemented groups [89].

Large Intestine

FOS supplementation (1.5%) induced a shorter leading edge (distance between base and highest labelled cells in crypt) and a smaller cell proliferation zone in the proximal colon of dogs compared to Solka floc (6%), beet pulp (6%) and a fibre blend (6% beet pulp, 2% gum talha and 1.5% FOS) supplementation. Crypt depth and cell density were not altered. An increasing zone of cell differentiation was suggested to maintain a normal colonic mucosal

[1] Fiber Sales and development Corp., St. Louis, MO, USA

development after a decreased proliferation zone and shorter leading edge in the proximal colon. In the distal colon, effects on cell proliferations and morphometry were not seen.

FOS also temporarily increased colonic blood flow measured by a surgically fitted ultrasonic blood flow probe [88]. The authors suggested that this was attributed to the SCFA absorption, due to the FOS fermentation.

Potential Side Effects

In rats, acute and subacute gavage and subacute feeding studies showed no toxicity for FOS and inulin. Chronic and carcinogenicity studies showed that the incidence of neoplasms was not affected by FOS treatment. Developmental and reproduction tests showed no adverse effects except for a moderate reduction in body weight of the dams (rats). The non-clinical toxicology test showed no evidence of increased morbidity, mortality or target organ toxicity [23]. However, the real issue is not that of safety but rather of GI tolerance. In humans signs of intolerance have been noted with doses of 20-30g. Gastrointestinal symptoms of intolerance are flatulence, bloating, abdominal distension and rumbling. Inulin has a better GI tolerance than FOS (average DP3). Inulin is fermented slower than FOS: slower fermented compounds are more easily tolerated and smaller molecules have a higher osmotic pressure. Fewer signs of intolerance are also seen when doses are divided in several smaller doses [23]. Undigested carbohydrates are fermented by the colonic flora resulting in the production of gas and therefore flatulence. When the capacity of the flora to ferment carbohydrates is exceeded, diarrhoea may develop [23].

Low doses are usually tolerated very well but prebiotics can induce diarrhoea or increase intestinal gas production [90 in 91].

In dogs, 2g lactulose /kg BW induced diarrhoea [38]. Ten % (DM) of FOS supplementation was associated with runny faeces in dogs [41].

Effect on Metabolism

NDO may also influence metabolism. Lipid metabolism might be influenced by inulin in rats. Results of human studies are still inconsistent but indicate that inulin or oligofructose may affect lipid metabolism [12]. Inulin may also influence glycaemia and insulinemia but may depend on physiological (fasted versus postprandial) or disease (diabetes) conditions [92]. In normal and nephrectomised rats, inulin increased faecal nitrogen excretion and decreased urinary nitrogen excretion. At the same time, plasma urea levels were decreased [93].

If these effects also exist in dogs and cats, there is a potential use for these NDO in cases of renal failure, liver failure, diabetes mellitus and hyperlipidemia. Some pet food companies already include FOS in diets for renal and liver failure and diabetes mellitus.

Lipid Metabolism

In rats, decreased triglyceridemia has been shown in both the fasted and the fed state. Two indirect effects are suggested to explain the modulation of triglyceride metabolism:

1) modification of glucose and/or insulin levels
2) an increased portal concentration of acetate and propionate: propionate as an inhibitor of fatty acids synthesis and acetate as a lipogenic substance [7].

The effect on cholesterolemia in humans is controversial. Moderate levels of inulin or oligofructose may affect human lipid metabolism but the available data are still inconsistent [12].

Pre- and postprandial plasma cholesterol and triglyceride concentrations were not changed after inulin supplementation (7%) in dogs [46].

However, FOS plus beet fibre supplementation (8.2% FOS + 2% beet fibre) significantly reduced triglyceride concentration during a 6-hour postprandial period in healthy (non hyperlipidemic) dogs. Weekly (6 weeks) preprandial cholesterol and triglyceride concentrations were also reduced compared to the control diet. At a lower inclusion rate (4% FOS + 1% beet fibre) only preprandial triglyceride concentration was significantly reduced [41]. Energy intake and fat digestibility were similar. It was speculated that the hypocholesterolemic effect was mediated through an increased propionate production after the addition of fermentable fibre. The fat content of the control diet was 22.5g/1000kcal [41], which was considerably lower compared to the experiment (35.9g/1000kcal or 14.35%DM) where no effects on fat metabolism were found [46]. However, in Diez et al. [41] FOS was supplemented wereas inulin was used in Diez et al. [46] which makes it difficult to compare both experiments. Fructans supplementation in combination to a low fat diet might be needed before an effect on lipid metabolism can be expected.

Glucose Metabolism

Fructans might modulate glycaemia and insulinemia although effects may depend on physiological (fasting versus postprandial) or pathologic (diabetes) conditions [7]. Two hypotheses are presented:

1) influence on digestion of macronutrients by delaying gastric emptying and/or by shortening small intestinal transit time.
2) modification of the hepatic glucose metabolism: reduced hepatic gluconeogenesis mediated by SCFA, especially propionate and/or enhanced glycolysis. Hepatic gluconeogenesis may also be influenced indirectly by lowering plasma fatty acids [7].

The incremental area under the curve (AUC) for plasma glucagon-like peptide-1 (GLP-1) and insulin was significantly increased by a diet containing fermentable fibre (beet pulp 6%, gum arabica 2% and FOS 1.5% as fed basis) compared to a cellulose supplemented (7%) diet in healthy dogs [89]. At the same time, AUC for glucose was decreased by the fermentable fibre diet. GLP-1 is considered as an anti-diabetogenic agent due to stimulation of insulin secretion, inhibition of glucagon and delayed gastric emptying. Dietary fibre type did not influence blood glucose concentrations during an oral glucose tolerance test [89]. Glucose intestinal transporter quantity and activity were also greater in the dogs consuming a diet with added fermentable fibre.

Diez et al. [46] noted no significant effects on fasting glucose concentration or postprandial glucose curve by the addition of inulin (7%DM) in healthy dogs. Pre- and postprandial insulin concentrations did not change [46]. With rather low inclusion rates of FOS, MOS or XOS (0.5%) effects on postprandial glucose concentrations were not seen in the dog [31].

Postprandial glucose concentrations were decreased significantly after FOS + beet fibre supplementation (8.2% FOS+ 2% beet fibre) in healthy dogs. Preprandial glucose concentrations were not changed as they are maintained within narrow ranges. Pre- and postprandial insulin concentrations were not changed [41]. IMO supplementation (10%) significantly decreased post-prandial glucose concentrations in healthy dogs [40].

More research into this field is necessary before conclusions on modulation of glucose concentrations can be made. Experiments with diabetic dogs are needed before prebiotics can be added to diets for diabetic dogs.

Nitrogen Metabolism

In rats fed a 10% casein diet supplemented with inulin (15%), faecal N excretion was increased and urinary N excretion decreased. In healthy rats plasma urea concentrations were decreased by 50%; in nephrectomised rats the plasma urea decrease was 30% [93]. Similarly, a 10% FOS supplementation decreased plasma urea by 30% in uremic rats [94].

Intestinal bacterial growth not only requires an energy source (fermentable carbohydrates) but also an N source for protein synthesis. When fermentable carbohydrate intake is high, nitrogen required to sustain maximum bacterial growth may become limiting and blood urea, by diffusion through the intestinal wall, may then become a nitrogen source for bacterial protein synthesis. Propionate may also inhibit urea synthesis in the liver [7].

In dogs, urinary urea excretion decreased linearly ($p=0.048$) by the addition of 0.1 and 0.3g lactulose/MJ ME to a meat-based dog diet. Urinary production, pH and creatinine excretion were not changed. A numerical but NS 22% increase in faecal N excretion and a decrease of 6% in urinary N excretion were noted on the high lactulose dose compared to the control diet. The apparent absorption of N significantly decreased by 2% units on the high lactulose diet [47].

Despite an increased faecal bacterial N excretion (estimated by purine content of faeces and bacterial isolates) ($p<0.1$) after 1.5% scFOS supplementation, urinary N excretion was not reduced ($p>0.1$). A high crude protein concentration of the diet, could have exceeded the capacity of FOS to trap N. The authors also suggest that a considerable amount of N can return to the circulation through ammonia absorption when highly fermentable fibres are used to increase urea flux into the caecum [29]. However, highly fermentable fibres may decrease intestinal pH and thus reduce ammonia absorption. Nitrogen excretion in faeces and urine was not influenced by 1% of oligofructose addition in dogs [51]. On the other hand, faecal bacterial protein excretion was probably not increased since total bacterial counts were not increased in this study. Moreover, the basal diet contained rice, corn and beet pulp and was probably already rich in non-digestible fermentable carbohydrates. The faecal N excretion was greater than that found in a previous study of the same author using a meat-based diet and dogs of comparable body weight [47] (1.3-1.4g N/day compared to 0.86-1.05g N/day). As a consequence, the trapping of colonic N may have been already substantial with no extra influence of supplemental oligofructose [51]. In both experiments [47,51] diets with high protein content were used (35.3 and 28.8% DM). Not N but energy will probably have been the limiting factor for bacterial synthesis in these experiments.

Renal N, urea and indican excretion were not changed by the supplementation of MOS, TGOS, lactose or lactulose (5.88%) in dogs when fed a high protein diet (36.6%) [38].

Diez et al. [46] measured pre- and postprandial plasma urea and α-amino-nitrogen in dogs but concentrations were not changed after inulin supplementation (7%) compared to the control diet (24.4% DM). However, pre- and postprandial plasma urea concentrations decreased after FOS and beet fibre supplementation compared to the control diet (FOS 4 or 8.2% + 1 or 2% beet fibre) (65.3g protein / 1000kcal) [41].

In cats supplemented with FOS (2%DM), faecal N excretion increased by 26% compared to the control diet ($p<0.05$). Urinary N excretion was decreased by 5% in the FOS supplemented cats but this difference did not reach statistical significance. N balance was not changed by the supplementation. The calculated N absorption was significantly decreased by FOS supplementation [34]. After injection of labelled urea, faecal ^{15}N excretion tended to increase whereas urinary ^{15}N excretion tended to decrease by FOS supplementation (3.1%DM) to a low protein diet. There was a trend for a 35% increase in faecal N excretion and a numerical reduction in urinary N excretion of 33%. The lower urinary N excretion can be the consequence of a lower ammonia absorption because N is used for bacterial protein synthesis and/or due to increase entrance of urea to the gut [66].

More research is needed, before inclusion of NDO's in diets for patients with chronic renal and liver failure. Especially, experiments with normal to low protein diets such as renal and liver diets are needed because then N will become a limiting factor for bacterial synthesis and N trapping may be possible.

Immune System

Bifidobacteria may have several effects on the immune system such as modification of mitogenic activity and adjuvant activity, promotion of macrophages, stimulation of antibody production and anti-tumor effects [71].

The effects of an addition of FOS (0.5%), MOS (0.5%) or FOS + MOS (0.5% of each) on immune system was tested in dogs [33]. Lymphocytes, expressed as a percentage of total WBC were significantly increased by MOS supplementation compared to control dogs. Total WBC and neutrophils were not influenced by the supplements, nor were serum Ig G, Ig M and Ig A and faecal Ig A ($p>0.1$). Ileal Ig A concentrations (on protein or DM basis, $p=0.052$, 0.062 respectively) tended to be increased on the combined FOS+MOS supplement, which could suggest an increased local immunity and greater protection against pathogens.

REFERENCES

[1] Rastall, R., Fuller, R., Gaskins, H., and Gibson, G., (2000). Colonic functional foods. In: Gibson, G., and Williams, C., eds. *Functional foods concept to product.* Cambridge, England: Woodhead publishing Limited and CRC press LLC, 71-95.

[2] Gibson, G., and Roberfroid, M., (1995). Dietary modulation of the human colonic microbiota: introducing the concept of prebiotics. *Journal of Nutrition, 125,* 1401-1412.

[3] Mul, A., and Perry, F., (1994). The role of fructo-oligosaccharides in animal nutrition. In: Gransworthy, P., ed. *Recent advances in animal nutrition.* Loughborough, UK, 57-79.

[4] Teitelbaum, J., and Walker, W., (2002). Nutritional impact of pre- and probiotics as protective gastrointestinal organisms. *Annual Review of Nutrition, 22,*107-138.

[5] Playne, M., and Crittenden, R., (1996). Commercially available oligosaccharides. *Bulletin of the International Dairy Federation, n° 313,* 10-22.

[6] Vijn, I., and Smeekens, S., (1999). Fructan: more than a reserve carbohydrate? *Plant Physiology, 120,* 351-359.

[7] Roberfroid, M., and Delzenne, N., (1998). Dietary fructans. *Annual Reviews in Nutrition, 18,* 117-143.

[8] Van Loo, J., Coussement, P., De Leenheer, L., Hoebregs, H., and Smits, G., (1995). On the presence of inulin and oligofructose as natural ingredients in the western diet. *Critical Reviews in Food Science and Nutrition, 35(6),* 525-552.

[9] Roberfroid, M., Van Loo, J., and Gibson, G., (1998). The bifidogenic nature of chicory inulin and its hydrolysis products. *Journal of Nutrition, 128,* 11-19.

[10] Hussein, H., Campbell, J., Bauer, L., Fahey, G., Hogarth, A., Wolf, B., and Hunter, D., (1998). Selected fructo-oligosaccharide composition of pet-food ingredients. *Journal of Nutrition, 128,* 2803S-2805S.

[11] Crittenden, R., and Playne, M., (1996). Production, properties and applications of food-grade oligosaccharides. *Trends in Food Science and Technology, 7,* 353-361.

[12] Van Loo, J., Cummings, J., Delzenne, N., Englyst, H., Franck, A., Hopkins, M., Macfarlane, G., Newton, D., Quigley, M., Roberfroid, M., van Vliet, T., and van den Heuvel, E., (1999). Functional food properties of non-digestible oligosaccharides: a consensus report from the ENDO project (DGXII AIRII-CT 94-1095). *British Journal of Nutrition, 81,* 121-132.

[13] Guillon, F., Champ, M., and Thibault, J., (2000). Dietary fiber functional products. In: Gransworthy, P., ed. *Functional foods: concept to product,* 315-364.

[14] Whistler, R., and Corbett, W., Polysaccharides, (1957). Part 1: general aspects and phyto and microbial polysaccharides. In: Pigman W. Ed. The carbohydrates, chemistry, biochemistry, physiology. New York: Academic press Inc., 669.

[15] Cummings, J., Macfarlane, G., and Englyst, H., (2001). Prebiotic digestion and fermentation. *American Journal of Clinical Nutrition, 73 (suppl.),* 415S-420S.

[16] Delzenne, N., (2003). Oligosaccharides: state of the art. *Proceedings of the Nutrition Society, 62,* 177-182.

[17] Cummings, J. and Macfarlane, G., (2002). Gastrointestinal effects of prebiotics. *British Journal of Nutrition, 87 (suppl.2),* S145-S151.

[18] Rumessen, J., Bodé, S., Hamberg, O. and Gudmand-Hoyer, E., (1990). Fructans of Jerusalem artichokes: intestinal transport, absorption, fermentation and influence on blood glucose, insulin and C-peptide responses in healthy subjects. *American Journal of Clinical Nutrition, 52,* 675-681.

[19] Rumessen, J., and Gudmand-Hoyer, E., (1998). Fructans of chicory: intestinal transport and fermentation of different chain lengths and relation to fructose and sorbitol malabsorption. *American Journal of Clinical Nutrition, 68,* 357-364.

[20] Zuo, Y., Fahey, G., Merchen, N., and Bajjalieh, N., (1996). Digestion response to low oligosaccharide soybean meal by ileally-cannulated dogs. *Journal of Animal Science, 74*, 2441-2449.

[21] Flickinger, E., Wolf, B., Garleb, K., Chow, J. Leyer, G., Johns, P., and Fahey, G., (2000). Glucose-based oligosaccharides exhibit different *in vitro* fermentation patterns and affect in vivo apparent nutrient digestibility and microbial populations in dogs. *Journal of Nutrition, 130 (5)*, 1267-1273.

[22] Gross, K., Wedekind, K., Cowell, C., Schoenherr, W., Jewell, D., Zicker, S., Debraekeleer, J., and Frey, R., (2000). Nutrients. In: Hand M., Thatcher C., Remillard R. and Roudebush P. (ed), Small Animal clinical nutrition 4th, Topeka, Kansas: Walsworth Publishing Company, 42-48.

[23] Carabin, I., and Flamm, W., (1999). Evaluation of safety of inulin and oligofructose as dietary fiber. *Regulatory Toxicology and Pharmacology, 30,* 268-282.

[24] Coussement, P., (1999). Inulin and oligofructose as dietary fiber: analytical, nutritional and legal aspects. In: S., Cho, L., Prosky, and M., Dreher, eds. *Complex carbohydrates in foods.* New York: Marcel Dekker, 203-212.

[25] Association of Analytical Communities, (1998). Official Method of Analysis 997.08, 16th ed. 4th review. AOAC International Gaithersburg, MD.

[26] Schneeman, B., (1999). Fibre, inulin and oligofructose: similarities and differences. *Journal of Nutrition, 129,* 1424S-1427S.

[27] Berk, Z., (1976). Pectic substances, plant gums. In: *Braverman's Introduction to the biochemistry of foods.* Elsevier Scientific Publishing Company, 131-143.

[28] Caspary, W., (1992). Physiology and pathophysiology of intestinal absorption. *American Journal of Clinical Nutrition, 55*, 299S-308S.

[29] Howard, M., Kerley, M., Sunvold, G., and Reinhart, G., (2000). Source of fiber fed to dogs affects nitrogen and energy metabolism and intestinal microflora populations. *Nutrition Research, 20(10),* 1473-1484.

[30] Silvio, S., Harmon, D., Gross, K., and McLeod, K., (2000). Influence of fiber fermentability on nutrient digestion in the dog. *Nutrition, 16,* 289-295.

[31] Strickling, J., Harmon, D., Dawson, K., and Gross, K., (2000). Evaluation of oligosaccharide addition to dog diets: influences on nutrient digestion and microbial populations. *Animal Feed and Technology*, *86 (3-4),* 205-219.

[32] Swanson, K., Grieshop, C., Flickinger, E., Bauer, L., Chow, J., Wolf, B., Garleb, K., and Fahey, G., (2002). Fructo-oligosaccharides and *Lactobacillus acidophilus* modify microbial populations, total tract digestibilities and fecal protein catabolite concentrations in healthy adult beagle dogs. *Journal of Nutrition, 132,* 3721-3731.

[33] Swanson, K., Grieshop, C., Flickinger, E., Bauer, L., Healy, H., Dawson, K., Merchen, N., and Fahey, G., (2002^{c}). Supplemental fructo-oligosaccharides and mannanoligosaccharides influence immune function, ileal and total tract nutrient digestibilities, microbial populations and concentrations of protein catabolites in the large bowel of dogs. *Journal of Nutrition, 132,* 980-989.

[34] Groeneveld, E., Kappert, H., Van der Kuilen, J., and Beynen, A., (2001). Consumption of fructo-oligosaccharides and nitrogen excretion in cats. *International Journal for Vitamin and Nutrition Research, 71 (4),* 254-256.

[35] Hesta, M., Janssens, G., Debraekeleer, J., and De Wilde, R., (2001). The effect of oligofructose and inulin on faecal characteristics and nutrient digestibility in healthy cats. *Journal of Animal Physiology and Animal Nutrition*, *85,* 135-131.

[36] Houpt, K., and Smit, S., (1981). Taste preferences and their relation to obesity in dogs and cats. *Canadian Veterinary Journal, 22*, 77- 81.

[37] Roberfroid, M., Gibson, G. and Delzenne, N., (1993). The biochemistry of oligofructose, a nondigestible fiber: an approach to calculate its caloric value. *Nutrition Reviews*, *51,* 137-146.

[38] Zentek, J., Marquart, B., and Pietrzak, T., (2002). Intestinal effects of mannanoligosaccharides, transgalacto-oligosaccharides, lactose and lactulose in dogs. *Journal of Nutrition*, *132,* 1682S-1684S.

[39] Hesta, M., Janssens, G., Debraekeleer, J., Millet, S., and De Wilde, R., (2003). Faecal odour components in dogs: nondigestible oligosaccharides and resistent starch do not decrease faecal H_2S emission. *Journal of Applied Research in Veterinary Medicine*, *1(3),* 225-232.

[40] Hesta, M., Debraekeleer, J., Janssens, G., and De Wilde R., (2001). The effect of a commercial high fibre diet and iso-malto-oligosaccharide supplemented diet on post prandial glucose concentrations in dogs. *Journal of Animal Physiology and Animal Nutrition*, *85*, 217-221.

[41] Diez, M., Hornick, J., Baldwin, P., and Istasse, L., (1997). Influence of a blend of fructo-oligosaccharides and sugar beet fiber on nutrients digestibility and plasma metabolite concentrations in healthy beagles. *American Journal of Veterinary Research, 58,* 1238-1242.

[42] Schneeman, B., (1987). Dietary fiber and gastrointestinal function. *Nutrition Reviews, 45 (5),* 129-132.

[43] Roberfroid, M., (1993). Dietary fiber, inulin and oligofructose: a review comparing their physiological effects. *Critical Reviews in Food Science and Nutrition, 33,* 103-148.

[44] Nyman, M., (2002). Fermentation and bulking capacity of indigestible carbohydrates: the case of inulin and oligofructose. *British Journal of Nutrition*, *87 suppl. 2,* S163-S168.

[45] Terada, A., Hara, H., Kataoka, M., and Mitsuoka, T., (1992). Effect of dietary lactosucrose on fecal flora and fecal metabolites of dogs. *Microbial Ecology in Health and Disease*, *5,* 43-50.

[46] Diez, M., Hornick, J., Baldwin, P., Van Eenaeme, C., and Istasse, L., (1998). Influence of sugar-beet fibre, guar gum and inulin on nutrient digestibility, water consumption and plasma metabolites in healthy beagle dogs. *Research in Veterinary Science, 64 (2),* 91-96.

[47] Beynen, A., Kappert, H. and Yu, S., (2001). Dietary lactulose decreases apparent nitrogen absorption and increases apparent calcium and magnesium absorption in healthy dogs. *Journal of Animal Physiology and Animal Nutrition*, *85* 67-72.

[48] Russell, T. (1998). The effect of natural source of non-digestible oligosaccharides on the fecal microflora of the dog and effects on digestion. Friskies R and D centre, Missouri.

[49] Hesta, M., Roosen, W., Janssens, G., Millet, S., and De Wilde, R., (2003). Prebiotics affect nutrient digestibility but not faecal ammonia in dogs fed increased protein levels. *British Journal of Nutrition, 90(6),* 1007-1014.

[50] Flickinger, E., Van Loo, J., and Fahey, G., (2003). Nutritional responses to the presence of inulin and oligofructose in the diets of domesticated animals: a review. *Critical Reviews in Food Science and Nutrition, 43 (1),* 19-60.

[51] Beynen, A., Baas, J., Hoekemeijer, P., Kappert, H., Bakker, M., Koopman, J., and Lemmens, A., (2002). Faecal bacterial profile, nitrogen excretion and mineral absorption in healthy dogs fed supplemental oligofructose. *Journal of Animal Physiology and Animal Nutrition, 86*, 298-305.

[52] Terada, A., Hara, H., Kato, S., Kimura, T., Fujimori, I., Hara, K., Maruyama, T., and Mitsuoka, T., (1993). Effect of lactosucrose on fecal fora and fecal putrefactive products of cats. *Journal of Veterinary Medical Science*, *55 (2)* 291-295.

[53] Sunvold, G., Fahey, G., Merchen, N., Titgemeyer, E., Bourquin, L., Bauer, L., and Reinhart, G., (1995[a]). Dietary fiber for dogs: IV. In vitro fermentation of selected fiber sources by dog fecal inoculum and in vivo digestion and metabolism of fiber-supplemented diets. *Journal of Animal Science*, *73,* 1099-1109.

[54] Sunvold, G., Fahey, G., Merchen, N., and Reinhart, G., (1995[b]). In vitro fermentation of selected fiber sources by dog and cat fecal inoculum: Influence of diet composition on substrate organic matter disappearance and short chain fatty acid production. *Journal of Animal Science, 73*, 1110-1122.

[55] Vickers, R., Sunvold, G., Russell, L., and Reinhart, G., (2001). Comparison of fermentation of selected fructo-oligosaccharides and other fiber substrates by canine colonic microflora. *American Journal of Veterinary Research*, *62 (4)*, 609-615.

[56] Bergman, E., (1990). Energy contribution of volatile fatty acids from the gastrointestinal tract in various species. *Physiological Reviews*, *70 (2),* 567-590.

[57] Blottière, H., Buecher, B., Galmiche, J., and Cherbut, C., (2003). Molecular analysis of the effect of short chain fatty acids on intestinal proliferation. *Proceedings of the Nutrition Society, 62,* 101-106.

[58] Drackly, J., Beaulieu, A., and Sunvold, G. (1998). Energy substrate for intestinal cells. In: Reinhart, G., Carey, D., eds. *Recent advances in canine and feline nutrition.* Ohio: Orange Frazer press, 463-472.

[59] Lupton, J., and Marchant, L., (1989). Independent effects of fiber and protein on colonic luminal ammonia concentration. *Journal of Nutrition*, *119,* 235-241.

[60] Fuller, M., and Reeds, P., (1998). Nitrogen cycling in the gut. *Annual Review of Nutrition, 18,* 385-411.

[61] Martineau, B., and Laflamme, D., (2002). Effect of diet on marker of intestinal health in dogs. *Research in Veterinary Science*, *72*, 223-227.

[62] Swanson, K., Grieshop, C., Flickinger, E., Merchen, N., and Fahey, G., (2002). Effects of supplemental fructo-oligosaccharides and mannanoligosaccharides on colonic microbial populations, immune function and fecal odor components in the canine. *Journal of Nutrition, 132,* 1717S-1719S.

[63] Reddy, B., Hamid, R., and Rao, C., (1997). Effect of dietary oligofructose and inulin on colonic preneoplastic aberrant crypt foci inhibition. *Carcinogenenis*, *18 (7),* 1371-1374.

[64] Hughes, R., and Rowland, I., (2001). Stimulation of apoptosis by two prebiotic chicory fructans in the rat colon. *Carcinogenesis*, *22 (1),* 43-47.

[65] Hussein, H., and Sunvold, G., (2000). Dietary strategies to decrease dog and cat faecal odour components. In: Reinhart, G., Carey, D., eds. *Recent advances in canine and feline nutrition.* Ohio: Orange Frazer press, 153-168.

[66] Hesta, M., Hoornaert E., Verlinden, A., Janssens, G., (2005). The effect of oligofructose on urea metabolism and faecal odour components in cats. *Journal of Animal Physiology and Animal Nutrition, 89 (3-6)*, 208-214.

[67] O'Neill, D., and Phillips, V., A., (1992). Review of the control of odor nuisance from livestock buildings: part 3, Properties of the odorous substances which have been identified in livestock wastes or in the air around them. *Journal of Agricultural Engineering Research*, *53,* 23-50.

[68] Sunvold, G., (1996). Dietary fiber for dogs and cats: an historical perspective. In: Carey, D., Norton, S., and Bolser, S., eds. *Recent advances in canine and feline nutritional research. Proceedings of the 1996 Iams International Nutrition Symposium.* Orange Frazer Press, 3-14.

[69] Tomomatsu, H., (1994). Health effects of oligosaccharides. *Feed Technology*, *48,* 61-65.

[70] Center, S., (1996). Pathophysiology of liver disease: normal and abnormal function. In: Guilfort, W., Center, S., Strombeck, D., Williams, D., and Meyer, D., eds. *Strombeck's Small Animal Gastroenterology.* Third ed., WB Saunders Company, Philadelphia, 592.

[71] Bornet, F., and Brouns, F., (2002). Immune-stimulating and gut health-promoting properties of short-chain fructo-oligosaccharides. *Nutrition reviews*, 60 *(11),* 326-334.

[72] Davis, C., Cleven, D., Balish, E. and Yale, C., (1977). Bacterial association in the gastrointestinal tract of beagle dogs. *Applied and Environmental Microbiology*, 34 *(2),* 194-206.

[73] Benno, Y., Nakao, H., Uchida, K., and Mitsuoka, T., (1992). Impact of the advances in age on the gastrointestinal microflora of beagle dogs. *Journal of Veterinary Medical Science, 54 (4),* 703-706.

[74] Sparkes, A., Papasouliotis, K., Sunvold, G., Werrett, G., Clarke, C., Jones, M., Gruffydd-Jones, T., and Reinhart, G., (1998). Bacterial flora in the duodenum of healthy cats, and effect of dietary supplementation with fructo-oligosaccharides. *American Journal of Veterinary Research, 59,* 431-435.

[75] Papasouliotis, K., Sparkes, A., Werrett, G., Egan, K., Gruffydd-Jones, E., and Gruffydd-Jones, T., (1998). Assessment of bacterial flora of the proximal part of the small intestine in healthy cats, and the effect of sample collection method. *American Journal of Veterinary Research, 59 (1),* 48-51.

[76] Greetham H., Giffard C., Hutson R., Collins M. and Gibson G., (2002). Bacteriology of the Labrador dog gut: a cultural and genotypic approach. *Journal of Applied Microbiology 93*, 640-646.

[77] Mitsuoka T. and Kaneuchi C., (1977). Ecology of the Bifidobacteria. *American Journal of Clinical Nutrition 30,* 1799-1810.

[78] Itoh K., Mitsuoka T., Maejima K., Hiraga C. and Nakano K., (1984). Comparison of faecal flora of cats based on different housing conditions with special reference to Bifidobacterium. *Laboratory Animals 18*, 280-284.

[79] Johnston, K., Lamport, A., and Batt, R., (1993). An unexpected bacterial flora in the proximal small intestine of normal cats. *Veterinary Record*, *132,* 362-363.

[80] Zentek, J., (2000). Bacterienflora des caninen Intestinaltrakts. *Kleintierpraxis, 45 (7),* 523-534.

[81] Willard, M., Simpson, R., Delles, E., Coben, N., Fossum, T., Kolp, D., and Reinhart, G., (1994). Effect of dietary supplementation of fructo-oligosaccharides on small intestinal bacterial overgrowth in dogs. *American Journal of Veterinary Research, 55 (5),* 654-659.

[82] Willard, M., Simpson, R., Cohen, N., and Clancy, J., (2000). Effects of dietary fructo-oligosaccharide on selected bacterial populations in feces of dogs. *American Journal of Veterinary Research, 16,* 820-825.

[83] Oyarzabal, O., Conner, D., and Blevins, W., (1995[a]). Fructo-oligosaccharide utilisation by Salmonellae and potential direct-fed microbial bacteria for poultry. *Journal of Food Protection, 58 (11*), 1192-1196.

[84] Oyarzabal, O., and Conner, D. (1995[b]). In vitro fructo-oligosaccharide utilisation and inhibition of Salmonella spp. by selected bacteria. *Poultry Science*, *74,* 1418-1425.

[85] Heijnen, A., Brink, E., Lemmens, A., and Beynen, A., (1993). Ileal pH and apparent absorption of magnesium in rats fed on diets containing either lactose or lactulose. *British Journal of Nutrition, 70*, 747-756.

[86] Otha, A., Ohtsuki, M., Baba, S., Adachi, T., Sakata, T., and Sakaguchi, E., (1995). Calcium and magnesium absorption from the colon and rectum are increased in rats fed fructo-oligosaccharides. *Journal of Nutrition*, *125*, 2417- 2424.

[87] Buddington, R., Buddington, K., and Sunvold, G., (1999). Influence of fermentable fibre on small intestinal dimensions and transport of glucose and proline in dogs. *American Journal of Veterinary Research, 60 (3),* 354-358.

[88] Howard, M., Kerley, M., Mann, F., Sunvold, G., and Reinhart, G., (1999). Blood flow and epithelial cell proliferation of the canine colon are altered by source of dietary fibre. *Veterinary Clinical Nutrition, 6 (2),* 8-15.

[89] Massimino, S., McBurney, M., Field, C., Thomson, A., Keelan, M., Hayek, M., and Sunvold, G., (1998). Fermentable dietary fibre increases GLP-1 secretion and improves glucose homeostasis despite increased intestinal glucose transport capacity in healthy dogs. *Journal of Nutrition*, *128,* 1786-1793.

[90] Marteau, P., and Flourie, B., (2001). Tolerance to low-digestible carbohydrates: symptomatology and methods. *British Journal of Nutrition*, *85 (suppl.1),* S17-S21.

[91] Marteau, P., and Boutron-Ruault, M., (2002). Nutritional advantages of probiotics and prebiotics. *British Journal of Nutrition*, *87 (suppl.2),* S153-S157.

[92] Roberfroid, M., and Slavin, J., (2000). Non-digestible oligosaccharides. *Critical Reviews in Food Science and Nutrition*, *40*, 461-480.

[93] Younes, H., Rémésy, C., Berh, S., and Demigné, C., (1997). Fermentable carbohydrate exerts a urea-lowering effect in normal and nephrectomised rats. *American Journal of Physiology - Gastrointestinal and Liver Physiology*, 272: G515-G521.

[94] Younes, H., Alphonse, J., Abdelkader, M., and Rémésy, C., (2001). Fermentable carbohydrate and digestive nitrogen excretion. *Journal of Renal Nutrition*, *11 (3),* 139-148.

[95] Sparkes, A., Papasouliotis, K., Sunvold, G., Werrett, G., Gruffydd-Jones, E., Egan, K., Gruffydd-Jones, T., and Reinhart, G., (1998). Effect of dietary supplementation with fructo-oligosaccharides on fecal flora of healthy cats. *American Journal of Veterinary Research*, *59,* 436-440.

INDEX

A

acceptance, 143
access, 35, 110, 207
acclimatization, 142, 143, 165, 167, 168, 171, 175
accounting, 26, 28, 29, 112
accumulation, 62, 63, 166, 167, 170
acetic acid, 193
acetylcholine, 169, 173, 174, 176
acid, x, 38, 101, 104, 105, 109, 112, 116, 117, 119, 127, 131, 133, 136, 180, 183, 184, 187, 188, 192, 193, 194, 207, 208, 217
acidity, 42, 111
ACTH, 75, 76, 83
activation, 72, 74, 83, 85, 88, 101
acute mountain sickness, 176
acylation, 70
adaptation, 175, 191
ADC, 205
adhesion, 56, 64
adipocyte, 67, 70
adiponectin, 70
adipose, 56, 62, 65, 69, 101
adipose tissue, 62, 65, 69
adiposity, 33, 35, 37, 51
adjustment, 59, 75
adolescence, viii, 23, 27, 33, 34, 35, 38, 48, 49
adolescent female, 3, 4, 7, 9, 27
adolescents, viii, 3, 4, 9, 10, 20, 22, 23, 26, 27, 28, 29, 32, 33, 34, 36, 38, 44, 45, 46, 47, 48, 49, 50, 51, 52
adrenaline, ix, 71, 75, 76, 80, 83, 85
adult obesity, 33, 34
adulthood, 10, 49
adults, vii, 1, 2, 3, 4, 9, 11, 12, 13, 14, 15, 16, 17, 18, 19, 20, 22, 27, 33, 36, 41, 45, 48, 59, 67, 68, 69, 104, 171
aerobe, 199
aerobic bacteria, 199
affect, ix, x, 10, 33, 39, 46, 58, 63, 68, 72, 77, 83, 84, 85, 110, 127, 131, 187, 193, 197, 208, 210, 211, 215, 217
Africa, 23, 30, 31, 34, 47, 48, 50, 53
African Americans, 3
agar, 201
age, vii, viii, 1, 2, 3, 4, 5, 6, 7, 8, 9, 10, 13, 16, 20, 23, 27, 28, 29, 30, 31, 32, 33, 34, 35, 37, 38, 40, 43, 44, 45, 46, 62, 73, 143, 156, 163, 170, 198, 204, 209, 218
agent, 100, 107, 211
agglutination, 206
alanine, 147
alanine aminotransferase, 147
alcohol, 4, 25, 73, 104
aldolase, 169
algae, 183
ALT, 147, 155, 161, 162, 169, 170
alternative, 10, 36, 64, 66
alternatives, 36
alters, 72
amines, 171, 196, 197, 198, 204
amino acids, x, 104, 110, 111, 112, 128, 129, 130, 131, 137, 138, 193
ammonia, x, 109, 110, 111, 125, 131, 132, 134, 135, 136, 137, 193, 195, 198, 204, 212, 213, 217
ammonium, 111, 193, 195
anabolism, 67
anaerobe, 199
anaerobic bacteria, 199
animals, ix, xi, 41, 57, 64, 65, 91, 112, 134, 138, 141, 142, 143, 144, 145, 146, 147, 156, 163, 165, 167, 169, 170, 179, 191, 198, 201, 203, 204, 217
anorexia, 142, 163, 164, 165, 171
ANOVA, 75, 118, 148
antibody, 213
aphasia, 168

apoptosis, 87, 187, 192, 209, 217
appetite, 36, 37, 58, 175
apraxia, 168
assessment, 42, 47, 67
assimilation, 185
association, viii, 11, 23, 33, 36, 37, 39, 40, 51, 57, 64, 118, 169, 218
atherogenesis, 65, 167, 170
athletes, ix, 72, 73, 85, 86, 87, 88, 103
atmospheric pressure, 144, 167, 172
ATP, 62, 128
attention, 34, 168, 171
attitudes, 46
Australia, 26, 37, 52
Austria, 75
availability, ix, 33, 52, 72, 83, 85, 112, 129, 130, 134, 135, 136, 137, 164, 168, 195, 208
avoidance, 144, 145
awareness, 2, 14

B

bacteria, x, xi, 38, 110, 111, 118, 123, 127, 128, 130, 131, 132, 135, 137, 138, 139, 179, 180, 181, 185, 187, 188, 193, 195, 196, 197, 198, 199, 201, 203, 204, 219
beams, 144
behavior, x, 92, 133, 139, 141, 142
beneficial effect, ix, 55, 58, 60, 64, 164, 179, 180
beverages, vii, viii, 2, 4, 6, 7, 8, 9, 10, 12, 14, 20, 22, 23, 28, 29, 30, 31, 32, 35, 36, 38, 46, 48, 52, 65
bicarbonate, 115, 116
bile, 180, 185, 186, 198
bile acids, 180, 185, 186, 198
binding, 96, 101, 183, 185, 187, 188, 205, 206, 208
bioavailability, 92
biodiversity, 111
biological systems, 92, 93
biomarkers, viii, 55, 57, 58, 60, 63, 64, 65, 68
biomass, 205, 207
birth, 28
bladder, 74
blocks, 3
blood, ix, xi, 24, 35, 56, 58, 64, 65, 66, 68, 70, 71, 72, 74, 75, 76, 83, 84, 86, 87, 92, 93, 94, 95, 98, 99, 100, 101, 105, 111, 112, 114, 130, 135, 136, 141, 145, 152, 158, 164, 165, 166, 167, 168, 169, 170, 171, 172, 175, 176, 177, 193, 210, 211, 212, 214
blood flow, 95, 130, 136, 172, 175, 210
blood plasma, 101, 111
blood pressure, 58, 64, 66
blood stream, 92, 93
blood-brain barrier (BBB), 56, 65, 70
body, viii, ix, x, 2, 11, 22, 23, 24, 33, 34, 36, 37, 44, 48, 49, 55, 56, 58, 60, 62, 64, 65, 66, 67, 69, 73, 74, 75, 76, 91, 92, 93, 94, 95, 96, 98, 99, 100, 103, 104, 105, 110, 114, 141, 142, 143, 145, 146, 150, 156, 164, 166, 167, 169, 170, 171, 172, 175, 176, 177, 186, 189, 209, 210, 212
body composition, 34, 164, 171, 175, 176
body fat, 11, 36, 37, 65, 69, 166
body fluid, 92
body mass index (BMI), viii, 11, 24, 33, 34, 35, 36, 37, 48, 49, 56, 66
body weight, viii, x, 2, 11, 22, 33, 37, 44, 55, 58, 60, 64, 65, 67, 69, 104, 114, 141, 142, 143, 145, 146, 150, 156, 164, 166, 167, 169, 170, 172, 177, 186, 189, 209, 210, 212
Bolivia, 169
bonds, 181, 182, 183
bone marrow, 84, 86
bowel, 47, 215
boys, 26, 33, 104
brain, 65, 95, 101, 103, 168, 169, 171
brain chemistry, 169
Brazil, 34
breakdown, 110, 111, 130, 138
breakfast, 32, 37, 48, 50, 51, 73
buildings, 218

C

caecum, 195, 198, 201, 212
caffeine, 12, 13, 38
calcium, 9, 10, 13, 14, 22, 29, 38, 42, 74, 87, 88, 115, 179, 208, 209, 216
caloric intake, 59, 60, 65, 164, 176
caloric restriction, 56, 60
calorie, 20, 59, 103, 104, 143
Canada, 36, 175
cancer, 33, 100, 107
cancer cells, 100
candidates, 83
carbohydrate, vii, viii, ix, x, xi, 1, 2, 3, 4, 5, 9, 11, 12, 13, 15, 16, 17, 18, 19, 20, 23, 24, 25, 26, 30, 31, 32, 35, 37, 38, 41, 42, 44, 46, 55, 56, 57, 58, 59, 60, 61, 62, 63, 64, 65, 66, 67, 68, 69, 70, 71, 72, 78, 85, 86, 87, 109, 112, 118, 120, 122, 123, 124, 125, 126, 132, 133, 134, 135, 136, 137, 138, 139, 141, 142, 143, 168, 172, 173, 174, 175, 176, 179, 183, 184, 185, 188, 189, 207, 208, 212, 214, 219
carbohydrate metabolism, 174, 175
carbon, 73, 104, 105, 110, 111, 181, 182, 186, 188
carbon atoms, 188

carbon dioxide, 73, 186
carcinogenesis, 187
cardiovascular disease, 11, 36, 49, 64, 65, 67, 68, 69
cardiovascular risk, ix, 35, 55, 58, 60, 70
caregivers, 43
carrier, 209
casein, 131, 138, 212
catabolism, 58
catecholamines, 83, 168, 176
cation, 208
causal relationship, 42
causation, 41
cell, ix, 56, 64, 72, 73, 74, 83, 84, 101, 111, 184, 185, 188, 191, 192, 193, 207, 209, 219
cell metabolism, 191
cellulose, vii, 25, 105, 184, 186, 187, 188, 192, 195, 199, 201, 202, 204, 205, 207, 208, 209, 211
central nervous system, 95, 173
cerebrospinal fluid, 65
chemical properties, 42, 185
chemiluminescence, 72, 75, 87
chemotherapy, 100
chicken, 11, 31
childhood, 10, 22, 27, 34, 36, 43, 47, 49, 50
children, vii, viii, 1, 2, 3, 6, 9, 10, 20, 22, 23, 26, 27, 28, 29, 30, 31, 32, 33, 34, 35, 36, 37, 38, 40, 41, 43, 44, 45, 46, 47, 48, 49, 50, 51, 52, 53, 103, 104, 107
China, 34
cholesterol, vii, xi, 2, 11, 12, 13, 24, 29, 56, 58, 63, 64, 66, 67, 68, 69, 141, 147, 166, 172, 173, 176, 185, 211
chronic hypoxia, 172, 175
chyme, 185
circulation, 62, 72, 83, 84, 92, 93, 95, 185, 212
classes, 93
classification, 24, 180
cleavage, 183
clinical trials, 42, 58
cluster, 3
CNS, 56, 65
CO2, 110, 187
coding, 4
coefficient of variation, 75
cognitive deficit, 170
cognitive dysfunction, 173
cognitive function, 168, 171
cognitive impairment, 175
cognitive performance, 168, 169
cohort, 11, 22, 28, 33, 45, 52
colon, 24, 180, 185, 186, 191, 193, 195, 196, 198, 199, 200, 201, 204, 209, 217, 219
colonisation, 187
communication, 137
community, 31, 32, 47, 50, 57
compensation, 29, 46
competition, 201
complex carbohydrates, 35, 44, 57
complexity, vii, 39
components, viii, 23, 24, 33, 34, 35, 38, 42, 116, 134, 144, 171, 173, 177, 180, 185, 196, 197, 204, 216, 217, 218
composition, 12, 26, 33, 34, 35, 39, 56, 58, 69, 104, 113, 114, 127, 128, 134, 136, 137, 139, 143, 174, 191, 193, 198, 203, 214
compounds, 105, 111, 193, 196, 198, 204, 210
concentration, ix, x, 57, 66, 71, 72, 74, 75, 78, 83, 85, 91, 92, 93, 94, 95, 96, 98, 99, 101, 109, 110, 111, 112, 113, 116, 117, 118, 119, 121, 122, 124, 127, 128, 130, 131, 133, 137, 165, 167, 174, 182, 184, 185, 192, 193, 195, 196, 197, 202, 211, 212, 217
conditioning, 145
confidence, 124
confidence interval, 124
confusion, 57
consensus, 214
consumers, 14, 20, 29, 31
consumption, vii, viii, 3, 9, 10, 12, 13, 21, 22, 23, 24, 25, 26, 27, 28, 29, 30, 31, 32, 35, 36, 37, 38, 39, 40, 41, 42, 43, 45, 46, 47, 48, 50, 51, 52, 53, 57, 60, 65, 67, 143, 164, 166, 172, 188, 191, 216
consumption patterns, viii, 9, 12, 24, 26, 27, 40, 42, 45
context, 26, 60
control, ix, x, 2, 9, 10, 36, 37, 41, 64, 91, 92, 109, 111, 117, 127, 129, 139, 141, 143, 144, 145, 151, 152, 158, 165, 170, 187, 188, 189, 190, 191, 192, 193, 195, 197, 199, 202, 206, 207, 208, 211, 212, 213, 218
control group, 170
controlled studies, 58
conversion, 62, 112, 164, 195
conversion rate, 62
cooking, 11
copper, 9, 10
corn, vii, x, 4, 9, 13, 22, 28, 30, 57, 109, 113, 116, 117, 122, 125, 126, 127, 128, 132, 134, 136, 182, 212
coronary heart disease, viii, 11, 22, 49, 55, 56, 58, 60, 66, 67
correlation, 57, 63, 131, 195
cortex, 174
cortisol, ix, 71, 75, 77, 80, 83, 84, 86, 176
costs, 66
creatinine, 212

critical period, 33
CRP, 56, 63, 64
cultivation, 43
culture, 50, 110, 135, 137
cycling, ix, x, 71, 73, 74, 84, 85, 86, 87, 110, 111, 131, 217
cytokines, viii, 55, 58
cytometry, 84

D

damage, 88, 100, 172
data set, 27
death, 49
decay, 52, 118
deficit, 181
definition, 41, 184
deformability, 88
degradation, 114, 127, 138, 196
degradation rate, 114, 127
dehydration, 86
delivery, 100, 107
dementia, 174
demographic transition, 43
demographics, 50
density, 13, 25, 29, 35, 46, 50, 56, 68, 69, 173, 174, 209
dental caries, viii, 23, 24, 32, 37, 38, 39, 40, 41, 42, 43, 51, 52
Department of Health and Human Services, 21, 47
deposition, 34, 48, 111
depression, 164, 170, 175
derivatives, 133
detection, 69, 130
detergents, 116
developed countries, viii, 23, 26, 27, 34, 36, 38, 112
diabetes, viii, 11, 36, 48, 55, 56, 57, 64, 69, 210
diabetic patients, 63, 67
diaphragm, 171
diastolic blood pressure, 62
diet, vii, viii, x, 1, 2, 3, 4, 9, 10, 11, 12, 13, 14, 20, 21, 23, 24, 25, 27, 28, 29, 30, 32, 33, 35, 36, 37, 38, 39, 40, 41, 42, 43, 44, 45, 46, 50, 51, 52, 53, 55, 57, 58, 59, 60, 62, 63, 64, 65, 66, 67, 68, 69, 70, 91, 102, 103, 104, 105, 107, 109, 110, 112, 113, 114, 116, 117, 119, 121, 123, 127, 128, 129, 130, 131, 133, 135, 137, 141, 143, 144, 163, 164, 167, 168, 170, 173, 175, 177, 180, 184, 187, 188, 189, 190, 191, 193, 194, 195, 196, 197, 198, 199, 201, 202, 203, 204, 205, 206, 207, 208, 209, 211, 212, 213, 214, 216, 217
diet composition, 50, 69, 217
dietary fat, 35, 66
dietary fiber, vii, 1, 2, 3, 9, 11, 13, 22, 66
dietary habits, 43
dietary intake, 21, 26, 37, 42, 47
dietary supplementation, 184, 218, 219
differentiation, 191, 192, 209
diffusion, 142, 185, 193, 212
digestibility, xi, 179, 184, 188, 189, 193, 195, 196, 204, 205, 206, 207, 208, 211, 215, 216, 217
digestion, 24, 105, 110, 134, 135, 138, 183, 184, 185, 197, 207, 211, 214, 215, 216, 217
discomfort, 164
disorder, 34
distilled water, 117
distribution, 28, 60, 92, 93, 94, 95, 96, 118
diversity, 198
division, 191
DNA, 101
dogs, xi, 170, 173, 174, 179, 184, 186, 187, 188, 189, 190, 191, 192, 193, 195, 196, 197, 198, 199, 200, 201, 202, 203, 204, 205, 206, 207, 208, 209, 210, 211, 212, 213, 215, 216, 217, 218, 219
dosage, 91, 92
dosing, x, 100, 109, 117, 120, 127, 129
dressings, 13
drinking water, 137, 144
drought, 181
drug delivery, 107
drug treatment, 100
drugs, ix, 91, 92, 93, 94, 95, 96, 100
dry matter, 117, 135, 182, 186, 189, 190
duodenum, x, 110, 114, 128, 130, 199, 218
duration, ix, 31, 39, 55, 58, 72, 83, 88, 91, 92, 152, 167, 168, 170, 191

E

eating, viii, 2, 24, 25, 35, 39, 41, 42, 45, 46, 47, 164
edema, 176
egg, 4
elderly, 196
electrolyte, 188
ELISA, 75
emission, 137, 197, 216
encouragement, 142
endocrine, 177
endocrine system, 177
endoscopy, 199
endosperm, 11, 183
endurance, ix, x, 72, 73, 85, 86, 88, 141, 142, 144, 145, 146, 150, 152, 156, 167, 168, 170, 171
energy density, 36
energy supply, 137, 197
England, 213

environment, 34, 112, 173, 180, 198, 201
environmental impact, 111
enzymes, 63, 72, 84, 103, 105, 167, 171, 174, 182, 183, 185, 187, 193, 196
epidemic, 22, 33, 34, 36, 37, 67
epidemiology, 43, 50
epinephrine, 88
epithelial cells, 183
epithelium, 180
equilibrium, 95, 169
equipment, 145
essential fatty acids, 105
ester, 69
estimating, 102, 129
ethanol, 46
ethnic groups, 47
etiology, viii, 23, 34, 38, 39, 40, 42, 53
Europe, 11, 51, 52, 53
European Union, 26
evacuation, 122
evidence, 11, 27, 34, 36, 37, 39, 40, 41, 42, 43, 58, 66, 83, 174, 185, 210
evolution, 110
exclusion, 202
excretion, 24, 92, 94, 99, 111, 113, 118, 120, 121, 129, 131, 133, 134, 139, 185, 188, 189, 193, 195, 196, 206, 210, 212, 213, 215, 217
exercise, ix, x, 56, 57, 67, 71, 72, 73, 74, 76, 81, 82, 83, 84, 85, 86, 87, 88, 89, 141, 142, 143, 145, 166, 167, 168, 169, 170, 171, 173, 175, 177
exercise performance, xi, 141, 168, 171
exertion, 74, 75, 76, 87
expenditures, 175
experts, 57
exposure, xi, 39, 40, 96, 141, 142, 144, 145, 146, 149, 150, 151, 152, 153, 154, 155, 156, 157, 158, 159, 160, 161, 163, 164, 165, 166, 167, 168, 169, 170, 171, 172, 173, 174, 175, 176, 177, 196

F

failure, 164, 210, 213
fast food, 13, 35
fasting, 58, 62, 63, 68, 74, 165, 166, 167, 211, 212
fasting glucose, 212
fat, vii, viii, 1, 2, 3, 4, 5, 6, 7, 8, 9, 11, 12, 13, 14, 15, 16, 17, 18, 19, 20, 23, 25, 27, 28, 29, 32, 34, 35, 36, 45, 46, 48, 50, 51, 58, 59, 60, 63, 64, 65, 67, 68, 69, 70, 104, 105, 139, 142, 143, 144, 164, 168, 175, 176, 185, 207, 211
fatigue, 84, 86, 168
fatty acids, 5, 15, 16, 17, 58, 62, 63, 104, 105, 110, 143, 165, 184, 191, 196, 209, 211, 217
feces, 111, 134, 219
feed additives, 179
feet, 177
females, vii, 1, 3, 8, 13, 22, 37
fermentable carbohydrates, 38, 39, 198, 212
fermentation, x, 109, 110, 112, 117, 120, 122, 127, 131, 133, 134, 135, 136, 137, 138, 184, 185, 186, 188, 189, 191, 192, 197, 198, 204, 205, 207, 209, 210, 214, 215, 217
fertilization, 111
fibers, vii
Finland, 135
fish, vii, 1, 2, 6, 7, 8, 11, 14, 18, 19
flora, xi, 179, 198, 199, 200, 203, 210, 216, 218, 219
fluctuations, 156, 164
fluid, x, 4, 39, 86, 109, 119, 120, 121, 122, 129, 130, 199
folate, 9, 10
food, vii, viii, x, xi, 2, 4, 6, 7, 8, 9, 10, 11, 12, 13, 14, 18, 19, 20, 22, 23, 24, 25, 26, 27, 28, 29, 30, 31, 32, 34, 36, 37, 39, 41, 42, 43, 44, 45, 46, 47, 48, 50, 51, 52, 53, 57, 58, 64, 65, 91, 102, 103, 104, 105, 141, 142, 144, 145, 146, 148, 149, 156, 164, 169, 170, 177, 180, 181, 182, 184, 185, 186, 189, 197, 204, 210, 214
food industry, 181
food intake, 11, 12, 20, 31, 36, 37, 44, 45, 46, 50, 51, 65, 142, 145, 146, 148, 149, 156, 164, 169, 170, 189
food production, 47
food products, 185
forgetting, 27
fractures, 32
France, 75, 133, 134, 135, 172
free radicals, 88
freedom, 75
frost, 181
fructose, 9, 22, 24, 25, 29, 51, 57, 62, 63, 65, 67, 70, 181, 182, 183, 201, 203, 214
fruits, vii, 2, 4, 6, 7, 8, 9, 11, 14, 19, 20, 28, 35, 41
fuel, 143, 192, 209

G

gastrointestinal tract, 24, 179, 180, 197, 217, 218
gender, vii, 1, 2, 3, 4, 5, 13, 16, 20, 27, 37
gender differences, 13
gene, 68
generation, 86
genetic factors, 42
Germany, 45, 48, 75, 138
girls, 26, 34, 35, 48, 104
gland, 130

glucagon, 211
gluconeogenesis, 167, 174, 211
glucose, ix, xi, 24, 25, 35, 48, 57, 58, 59, 62, 63, 64, 65, 69, 70, 71, 72, 75, 78, 80, 83, 85, 88, 100, 101, 105, 120, 122, 128, 137, 138, 141, 144, 145, 147, 152, 158, 164, 165, 168, 169, 170, 171, 172, 174, 175, 176, 181, 182, 183, 184, 185, 186, 192, 203, 207, 209, 211, 212, 216, 219
glucose regulation, 48, 88
glucose tolerance, 48, 164, 165, 172, 176, 211
glucose tolerance test, 211
glutamate, 129
glycerol, 143
glycogen, xi, 141, 143, 145, 147, 156, 163, 167, 168, 172, 174, 177
glycolysis, 171
goals, 143
government, vii, 1, 2, 32
government policy, 32
grains, vii, x, 2, 11, 14, 18, 20, 25, 27, 28, 29, 33, 35, 46, 109, 115, 127, 128, 137, 139, 183
granules, 72
granulocytosis, 87
grass, 129, 133, 134, 135, 137
groundwater, 111
groups, vii, viii, x, 1, 2, 3, 4, 5, 6, 7, 8, 9, 10, 11, 13, 14, 18, 19, 20, 23, 25, 27, 28, 29, 30, 31, 32, 38, 45, 46, 59, 60, 64, 141, 143, 144, 145, 149, 150, 152, 153, 155, 156, 158, 159, 160, 163, 164, 165, 166, 167, 168, 169, 170, 189, 190, 197, 198, 199, 208, 209
growth, x, 33, 43, 75, 80, 86, 87, 88, 91, 102, 103, 111, 112, 127, 128, 137, 164, 170, 171, 176, 180, 196, 198, 201, 212
growth factor, 86
growth hormone, 75, 80, 86, 87, 88
growth rate, 164, 170, 201
guidance, vii, 1, 2, 20
guidelines, 2, 25, 48, 50, 53, 87, 114, 143
gut, 183, 209, 213, 217, 218

H

HE, 143, 144, 146, 148, 149, 150, 151, 152, 157, 158, 163, 164, 165, 166, 168, 169
headache, 142
headache, 142
health, vii, viii, 1, 2, 10, 23, 32, 33, 34, 35, 38, 39, 41, 43, 44, 46, 47, 48, 49, 51, 52, 53, 56, 60, 67, 69, 111, 136, 179, 180, 185, 196, 197, 198, 217, 218
health care, 56
health effects, 44
health problems, viii, 23, 32, 33, 41
health status, 48
heart disease, viii, 20, 32, 55, 62, 68
heart rate, 73, 75, 84
height, 11, 33, 34, 73, 209
hematocrit, 165
hematology, 74
hemicellulose, 25, 184
hemoglobin, 59
hemorrhagic stroke, 11
hepatocytes, 63
high blood cholesterol, 69
high density lipoprotein, 56, 69
high fat, 59, 63, 64
hip, viii, 24
Hispanic population, 62
Hispanics, 62
homeostasis, 65, 67, 70, 85, 172, 219
homogeneity, 75
hormone, ix, 71, 75, 80, 83, 85, 177
host, 72, 110, 111, 180, 191
housing, 218
human milk, 182
human neutrophils, 87, 88
hydrogen, 104, 105, 186, 197
hydrolysis, 101, 181, 182, 183, 185, 196, 214
hyperglycemia, 62
hyperinsulinemia, 62
hyperlipidemia, 57, 59, 64
hypertension, 32, 57
hypoglycemia, 83
hypothermia, 175
hypothesis, 36, 37, 73, 96, 127, 130
hypoxia, x, 141, 142, 144, 145, 146, 150, 151, 152, 156, 157, 158, 164, 165, 166, 167, 168, 169, 170, 171, 172, 173, 174, 175, 176, 177

I

identification, viii, 24
IL-6, 56, 64, 73, 74, 75, 78, 83, 85
ileostomy, 184
ileum, 184, 185, 198, 199, 207
immune function, 72, 197, 215, 217
immune system, xi, 86, 87, 179, 198, 213
immunity, 72, 213
immunosuppression, 86
in vitro, ix, 65, 71, 72, 84, 88, 107, 128, 135, 136, 181, 192, 195, 203, 208, 215
incidence, viii, 33, 39, 40, 51, 52, 55, 57, 210
inclusion, 187, 188, 192, 195, 199, 201, 202, 203, 206, 207, 209, 211, 212, 213
income, 3

incubation period, 193, 195
independent variable, 118
India, 91, 141, 147, 148
Indians, 30
indication, 168, 196
indices, 100
indirect effect, 210
industrialized countries, 40, 41
infancy, 33, 43
infants, 30, 31, 104
infectious disease, viii, 23
inflammation, 58, 64, 67
influence, 10, 35, 42, 52, 58, 65, 84, 85, 133, 168, 174, 186, 195, 199, 203, 205, 209, 210, 211, 213, 214, 215
information processing, 168
informed consent, 73
ingest, 72
ingestion, ix, 38, 42, 57, 67, 71, 73, 74, 83, 84, 85, 86, 87, 103, 163, 172, 177, 184
inhibition, 211, 217, 219
inhibitor, 211
initial state, 93
initiation, 38, 116, 117
innate immunity, 72
inoculation, 192
inoculum, 192, 193, 217
input, 101
insomnia, 142
insulin, viii, 9, 35, 55, 56, 57, 58, 59, 62, 63, 64, 65, 66, 67, 69, 70, 173, 175, 184, 211, 212, 214
insulin resistance, ix, 56, 57, 62, 63, 64, 66
insulin sensitivity, viii, 55, 57, 64, 66, 69
intelligence, 169
intensity, x, 57, 67, 75, 76, 86, 87, 88, 91, 92, 144, 167, 170, 176
interaction, 43, 76, 78, 81, 82, 88, 120, 203
interactions, 88
interest, 35, 57, 179, 180
interpretation, 60
interval, ix, 71, 74, 83, 84, 85, 87, 97, 119, 145, 146
intervention, ix, 11, 39, 43, 44, 55, 59, 63, 64, 66
interview, 2
intestinal flora, 180
intestinal tract, 201
intestine, xi, 102, 111, 179, 180, 182, 184, 186, 187, 191, 193, 196, 198, 205, 209
inversion, 74
investment, 44
Ireland, 75
iron, 9, 10, 13, 29
ischaemic heart disease, 69
isolation, 85, 201
isotope, 117, 124, 130
Israel, 49

J

Japan, 182
jejunum, 198
junior high school, 33
justification, 43

K

kidneys, 95
kinetics, 92, 93, 94, 98, 100, 107
knowledge, 44, 46, 47
KOH, 147

L

labeling, 117
lactate dehydrogenase, 148, 156
lactation, x, 104, 109, 114, 131, 133, 136, 139
lactic acid, 191
lactobacillus, 199
lactose, 26, 29, 182, 187, 191, 193, 195, 205, 206, 207, 208, 209, 213, 216, 219
laparotomy, 199
large intestine, 181, 183, 193, 196, 198, 203, 205, 207, 208
later life, 34
LDL, xi, 11, 56, 58, 59, 60, 61, 63, 66, 67, 68, 69, 141, 147, 154, 159, 165, 166, 170
lead, 2, 34, 38, 62, 65, 143
lean body mass, 166
learning, 145, 147, 168, 172
leptin, viii, 9, 55, 65, 70
leukocytosis, ix, 71, 83, 85
lifestyle, 35, 37, 43, 46, 48, 66
lifetime, 177
lignin, 184, 185
likelihood, 36
limitation, 59, 138
linkage, 180, 183, 185
links, 184
lipase, 63, 69
lipemia, 58, 68
lipids, ix, 50, 55, 58, 59, 60, 65, 66, 67, 68, 69, 142, 166, 170, 172, 175, 177, 185
lipolysis, 58, 85
lipoproteins, 58, 172, 174, 175, 177
lithium, 74

liver, xi, 58, 62, 63, 93, 95, 102, 111, 112, 129, 141, 145, 147, 156, 163, 167, 172, 185, 210, 212, 213, 218
liver disease, 62, 218
liver failure, 210
livestock, 218
localization, 93
location, 144
long run, 98
longitudinal study, 37
loss of appetite, 164
low fat diet, 59, 60, 64, 66, 211
lymphocytes, 78, 83
lymphocytosis, ix, 71, 83
lysozyme, 87

M

macronutrients, 4, 5, 12, 13, 30, 57, 64, 211
macrophages, 213
magnesium, 9, 10, 13, 74, 208, 209, 216, 219
males, vii, 1, 3, 7, 8, 13, 27, 62
malnutrition, 50
management, 56, 57, 139
manipulation, 29, 135
manure, 112, 136, 139
market, 35
marrow, 84, 87
masking, 203
mass, 24, 49, 73, 74, 75, 76, 97, 102, 164, 188, 209
mass loss, 75, 76
mass media, 49
matrix, 176
maturation, 192, 209
meals, 4, 20, 32, 36, 39, 50, 65, 70
measures, 37, 41, 75, 143, 208
meat, vii, 1, 2, 6, 7, 8, 11, 13, 14, 18, 19, 20, 29, 36, 190, 207, 212
media, 47, 101, 110, 128
medication, 73
membrane permeability, 170
membranes, 207
memory, 145, 147, 168, 169, 171, 172, 174, 176
men, 3, 14, 50, 58, 59, 62, 68, 69, 143, 166, 168, 171, 173
meta analysis, 58
metabolic disturbances, 57
metabolic syndrome, viii, 33, 34, 48, 55, 56, 62, 69
metabolism, xi, 57, 58, 65, 67, 70, 92, 93, 99, 101, 103, 111, 114, 133, 134, 135, 136, 137, 138, 143, 164, 166, 170, 172, 174, 175, 176, 177, 179, 185, 187, 210, 211, 215, 217, 218
metabolites, 92, 103, 198, 216
methodology, 3
methylation, 186
mice, 63, 65, 69, 171
milk, vii, x, 1, 2, 4, 6, 7, 8, 9, 10, 11, 14, 19, 20, 22, 25, 27, 28, 29, 30, 31, 36, 65, 109, 110, 111, 112, 113, 114, 117, 118, 119, 121, 123, 124, 126, 129, 130, 131, 132, 133, 134, 135, 136, 137, 139, 180
mixing, 74, 117
model system, 42
modeling, 100
models, vii, 2, 13, 42, 93, 100, 108, 118, 119, 128, 172, 173
moisture, 188, 189, 190, 191, 197
moisture content, 188, 189, 190, 191
molasses, x, 109, 127
molecular weight, 24, 187
molecules, viii, 55, 58, 93, 104, 183, 184, 185, 210
monitoring, vii, 1, 2, 92
monomers, 181
monounsaturated fatty acids, 173
mood, 168, 176
morbidity, 210
Morocco, 35
mortality, 210
Moscow, 109
mothers, 103
mountains, 142, 175
movement, 101
MRS, 172
mucosa, 63, 111, 185, 192
mucus, 187
muscles, 62, 147, 168, 170

N

NaCl, 115, 116
needs, viii, 23, 33, 64, 68, 93, 104, 112, 142, 143, 209
nervous system, 56, 101
Netherlands, 133, 138, 139
neurotransmitter, 174
neurotransmitters, 168
neutrophils, ix, 71, 73, 75, 78, 83, 84, 86, 87, 88, 213
nitrogen, x, xi, 109, 110, 111, 119, 120, 122, 131, 133, 134, 135, 136, 137, 138, 139, 176, 179, 193, 205, 206, 210, 212, 213, 215, 216, 217, 219
nitrous oxide, 135, 173
North Africa, 34
Norway, 49, 52
nutrients, viii, 4, 14, 15, 24, 25, 26, 29, 30, 36, 44, 46, 110, 115, 116, 129, 164, 179, 180, 188, 193, 204, 216

nutrition, vii, viii, 1, 2, 23, 24, 26, 32, 34, 35, 38, 43, 44, 49, 50, 51, 53, 138, 142, 179, 199, 214, 215, 217, 218

O

obesity, viii, 9, 10, 11, 20, 22, 23, 24, 29, 32, 33, 34, 35, 36, 37, 43, 48, 49, 50, 51, 55, 56, 57, 58, 59, 62, 63, 65, 66, 68, 69, 143, 174, 175, 216
observations, 86, 113, 129, 175
oil, 69
oils, 35, 105, 106, 107
oligomers, 181
oligosaccharide, 181, 183, 184, 186, 188, 189, 190, 192, 195, 201, 202, 204, 205, 206, 207, 214, 215, 216, 219
optimization, 111
organ, 95, 210
organic compounds, 104
organic matter, 120, 121, 122, 135, 138, 189, 205, 217
organism, 108, 180
osmotic pressure, 210
osteoporosis, 32
output, 119, 130, 136, 138, 188, 189, 190, 199, 204
overweight, viii, 2, 9, 11, 22, 33, 34, 35, 36, 37, 49, 50, 51, 55, 56, 58, 59, 60, 64, 66, 67, 68, 69
overweight adults, 34
oxalate, 208
oxidation, 60, 63, 164, 192
oxygen, 73, 104, 105, 110, 142, 168, 172, 173

P

packaging, 63
parameter, 60, 94, 96, 118, 119, 126, 132
parents, 10, 22, 43
particles, 58, 136, 177
passive, 145, 193
pathogens, 72, 187, 213
pathophysiology, 215
pathways, 59, 85
peptides, 111, 193
percentile, 33, 34, 37
perspective, 67, 218
Peru, 166, 169
pH, x, 40, 42, 74, 101, 109, 110, 112, 119, 120, 122, 127, 128, 139, 184, 188, 191, 193, 195, 197, 198, 204, 208, 212, 219
phagocytosis, 72, 86
pharmacokinetics, 92, 93
pharmacology, 93
phenol, 196, 197
phenotype, 68
phospholipids, 185
phosphorus, 9, 10, 13, 131, 137, 208, 209
phosphorylation, 174
photosynthesis, 181
physical activity, vii, 1, 2, 20, 34, 46, 48, 49, 173
physical properties, 93
physiology, 173, 214
pilot study, 64
placebo, ix, 71, 72, 74, 196
plants, 180, 181, 185
plasma, viii, ix, xi, 51, 55, 56, 57, 58, 59, 60, 62, 63, 64, 65, 66, 69, 71, 72, 73, 74, 75, 76, 78, 80, 83, 84, 85, 86, 87, 94, 95, 96, 102, 141, 145, 147, 148, 153, 154, 155, 158, 159, 160, 161, 163, 165, 166, 169, 170, 171, 172, 173, 174, 175, 177, 210, 211, 212, 213, 216
plasma levels, 83
plasma proteins, 96
plexus, 145
PM, 44, 46, 69, 70, 172, 173, 177, 190
pollution, 111, 135, 139
polymerization, 24, 25
polymers, 181, 182
polypropylene, 143
pools, 84, 118, 121, 132
poor, ix, 32, 33, 43, 55, 184
population, vii, ix, 1, 2, 3, 25, 27, 28, 32, 34, 35, 38, 40, 44, 49, 50, 55, 56, 118, 198, 199
portal vein, 62
Portugal, 136
positive relation, viii, 24
potassium, 13, 209
potatoes, 28, 30, 31
poultry, vii, 1, 2, 6, 7, 8, 11, 13, 14, 18, 19, 35, 190, 219
power, 42
prediction, 41, 70
predictors, 34, 37
preference, 67, 142
pregnancy, 104
preparation, 64, 147
preschool children, 28, 40, 46, 47, 50, 52
preschoolers, 9, 21, 30
pressure, 142, 144, 145, 176
prevention, 20, 40, 47, 51, 53, 56, 66, 171, 179
prices, 67
primary school, 30, 47
priming, 86, 88
probability, 2
probe, 210
probiotic, 180, 197, 201

production, x, 9, 58, 62, 63, 65, 72, 84, 85, 103, 110, 111, 112, 114, 117, 128, 130, 131, 134, 137, 139, 169, 181, 182, 184, 188, 189, 190, 191, 192, 193, 195, 196, 197, 204, 209, 210, 211, 212, 213, 217
productivity, 111
program, 56
proliferation, 193, 201, 206, 209, 217, 219
proportionality, 94
protective factors, 42
protein kinase C, 85
protein synthesis, x, 109, 110, 111, 112, 114, 122, 124, 129, 130, 131, 132, 134, 135, 138, 139, 193, 212, 213
proteins, 65, 96, 104, 111, 113, 130, 134, 195, 206
protocol, ix, 71, 73, 77, 78, 83, 145, 146, 147, 148, 164, 165
puberty, 36
public health, 2, 33, 49, 56
pulse, x, 109
pumps, 144
pyridoxine, 176

Q

quality of life, 35
quartile, vii, 2, 3, 12, 13, 14, 20

R

race, 86
range, 14
ratings, 75
RDP, 112, 114
reaction time, 168, 177
reactive oxygen, 72, 88
reasoning, 168
recall, 2, 31, 168, 169
receptors, 183
recognition, 43
reconcile, 24
recovery, ix, x, 71, 73, 74, 83, 84, 85, 87, 88, 109, 123, 131, 167, 180
recreation, 142
rectum, 198, 201, 219
recycling, 114, 119, 130, 133, 135
redistribution, ix, 71, 73, 83
reduction, 10, 11, 36, 41, 58, 59, 60, 64, 65, 68, 70, 113, 114, 127, 128, 129, 165, 166, 167, 168, 170, 207, 210, 213
reflection, 37, 195
regression, vii, 2, 13, 60, 118, 119
regression analysis, 60
regulation, 24, 44, 48, 57, 58, 65, 84
relationship, ix, 2, 37, 40, 41, 42, 56, 60, 74, 93, 110, 135, 170
relationships, 92
reliability, 40
replacement, 104, 137
reproduction, x, 91, 102, 209, 210
reserves, 167
residuals, 118
resistance, viii, 48, 49, 55, 56, 57, 58, 62, 63, 64, 65, 67, 70, 183, 187
resources, 135
respiratory, 86
responsiveness, 88
retardation, 171
retention, ix, 42, 55, 176, 185
reticulum, 117
riboflavin, 13
rice, 4, 11, 30, 31, 115, 116, 182, 212
risk, vii, viii, 1, 2, 11, 22, 23, 29, 32, 34, 35, 36, 37, 38, 39, 40, 41, 43, 49, 52, 55, 56, 57, 58, 59, 60, 62, 64, 65, 66, 67, 68, 69, 72, 167, 170, 186
risk factors, viii, 2, 43, 49, 55, 58, 60, 69
rodents, 179
rods, 144, 199
rural areas, 47
Russia, 34

S

safety, 210, 215
saliva, 38, 111, 136
sample, 2, 27, 45, 74, 117, 123, 145, 147, 218
sampling, 75, 120, 127
saturated fat, vii, 1, 2, 5, 11, 12, 13, 14, 15, 20, 29, 33, 58, 60, 64
scatter, 144
school, 22, 30, 37, 47, 49, 51, 52, 104
scores, 187, 189
sea level, 165, 167, 168, 171, 175
sea-level, 145
search, 172
secretion, x, 9, 35, 58, 62, 63, 65, 67, 70, 86, 110, 118, 119, 123, 124, 126, 131, 132, 175, 211, 219
sedentary lifestyle, 49
selenium, 13
sensitivity, ix, 55
series, 24, 63
serotonin, 168
serum, 24, 35, 50, 58, 65, 66, 67, 68, 169, 171, 173, 174, 177, 184, 213
SES, 66
severity, 38, 40

SGOT, 169
SGPT, 169
shear, 86
sheep, 128, 129, 133, 136, 137, 138
shock, 144, 145, 147, 151, 156
shortage, 34
side effects, ix, 91
sign, 94
signalling, 85
signals, 37, 65
sites, 95, 180, 187
skeletal muscle, 63, 167, 170
skin, 11, 62
small intestine, 24, 111, 119, 127, 129, 130, 133, 183, 185, 186, 203, 209, 218
smoking, 49
sodium, 2, 12, 13, 29, 209
software, 3
solubility, 42, 135, 184, 185, 188, 205, 208
South Africa, 30, 31, 32, 34, 43, 47, 49
species, 72, 88, 128, 179, 190, 192, 199, 201, 203, 217
speed, 85, 145, 150, 151, 156
Sprague-Dawley rats, 143
SPSS, 118
stability, 100
stages, 2, 43
standard error, 75
starch, viii, x, 23, 25, 28, 29, 36, 41, 42, 50, 105, 109, 110, 113, 114, 115, 116, 117, 121, 122, 125, 126, 127, 128, 129, 131, 132, 133, 137, 181, 183, 185, 190, 197, 207, 216
starch polysaccharides, 25, 36, 115, 117, 185
starvation, 65, 143, 165, 174
statin, 59, 68
steel, 143
stimulus, 144
stomach, 110
storage, 43, 110, 136, 181
strain, 201, 202
strategies, 11, 20, 72, 87, 218
strength, 40
streptococci, 38
stress, ix, 71, 72, 73, 74, 83, 85, 87, 88, 142, 156, 170, 176, 177
stroke, 11, 22
students, 33, 47
subacute, 210
substitutes, 180
substitution, 183
substrates, xi, 110, 179, 180, 185, 192, 217
sucrose, 28, 29, 37, 39, 41, 42, 50, 51, 58, 128, 129, 135, 137, 181, 182, 203
sugar, vii, viii, 3, 9, 10, 20, 21, 23, 25, 26, 27, 28, 29, 30, 31, 32, 33, 35, 36, 37, 38, 39, 40, 41, 42, 44, 45, 46, 50, 51, 52, 53, 67, 127, 128, 143, 172, 180, 182, 187, 189, 206, 216
sulphur, 196, 197
supply, 24, 32, 37, 40, 43, 52, 111, 114, 117, 131, 133, 134, 138, 171
suppression, 70, 84
surface area, 103, 185
surface component, 63
survival, 88
susceptibility, 60, 69
Sweden, 73
sympathetic nervous system, 85
symptoms, ix, 44, 56, 88, 142, 176, 210
synchronization, 113, 138
syndrome, ix, 62, 63, 66, 69
synthesis, x, 39, 58, 62, 103, 109, 110, 111, 112, 113, 120, 129, 130, 131, 135, 137, 138, 168, 171, 173, 174, 181, 193, 211, 212, 213
systems, 88, 112, 168

T

Taiwan, 49, 71
task performance, 168
teachers, 43
teenagers, 41, 46
teeth, 38, 41, 52
temperature, 74, 110, 144, 181, 197
tenure, 142
theory, 37, 53, 56, 143
therapy, 44, 59, 68
threat, 41
threshold(s), 34, 42, 83, 85, 88, 113, 177
time, ix, 2, 12, 24, 26, 27, 32, 33, 37, 43, 45, 57, 60, 66, 75, 76, 78, 81, 82, 91, 92, 93, 94, 96, 98, 101, 112, 118, 119, 120, 122, 123, 144, 145, 146, 151, 152, 153, 155, 156, 157, 158, 161, 165, 184, 185, 186, 188, 195, 196, 199, 206, 207, 210, 211
time frame, 57
time periods, 66, 151, 153, 156
tissue, 56, 62, 69, 72, 100, 101, 103, 104, 147, 171, 199
TNF-α, 63
total cholesterol, xi, 35, 59, 66, 141, 166
total energy, vii, 2, 3, 4, 9, 10, 11, 12, 13, 15, 16, 17, 18, 19, 25, 26, 28, 29, 30, 31, 35, 36, 37, 57, 58, 60, 63, 66, 103, 105, 146
toxicity, 138, 210
toxicology, 210
toxin, 198
tracking, 49

training, 145, 166, 170, 171, 175, 177
transformation(s), 92, 94, 111, 122
transition, viii, 23, 34, 35, 38, 49, 137
translocation, 171
transport, 65, 93, 96, 138, 214, 219
trend, 12, 38, 59, 128, 153, 161, 188, 195, 199, 202, 203, 205, 213
trial, 59, 60, 68, 73, 75, 76, 78, 81, 82, 83, 84
triggers, 88
triglycerides, xi, 56, 63, 64, 68, 70, 141, 143, 147, 186
tumor, 56, 64, 100, 213
tumor growth, 100
tumor necrosis factor (TNF), 56, 63, 64
tumors, 100
type 2 diabetes, 64, 67, 69
tyramine, 196, 197
tyrosine, 169, 174, 175

U

underlying mechanisms, 168
United Kingdom (UK), 22, 28, 38, 45, 69, 71, 73, 74, 75, 214
United Nations, 24
United States, v, 1, 21, 22, 26, 34, 46, 49, 52, 67
upper airways, 87
urban areas, 31
urbanization, viii, 23
urea, 111, 112, 114, 129, 133, 135, 136, 137, 138, 193, 196, 210, 212, 213, 218, 219
urine, 111, 129, 133, 184, 206, 212

V

vacuum, 144
values, xi, 12, 75, 76, 77, 81, 84, 102, 122, 124, 126, 131, 141, 150, 151, 152, 153, 155, 156, 157, 158, 160, 161, 163, 164, 165, 167, 168, 169
variability, 113
variable(s), ix, 13, 37, 42, 56, 75,113, 117, 119, 121, 127, 128, 129, 130, 137, 147, 148, 150, 157, 144, 184
variance, 75, 119
variation, 35, 38, 40, 112, 131, 165, 177
VAT, 56, 62
vegetables, vii, 1, 2, 6, 7, 8, 9, 11, 14, 18, 20, 25, 28, 29, 31, 33, 35, 181
vein, 74
velocity, 34
viscosity, 184, 185, 186, 207, 208
visual stimulus, 144
vitamin A, 9, 10
vitamin B12, 9, 10, 13
vitamin B6, 9, 10, 13, 29
vitamin C, 9, 13
vitamin D, 29
vitamins, 10, 26, 105, 197
VLDL, 58, 61, 62, 63, 64, 154, 159, 165, 166
vulnerability, 173

W

waking, 103
walking, 86
war, 52
warrants, 73
water, xi, 4, 20, 74, 75, 76, 96, 105, 116, 136, 141, 142, 144, 145, 164, 172, 181, 184, 185, 188, 190, 191, 192, 205, 208, 216
wear, 104
weight control, 36, 51
weight gain, 2, 9, 12, 34, 35, 36, 57, 64, 65, 150, 164, 176
weight loss, viii, 10, 11, 12, 24, 36, 37, 51, 55, 56, 57, 60, 64, 65, 66, 67, 68, 69, 142, 143, 163, 164, 166, 171
weight management, 12, 20
weight reduction, 174
West Indies, 34
wheat, 11, 128, 182
women, 3, 11, 14, 22, 34, 49, 59, 60, 62, 64, 65, 66, 67, 68, 69, 70, 103, 173
words, 142
work, 73, 103, 104, 105, 106, 129, 142, 168, 173, 177
workers, 103, 165, 166, 168, 169, 170
working memory, 174
World Health Organization, 22, 24
World War I, 38

Y

yeast, 4, 14, 183
yield, 113, 130, 131, 134, 135, 137, 139
young adults, viii, 23, 33, 38, 169, 172

Z

zinc, 9, 13, 29